# Assessing Culturally and Linguistically Diverse Students

# THE GUILFORD PRACTICAL INTERVENTION
## IN THE SCHOOLS SERIES
### Kenneth W. Merrell, Series Editor

Books in this series address the complex academic, behavioral, and social–emotional needs of children and youth at risk. School-based practitioners are provided with practical, research-based, and readily applicable tools to support students and team successfully with teachers, families, and administrators. Each volume is designed to be used directly and frequently in planning and delivering clinical services. Features include a convenient format to facilitate photocopying, step-by-step instructions for assessment and intervention, and helpful, timesaving reproducibles.

# Assessing Culturally and Linguistically Diverse Students

## A Practical Guide

ROBERT L. RHODES
SALVADOR HECTOR OCHOA
SAMUEL O. ORTIZ

THE GUILFORD PRESS
New York      London

© 2005 The Guilford Press
A Division of Guilford Publications, Inc.
72 Spring Street, New York, NY 10012
www.guilford.com

Printed in Canada

This book is printed on acid-free paper.

Last digit is print number:  9   8   7   6   5

**Library of Congress Cataloging-in-Publication Data**

Rhodes, Robert L.
    Assessing culturally and linguistically diverse students : a practical guide / Robert L. Rhodes,
Salvador Hector Ochoa, Samuel O. Ortiz.
        p. cm.—(The Guilford practical intervention in the schools series)
    Includes bibliographical references and index.
    ISBN 1-59385-141-3 (pbk.: alk. paper)
    1. Minority students—United States—Ability testing—Handbooks, manuals,
etc.   2. Minorities—Education—United States—Handbooks, manuals, etc.   3. Linguistic
minorities—Education—United States—Handbooks, manuals, etc.   4. Educational tests and
measurements—United States—Handbooks, manuals, etc.   5. Multicultural education—United
States—Handbooks, manuals, etc.   6. Bilingual education—United States—Handbooks, manuals,
etc.   I. Ochoa, Salvador Hector.   II. Ortiz, Samuel O., 1958–   III. Title.   IV. Series.
    LC3731.R46 2005
    371.829—dc22
                                                                                    2005000319

*To our families, who have fulfilled and inspired us:*

*Elena, Jessica Lynn, Joshua Robert, and Julia Elena—R. L. R.*

*Maricela, Victoria Vianey, and Aaron Rafael—S. H. O.*

*Kathryn Anne, Samuel Benjamin, Gabriella Marie, Alisa Carmen, and Carlos Ayala*
*—S. O. O.*

*and*

*To those exceptional teachers who have inspired the hearts and stimulated*
*the intellect of those we love, our children:*

*Cindy Volkmer, from the Developmentally Delayed Preschool,*
*University Hills Elementary, Las Cruces Public Schools, New Mexico;*
*Pat Clark and Anna Marie Rios, from Highland Elementary,*
*Las Cruces Public Schools, New Mexico;*
*Janet Denmark, Pamela Homa, Celia Saucedo, and Christine Woods,*
*from Hillrise Elementary, Las Cruces Public Schools, New Mexico;*
*The Sixth Grade Science Magnet Team, Sierra Middle School,*
*Las Cruces Public Schools, New Mexico;*
*Erin Cain, Mary Jones, Vicki Murphy, Gayle Patranella, and Karen Steck,*
*from College Hills Elementary, College Station ISD Texas;*
*Beth Simple, from Longmire Learning Center, College Station, Texas;*
*Valerie Navarro, from Henry Foss High School,*
*Tacoma School District, Washington;*
*Lee Dash, from Longwood High;*
*Daniel Mrose, from Longwood Junior High;*
*and Amy Kelly and Mrs. DeNapoli, from Charles E. Walters Elementary,*
*Longwood Central School District, New York*

# About the Authors

**Robert L. Rhodes, PhD, NCSP,** is Chair of the Department of Special Education/Communication Disorders at New Mexico State University, as well as a school psychology faculty member. He received his doctorate in school psychology from the University of Northern Colorado and has experience working in public schools, child and adolescent psychiatric facilities, and an international school setting. Dr. Rhodes has served as President of the New Mexico Association of School Psychologists and state delegate to the National Association of School Psychologists, and is an associate editor of the *School Psychology Quarterly* journal for Division 16 of the American Psychological Association. His research has focused on intervention strategies for culturally and linguistically diverse students and neuropsychological applications in the schools.

**Salvador Hector Ochoa, PhD,** is an Associate Professor of Educational Psychology at Texas A&M University, where he has a joint appointment in school psychology and special education. Dr. Ochoa serves on various editorial boards of school psychology and special education journals, and has recently been named as an Associate Editor for the *American Educational Research Journal: Teaching, Learning and Human Development*. He is a past recipient of the Texas A&M Center for Teaching Excellence–Teaching Excellence Award. Dr. Ochoa also received the Association of Former Students Faculty Distinguished Achievement Award for Teaching. His research focuses on bilingual assessment, social status, and educational programming issues of Hispanic children.

**Samuel O. Ortiz, PhD,** is Associate Professor of Psychology at St. John's University in Queens, New York. He holds a doctorate in clinical psychology from the University of Southern California and a credential in school psychology with postdoctoral training in bilingual school psychology from San Diego State University. Dr. Ortiz has served as a Visiting Professor and Research Fellow at Nagoya University, Japan, and is currently Vice President for Professional Affairs of American Psychological Association (APA) Division 16 (School Psychology). He was recently appointed to APA's Committee on Psychological Testing and Assessment. He is widely published on topics such as CHC Cross-Battery Assessment, intelligence testing, nondiscriminatory assessment, cultural and linguistic issues in psychology, and learning disabilities.

# Preface

There has long been need for a book that focuses on the assessment of students who are culturally and linguistically diverse. Conducting assessments and interviews through the assistance of an interpreter, the selection of nondiscriminatory instruments and procedures, assessment of language proficiency, assessment of acculturation, and the examination of exclusionary factors are just some of the issues faced by school-based practitioners. The complex process of assessment is further complicated for many mental health and educational professionals because they have a limited knowledge of the students' culture and primary language. In the field of school psychology, for example, fewer than 6% of practitioners are members of a minority population. Similar disproportionate representation exists across all fields of psychology within the United States. As a result, many mental health and educational professionals involved in the assessment of school-age children are unfamiliar with the unique cultural and linguistic characteristics of their clientele.

In order to address this pressing need, a significant amount of research and theory-based literature has been produced during the past several years. Unfortunately, to date, no hands-on guide to the assessment of culturally and linguistically diverse students has been available to practitioners. Interested mental health and educational professionals have instead been forced to wade through available research and theory in order to develop a working approach to assessment strategies and procedures. This book represents an attempt to provide a practical and informative guide to the assessment of culturally and linguistically diverse students for practitioners in the fields of school psychology, special education, educational diagnostics, and other related areas.

*Assessing Culturally and Linguistically Diverse Students* is a nontechnical resource. Although the material in the book is based on established research and theory, it is generally free from technical jargon and language. The focus of the book is instead based on a practical, problem-solving approach to the assessment of culturally and linguistically diverse students. In order to accomplish this objective, a number of reproducible checklists and worksheets are included so that the reader has immediate hands-on application of the material discussed.

The topics covered were carefully chosen to address the activities and situations most commonly encountered by practitioners in the field. Step-by-step procedural guidelines are provided, for example, for the interview process, the use of interpreters, using informal and curriculum-based measures, and using norm-referenced or standardized measures. Specialized procedures of equal importance but sporadic implementation in everyday practice are also addressed, including the examination of exclusionary factors and the assessment of acculturation. The book also includes practical guidelines that should be carefully considered in each individual situation and used as a basis upon which to formulate an individual and appropriate assessment strategy. It should be noted, however, that the issues and procedures discussed within this book are complex and at times potentially controversial. It should be further noted that there are no simple answers or directives that will enable school-based practitioners to systematically meet the unique and varied needs of all the students with whom they work.

The book can be conceptualized as being divided into three sections, each containing four chapters. The first four chapters provide insight into key issues, demographics, and concerns related to assessing culturally and linguistically diverse students. The next four chapters address specific issues critical to the assessment process. The final four chapters provide step-by-step procedures and recommendations for the assessment of language proficiency, cognitive functioning, and academic achievement.

Although as authors we strove to present one "voice" throughout the various chapters of the book, there were times when it was important for the individual style, experience, perception, and opinion of the author(s) to be clearly represented. In addition, specific models of assessment are presented for the first time within this book, and we want to ensure that the original source for these models and recommendations is clear. The following is a brief description of the content of each chapter, and the accompanying author(s):

The first two chapters of the book, by Salvador Hector Ochoa, provide a comprehensive and detailed analysis of the linguistic diversity embodied within U.S. public schools, as well as the historic and current disproportionate representation of culturally and linguistically diverse students in special education. These two introductory chapters clearly establish the factual need for new and different approaches when working with a rapidly increasing number of culturally and linguistically diverse students, and provide invaluable insight into the rationale and practices that have led to misdiagnosis and inappropriate placement.

Chapter 3, by Robert L. Rhodes, builds upon the first two chapters by clearly delineating legal and ethical requirements when assessing students who are culturally and linguistically diverse. This chapter draws upon multiple sources to provide readers with an in-depth overview of court cases, consent decrees, federal law, and ethical guidelines related to the assessment of diverse learners.

Chapters 4 and 5, by Salvador Hector Ochoa, provide a step-by-step examination of the various forms of bilingual education and second-language acquisition, as well as the multiplicity of prereferral considerations pertaining to culturally and linguistically diverse students.

Chapters 6 and 7, by Robert L. Rhodes, detail practical guidelines for the use of interpreters during the assessment process and school-based practice and include a thorough guide for conducting interviews with parents, students, and teachers.

Chapter 8, by Samuel O. Ortiz, summarizes the acculturation factors that often influence the performance of culturally and linguistically diverse students during psychoeducational assessment procedures. This is an often ignored area of assessment that has a profound impact on student performance.

Chapter 9, by Salvador Hector Ochoa and Samuel O. Ortiz, focuses on language proficiency assessment as a foundation for psychoeducational assessment of culturally and linguistically diverse students. This is the first of four specialized chapters focusing on particular components of the assessment process.

Chapters 10 and 11, by Samuel O. Ortiz and Salvador Hector Ochoa, provide a two-part analysis and guide for the cognitive assessment of culturally and linguistically diverse students. The Multidimensional Assessment Model for Bilingual Individuals introduced in this book is the authors' attempt to provide a comprehensive and detailed analysis of the assessment of diverse students.

The final chapter of the book, written by Robert L. Rhodes, focuses on practical guidelines for the assessment of academic achievement. Curriculum-based and formal measures are discussed as well as recommendations for an integrated and comprehensive approach to academic achievement assessment.

# Acknowledgments

We would like to acknowledge the following individuals and groups for their generous assistance in the completion of this project: Kenneth W. Merrell, Series Editor of The Guilford Practical Intervention in the Schools Series, for his guidance and insight; Dawn Flanagan, Celeste Roseberry-McKibben, Larry Mattes, Wayne Thomas, and Virginia Collier, from whose work we were able to draw and build upon; Connie Fournier, for her review of the manuscript; and the American Psychological Association, the Council for Exceptional Children, and the National Association of School Psychologists, for use of excerpts from their publications in this practitioner-focused effort.

Moreover, we would like to acknowledge the work of individuals whose scholarship has greatly influenced our work and has had a significant impact within the school psychology, special education, and speech and language pathology fields with regard to English language learners. They are, in no particular order: Richard Woodcock, Ana Muñoz-Sandoval, Richard Figueroa, Leonard Baca, Alba Ortiz, Thomas Oakland, Jonathan Sandoval, Criselda Alvarado, Jim Cummins, Ena Vazquez-Nuttall, Alfredo Artiles, Hortencia Kayser, Celeste Roseberry-McKibben, Larry Mattes, and Elizabeth Pena.

And last, but certainly not least, we would like to express our appreciation and gratitude to our graduate assistants, research assistants, and secretarial and office staff for their invaluable efforts in bringing all of this together: Agnieszka Dynda, Erin Lindemann-Labuhn, Roman Garcia de Alba, Sandra Romero, and Adam Schaer.

# Contents

# List of Forms, Tables, and Figures

## FORMS

## TABLES

## FIGURES

# 1

# English-Language Learners in U.S. Public Schools

## A Heterogeneous Population

This book examines and addresses many factors associated with assessing school-age students in U.S. schools who are culturally and linguistically diverse. Many of these students do not have sufficient English-language skills. Many terms are used to identify these students; some of the more commonly used terms include "limited English proficient" (LEP), "second-language learner" (SLL), "English-language learner" (ELL), "culturally and linguistically diverse" (CLD), and "bilingual." Moreover, states use different definitions to operationally define which students comprise this population (Anstrom, 1996). This multiplicity leads to confusion and differences of opinion about who is LEP and what is the number of LEP students in the United States.

The purpose of this chapter is to provide a set of definitions with which to identify LEP students, and to discuss the incidence of this particular student population. With a more comprehensive understanding of these issues, school-based practitioners can better understand the challenges faced by LEP children and recognize the increasing probability that they will need to provide assessment services for these children. The implications of this information for school psychologists and other school personnel are also addressed.

## DEFINITIONS

### Federal Definition

Title VII of the Improving America's School Act of 1994 (Public Law 103-382) provides the following definition to identify LEP students. The LEP individual is defined as someone who

has sufficient difficulty speaking, reading, writing, or understanding the English language and whose difficulties may deny such individual the opportunity to learn successfully in classrooms where the lan-

---

This chapter is by Salvador Hector Ochoa.

1

guage of instruction is in English or to participate fully in our society due to one or more of the following reasons:

[1] was not born in the United States or whose native language is a language other than English and comes from an environment where a language other than English is dominant;

[2] is a Native American or Alaska Native or who is a native resident of the Outlying Areas and comes from an environment where a language other than English has had significant impact on such individual's level of English language proficiency; or

[3] is migratory and whose native language is other than English and comes from an environment where a language other than English is dominant. (sec. 7501)

## State-Level Definitions

The manner in which this federal definition is operationally defined by states varies considerably. Henderson, Abbott, and Strang (1993, as cited in Hopstock & Bucaro, 1993) surveyed state and U.S. territories education agencies in order to determine how each defined LEP. From the 52 education agencies that responded to the survey, they found that the definitions of LEP contained the "following criteria: a non-English language background (44 cases); difficulty in understanding, speaking, reading, and/or writing English (29 cases); percentile cutoffs on language or achievement tests (17 cases); local determination (9 cases); and other criteria such as grade reports and teacher judgements (13 cases)" (pp. 27–28).

Each state agency's definition of LEP will impact the methods used to identify LEP students. Macias (1998) researched the different methods employed by each state agency in order to identify LEP students. Table 1.1 lists the top 11 methods and an "other" category used by states to achieve this task. These methods include the use of student records, teacher observation, teacher interview, referral, parent information, student grades, home language survey, informal assessment, language proficiency test, achievement tests, and criterion-referenced test. Data for four states (Nebraska, Pennsylvania, Virginia, and West Virginia) are not provided. The data in Table 1.1 reveal that there is considerable variation in how states identify LEP students. The number of methods used by states ranged from 4 (Florida and Texas) to 12 (Louisiana, Maine, Oklahoma, and South Carolina). All states (with the exception of Hawaii) used home language surveys as a method to identify LEP students. A home language survey usually asks the parent to identify what language is spoken at home and/or if anyone in the home speaks a language other than English. Moreover, all but two states (Kentucky and Tennessee) used a language proficiency test as part of their data collection process to identify LEP children.

It is important that school-based practitioners know which methods are used by their respective states to identify LEP students for several reasons. First, knowing what data to look for in the child's cumulative education record will help to ensure whether or not the child was appropriately identified as LEP. Second, data for the various methods can provide the school-based practitioner with critical information regarding the child's family background and history (38 states obtain parent information) as well as his or her educational achievement (36 states obtain achievement test data and 20 collect criterion-referenced test data). Third, the practitioner can ascertain if educational progress has occurred from initial LEP identification by comparing achievement results from initial placement tests with the practitioner's own data obtained from formal and informal achievement testing. Fourth, the information obtained by the various methods used to identify LEP students can help the practitioner identify factors that might have been overlooked during the prereferral process.

## Practical Definitions

There are several practical definitions of LEP students that are helpful to consider while assessing these pupils. These three definitions/constructs help to illustrate the different types of LEP students that exist in the United States:

1. Variations in degrees of proficiency across both languages
2. Sequential versus simultaneous bilingualism
3. Elective versus circumstantial bilingualism

### Variations in Degrees of Proficiency across Both Languages

It is important to recognize that LEP students are very heterogeneous with respect to their linguistic abilities in both their first (native) language and in their second language, English. Valdéz and Figueroa (1996) contend that "it is important to view bilingualism as a continuum and bilingual individuals as falling along this continuum at different points to each other, depending on the varying strength and cognitive characteristics of their two languages" (p. 8). Moreover, this continuum should be noted across oral language skills, reading, writing, and listening (Hamayan & Damico, 1991b).

One way to understand this continuum is to consider the five levels of language proficiency that can be obtained from the Woodcock–Muñoz Language Survey (Woodcock & Muñoz-Sandoval, 1993): *negligible, very limited, limited, fluent,* and *advanced.* The Woodcock–Muñoz Language Survey provides information on a student's language skills across oral language and reading/writing domains in both English and Spanish.

To understand how variation can exist within the LEP population, three scenarios are provided. In the first scenario, an LEP student is at the *fluent* level in the oral language domain in Spanish and *very limited* in the reading/writing domain; at the same time, he or she is at the *limited* level in the oral language domain in English and *negligible* in the reading/writing domain. This scenario could possibly describe an LEP student who comes from a Spanish-speaking home with parents who have limited literacy skills; or a student who has yet to receive academic instruction in his or her first language, who has learned some English by watching television and/or playing with friends in the community, and who has no formal academic instruction in English.

In a second scenario, the LEP student is at the very limited level in the oral language domain in Spanish and negligible in the reading/writing domain; at the same time, he or she is at the negligible level in both the oral language and reading/writing domains in English. This student has little or no linguistic abilities in either domain in both languages. This scenario could possibly describe an LEP student who has recently immigrated to the United States or who has been in the United States for several years but who has not received sufficient instruction in his or her first language to adequately develop his or her English skills.

In a third scenario the LEP student is at the advanced proficiency level in the oral language domain in Spanish and at the fluent level in the reading/writing domain; at the same time, he or

TABLE 1.1. Methods Used to Identify LEP Students, by State, 1995–1997

| State | Student records | Teacher observation | Teacher interview | Referral | Parent information | Student grades | Home language survey | Informal assessment | Language proficiency test | Achievement test | Criterion-referenced test | Other | Total |
|---|---|---|---|---|---|---|---|---|---|---|---|---|---|
| Alabama | X | X | X | X | X | X | X | X | X | X | | X | 11 |
| Alaska | X | X | | | X | | X | | X | X | X | | 7 |
| Arizona | | | | X | X | X | X | | X | X | | X | 7 |
| Arkansas | X | X | X | X | X | X | X | X | X | X | X | | 11 |
| California | | | | | | | X | X | X | X | X | | 5 |
| Colorado | X | X | X | X | | | X | X | X | X | | X | 9 |
| Connecticut | X | X | X | | | X | X | X | X | | | | 7 |
| Delaware | X | X | X | X | X | X | X | X | X | | | | 9 |
| District of Columbia | | | | | X | X | X | | X | X | | X | 6 |
| Florida | | | | | | | X | | X | X | | X | 4 |
| Georgia | X | X | X | X | X | X | X | X | X | X | | | 10 |
| Hawaii | X | X | | X | X | X | | X | X | X | | | 8 |
| Idaho | X | X | X | X | X | X | X | X | X | X | | | 10 |
| Illinois | X | X | X | X | X | X | X | X | X | X | X | | 11 |
| Indiana | X | | | | | | X | X | X | | | | 4 |
| Iowa | X | X | X | X | | X | X | | | | | | 6 |
| Kansas | X | X | X | X | X | X | X | X | X | X | X | | 11 |
| Kentucky | X | X | X | X | X | X | X | X | | | | | 8 |
| Louisiana | X | X | X | X | X | X | X | X | X | X | X | X | 12 |
| Maine | X | X | X | X | X | X | X | X | X | X | X | X | 12 |
| Maryland | X | X | X | X | X | X | X | X | X | X | | | 9 |
| Massachusetts | X | X | X | X | X | X | | X | X | | | | 9 |
| Michigan | X | X | X | X | X | X | X | | | | | | 6 |

| State | | | | | | | | | | | | | Total |
|---|---|---|---|---|---|---|---|---|---|---|---|---|---|
| Minnesota | × | × | × | × | × | × | × | × | × | × | × | | 11 |
| Mississippi | × | × | × | × | × | × | × | × | × | × | | | 10 |
| Missouri | × | × | | × | × | × | × | × | × | × | | | 8 |
| Montana | × | × | | × | × | × | × | | × | | × | | 8 |
| Nebraska | | | | | | | | | | | | | |
| Nevada | × | × | × | × | × | × | × | × | × | × | | | 10 |
| New Hampshire | × | × | | | × | × | × | × | × | × | | × | 9 |
| New Jersey | × | × | | | × | × | × | × | × | × | | × | 9 |
| New Mexico | | × | | | × | × | × | | × | × | | | 5 |
| New York | × | × | | × | × | × | × | × | × | × | | | 9 |
| North Carolina | × | × | × | × | × | × | × | × | × | × | | | 11 |
| North Dakota | × | × | × | × | × | × | × | × | × | × | × | × | 11 |
| Ohio | × | × | × | × | × | × | × | × | × | × | × | | 11 |
| Oklahoma | × | × | × | × | × | × | × | × | × | × | × | × | 12 |
| Oregon | × | × | × | × | × | × | × | × | × | × | | | 11 |
| Pennsylvania | | | | | | | | | | | | | |
| Rhode Island | × | × | | | × | × | × | × | × | × | × | | 6 |
| South Carolina | × | × | × | × | × | × | × | × | × | × | × | × | 12 |
| South Dakota | × | × | × | × | × | × | × | × | × | × | × | | 11 |
| Tennessee | × | × | × | | | | × | | × | | | | 7 |
| Texas | × | × | × | × | | × | × | × | × | × | × | | 4 |
| Utah | × | × | × | × | | × | × | × | × | × | × | | 8 |
| Vermont | | × | | | × | × | × | × | × | × | | | 9 |
| Virginia | | | | | | | | | | | | | |
| Washington | × | | | | × | | × | | × | × | × | | 6 |
| West Virginia | | | | | | | | | | | | | |
| Wisconsin | × | × | × | × | × | × | × | × | × | × | × | | 11 |
| Wyoming | × | × | × | × | × | × | × | × | × | × | | × | 10 |
| Total | 40 | 40 | 31 | 34 | 38 | 34 | 46 | 34 | 45 | 36 | 20 | 13 | 441 |

*Note.* From Macias (1998, Table A-6). Reprinted with permission from the National Clearinghouse for English Language Acquisition and Language Instruction Educational Programs.

5

she is at the very limited level in both the oral language domain and reading/writing domain in English. This scenario could possibly portray a student who is a recent immigrant, who received instruction in his or her native language (Spanish) in the home country, and who is beginning to learn English in a U.S. school. This scenario could possibly describe a young LEP student who has been in a dual-language instructional setting that has enabled him or her to develop his or her first language, which facilitates the acquisition of English skills. These three students are at different points of the continuum with respect to their proficiency skills across oral language and reading/writing domains in Spanish and English. Recognizing that LEP students possess varying degrees of proficiency across domains in both languages is critical to conducting a fair assessment process. The practical consequences of examining the levels of proficiency across both language domains are discussed in Chapter 9.

Information obtained on the student's language proficiency levels across domains in both languages can be used to determine if he or she is "nonbalanced," "balanced," or "mixed" bilingual (Hamayan & Damico, 1991b, p. 42). If an LEP student is stronger across all domains in the first language versus the second language, he or she would be described as a "nonbalanced bilingual" (Hamayan & Damico, 1991b). If an LEP student is stronger in one domain in one language (e.g., oral language skills in Spanish) and stronger in another domain in the second language (e.g., reading and/or writing skills in English), then he or she would be considered a "mixed" bilingual (Hamayan & Damico, 1991b). If an LEP pupil has commensurate levels of proficiency across domains (i.e., oral, reading, writing, and listening) in English and his or her native language, he or she would be characterized as a "balanced" bilingual (Hamayan & Damico, 1991b). As school-based practitioners, we will more likely be faced with assessing LEP students who are nonbalanced and mixed bilinguals.

## Sequential versus Simultaneous Bilingualism

The individual who initially was a monolingual speaker in his or her native language and was subsequently exposed to an additional language at a later time in his or her development is considered to have sequential bilingual ability (Valdés & Figueroa, 1996). Sequential bilingualism might develop in a student who recently immigrated to the United States or who came from a non-English-speaking home and is now entering public school. Simultaneous bilingualism tends to occur when someone comes from a home where two languages are used, or when a child is in a situation in which he or she was exposed to two languages at the same time at a very early age (Valdés & Figueroa, 1996). Simultaneous bilingualism could develop in a child whose parents are bilingual; one parent may speak to the child in one language, whereas the other parent interacts with the child in the other language. Simultaneous bilingualism could also develop in a child in a military family, for example, where the dominant language of one parent is English and the other parent's dominant language is a language other than English (e.g., Vietnamese); each parent speaks to the child in his or her dominant language. In both of these scenarios, the child learns both languages at the same time. School-based practitioners who assess LEP students can expect to assess a significant number of students who demonstrate sequential bilingualism.

## Elective versus Circumstantial Bilingualism

The elective/circumstantial bilingualism construct was developed by Valdés and Figueroa (1996). They describe individuals who develop circumstantial bilingualism as "individuals who because of their circumstances, find that they must learn another language in order to survive. . . . [T]hese individuals find themselves in a context which their ethnic language is not the majority, prestige, or national language" (p. 12). Many LEP students in U.S. public schools can be considered circumstantial bilinguals. These children typically come from families who have recently immigrated to this country or who live in homes where parents and other family members have primarily, if not exclusively, conversed in their native language. Elective bilingualism occurs when individuals have selected to learn an additional language—for example, a school-age child whose monolingual English-speaking parents elect to enroll him or her in a two-way bilingual program in a U.S. school. (This type of bilingual program is explained in Chapter 4.) School psychologists who conduct psychoeducational assessment with culturally and linguistically diverse students can expect to assess significant numbers of students who have circumstantial bilingualism compared with those who have elective bilingualism.

## DEMOGRAPHICS

The LEP student population is rapidly increasing. In order to understand the extent of this growth, demographic data are discussed on a national scale and at the levels of state, school, and classroom. These data clearly indicate that many school-based practitioners will encounter LEP children as part of their caseload.

### National Scale

The LEP student population accounts for 9.3% of the total school-age population (prekindergarten to 12th grade) in the United States for the 1999–2000 academic year (Kindler, 2002). The U.S. school-age population includes data from the 50 states, the District of Columbia, and seven U.S. territories (Guam, Marshall Islands, Micronesia, Northern Mariana Islands, Palau, Puerto Rico, and Virgin Islands). The LEP student population totaled 4,416,580 (Kindler, 2002). Approximately 95% of this population resided in the 50 states and the District of Columbia; 5% reside in the seven U.S. territories.

With regard to the 50 states and the District of Columbia, LEP students comprised 8% of the school-age population (Kindler, 2002) and totaled 3,730,966. In particular, LEP students constituted 10.3% of the elementary (prekindergarten to 6th grade) school-age population (Kindler 2002).

The LEP student population is increasing at a faster rate than the general student population in the United States. The National Clearinghouse for English Language Acquisition (2002c) and Language Instruction Educational Programs reported that the LEP student population in the United States increased 104.97% from 1989–1990 to 1999–2000, whereas the general student population increased only 24.21% during this same time period. Moreover, it should be noted that the U.S. Bureau of the Census (2001) reported that one in five children in the United States had at least one parent who was foreign born.

As noted, the U.S. LEP student population is quite heterogeneous. This population encompasses over 400 different languages (Kindler, 2002), of which 77% is Spanish speaking (National Clearinghouse for English Language Acquisition, 2002b). The other nine languages include Vietnamese (2.3%), Hmong (2.2%), Haitian Creole (1.1%), Korean (1.1%), Cantonese (1.0%), Arabic

(0.9%), Russian (0.9%), Navajo (0.9%), and Tagalog (0.8%). The remaining languages are spoken by 12% of the LEP student population.

## State Level

The school-age LEP population demonstrates interesting differences and trends on a state level. The differences include the number of LEP students in each state and the particular languages they speak. The trends include the emergence of language groups in certain regions of the country and the rapid growth of all LEP students in nearly every state.

Table 1.2 reveals that LEP pupils constitute at least 10%, or more, of the pupils in six states (California = 24.9%, New Mexico = 23.6%, Alaska = 14.8%, Arizona = 14.7%, Texas = 13.9%, Nevada = 12.4%). In contrast, this population comprises less than 2% of the overall enrollment in 12 states (Alabama, Indiana, Kentucky, Louisiana, Maine, Missouri, New Hampshire, Ohio, Pennsylvania, Tennessee, Vermont, West Virginia).

Differences also exist with respect to the most frequently spoken languages by LEP students in each state. Table 1.3 lists the top 5 languages for each state and the District of Columbia. Data for Colorado and North Dakota were not included. Other than English, Spanish is the most frequent language spoken by LEP students in 41 states and the District of Columbia. Spanish ranked second in 2 states and third in 3 states; it did not emerge in the top 5 languages spoken by LEP students in Montana and Hawaii. Vietnamese, the second largest LEP population subgroup, was among the top 5 languages spoken (other than English) in 31 states and the District of Columbia; it ranked second in 14 states and the District of Columbia, third in 9 states, fourth in 7 states, and fifth in 1 state. Although Spanish and Vietnamese differ considerably in their overall representation in the LEP student population (77% vs. 2.3%), these two languages are the most prevalent across many states and the District of Columbia.

Interesting trends also emerge for some of the other top 10 language groups in the United States. Hmong was the most frequent language spoken, other than English, by the LEP student population in Minnesota; it ranked second in Wisconsin, third in California, and fourth in Oregon and Michigan. Thus, there is a significant Hmong presence in the North-Central and West Coast regions of the United States. The fourth largest LEP subgroup, Haitian Creole, is concentrated in the Northeastern United States (Delaware, New Jersey, New York, Massachusetts) and Florida. Haitian Creole did not rank among the top five languages in any other states. Korean, which ranked fifth nationally, was among the top five languages spoken in 19 states. This language group ranked in either second or third in some Northeast coastal states (New Jersey, New York, Maryland, Virginia). Arabic is the seventh largest LEP language subgroup in the United States and is most prevalent in five states that border one another: Illinois, Michigan, Indiana, Ohio, and West Virginia. Arabic is either the second or third most common LEP language subgroup in these five states. Russian is the eighth largest LEP language subgroup in the United States and emerged in the top five languages spoken in 13 states and Washington, DC. Children from this language subgroup are prevalent in the Northwestern United States (Alaska, Washington, Oregon, Idaho). Lastly, Navajo-speaking children are most prevalent in the Western states of Arizona, New Mexico, and Utah, where they ranked as the second largest subgroup of LEP children.

The most important trend noted among the LEP population in the United States is its rapid growth. Table 1.4 lists the overall student population and LEP school-age population growth for every state and the District of Columbia from 1989–1990 to 1999–2000. It should be noted that

**TABLE 1.2. Pre-K–12 LEP Public School Enrollment, by State, 1999–2000**

| Jurisdiction | LEP enrollment, 1999–2000 | Total enrollment, 1999–2000[a] | Percent LEP, 1999–2000 |
|---|---|---|---|
| Total—United States | 4,416,580 | 47,356,089 | 9.3% |
| Subtotal—States and DC | 3,730,966 | 46,632,055 | 8.0% |
| Alabama | 7,260 | 740,732 | 1.0% |
| Alaska[b] | 19,721 | 133,047 | 14.8% |
| Arizona[b] | 125,311 | 850,840 | 14.7% |
| Arkansas | 9,102 | 451,034 | 2.0% |
| California[b] | 1,480,527 | 5,952,598 | 24.9% |
| Colorado | 60,031[c] | 708,109 | 8.5% |
| Connecticut[b] | 20,190 | 553,993 | 3.6% |
| Delaware | 2,284 | 112,836 | 2.0% |
| District of Columbia | 5,177 | 77,194 | 6.7% |
| Florida | 235,181 | 2,381,396 | 9.9% |
| Georgia[b] | 30,491 | 1,391,403 | 2.2% |
| Hawaii | 12,879 | 185,860 | 6.9% |
| Idaho | 17,732 | 245,331 | 7.2% |
| Illinois | 143,855 | 2,027,600 | 7.1% |
| Indiana | 13,079 | 988,702 | 1.3% |
| Iowa | 10,120 | 497,301 | 2.0% |
| Kansas | 18,672 | 472,188 | 4.0% |
| Kentucky | 4,847 | 648,180 | 0.7% |
| Louisiana | 6,906 | 756,579 | 0.9% |
| Maine | 2,748 | 209,253 | 1.3% |
| Maryland | 20,855 | 846,582 | 2.5% |
| Massachusetts | 45,065 | 971,425 | 4.6% |
| Michigan[b] | 44,471 | 1,701,044 | 2.6% |
| Minnesota[b] | 45,640 | 844,800 | 5.4% |
| Mississippi | 1,799 | 500,716 | 0.4% |
| Missouri | 10,238 | 914,110 | 1.1% |
| Montana[b] | 4,016 | 157,058 | 2.6% |
| Nebraska | 9,144 | 288,261 | 3.2% |
| Nevada | 40,469 | 325,610 | 12.4% |
| New Hampshire[b] | 2,471 | 205,072 | 1.2% |
| New Jersey[b] | 49,847 | 1,275,062 | 3.9% |
| New Mexico | 76,661 | 324,495 | 23.6% |
| New York[b] | 228,730 | 2,850,163 | 8.0% |
| North Carolina | 41,667 | 1,275,925 | 3.3% |
| North Dakota[b] | 8,324 | 112,104 | 7.4% |
| Ohio | 16,841 | 1,836,554 | 0.9% |
| Oklahoma | 38,823 | 627,032 | 6.2% |
| Oregon | 43,845 | 545,033 | 8.0% |
| Pennsylvania | 28,540 | 1,816,716 | 1.6% |
| Rhode Island | 10,245 | 156,454 | 6.5% |
| South Carolina[b] | 5,577 | 650,450 | 0.9% |
| South Dakota | 5,495 | 131,037 | 4.2% |
| Tennessee | 11,039 | 916,202 | 1.2% |
| Texas | 554,949 | 3,991,783 | 13.9% |
| Utah | 41,306 | 480,255 | 8.6% |
| Vermont | 936 | 104,559 | 0.9% |
| Virginia | 31,675 | 1,133,994 | 2.8% |
| Washington | 55,709 | 1,003,714 | 5.6% |
| West Virginia | 1,039 | 291,811 | 0.4% |
| Wisconsin | 27,184 | 877,753 | 3.1% |
| Wyoming[b] | 2,253 | 92,105 | 2.4% |

*Note.* From Kindler (2002, Table 1). Reprinted with permission from the National Clearinghouse for English Language Acquisition and Language Instruction Educational Programs.

[a]Total enrollment data from the NCES (2001).

[b]Includes K–12 data only (pre-K either not available or not reported).

[c]Jurisdictions did not respond to 1999–2000 State Educational Agency (SEA) Survey; total LEP enrollment figures are imputed from the most recently available data from SEAs.

**TABLE 1.3. Top Five Languages Spoken by LEP Students, by State, 1999–2000**

| Jurisdiction | #1 language | #2 language | #3 language | #4 language | #5 language |
|---|---|---|---|---|---|
| United States | Spanish | Vietnamese | Hmong | Haitian Creole | Korean |
| Alabama | Spanish | Vietnamese | Cambodian | Korean | Arabic |
| Alaska | Yup'ik | Inupiak | Spanish | Russian | Korean |
| Arizona | Spanish | Navajo | Apache | Vietnamese | O'Odham |
| Arkansas | Spanish | Lao | Vietnamese | Arabic | Korean |
| California | Spanish | Vietnamese | Hmong | Cantonese | Tagalog |
| Colorado | — | — | — | — | — |
| Connecticut | Spanish | Portuguese | Polish | Chinese (unspec.) | Albanian |
| Delaware | Spanish | Haitian Creole | Korean | Arabic | Cantonese |
| District of Columbia | Spanish | Vietnamese | Chinese (unspec.) | Russian | Arabic |
| Florida | Spanish | Haitian Creole | Portuguese | Vietnamese | French |
| Georgia | Spanish | Vietnamese | Korean | Chinese (unspec.) | Russian |
| Hawaii | Ilocano | Samoan | Tagalog | Marshallese | Cantonese |
| Idaho | Spanish | Native American | Serbo-Croatian | Russian | Vietnamese |
| Illinois | Spanish | Arabic | Korean | Cantonese | Russian |
| Indiana | Spanish | Japanese | Arabic | Vietnamese | Korean |
| Iowa | Spanish | Serbo-Croatian | Vietnamese | Lao | German |
| Kansas | Spanish | Vietnamese | Lao | Cambodian | Korean |
| Kentucky | Spanish | Serbo-Croatian | Vietnamese | Japanese | Arabic |
| Louisiana | Spanish | Vietnamese | Arabic | Cantonese | Korean |
| Maine | French | Spanish | Passamaquoddy | Cambodian | Somali |
| Maryland | Spanish | Korean | English Creole | Vietnamese | Cantonese |
| Massachusetts | Spanish | Portuguese | Cambodian | Vietnamese | Haitian Creole |
| Michigan | Spanish | Arabic | Chaldean | Hmong | Albanian |
| Minnesota | Hmong | Spanish | Vietnamese | Lao | Cambodian |
| Mississippi | Spanish | Vietnamese | Arabic | Korean | Tagalog |
| Missouri | Spanish | Serbo-Croatian | Vietnamese | Arabic | Somali |
| Montana | Salish | Cree | Crow | Dakota | Assiniboine |
| Nebraska | Spanish | Vietnamese | Arabic | Omaha | Navajo |
| Nevada | Spanish | Tagalog | Chinese (unspec.) | Vietnamese | Korean |
| New Hampshire | Spanish | Vietnamese | Portuguese | Lao | Russian |
| New Jersey | Spanish | Korean | Portuguese | Haitian Creole | Gujarati |
| New Mexico | Spanish | Navajo | Vietnamese | Arabic | Korean |
| New York | Spanish | Chinese (unspec.) | Russian | Haitian Creole | Urdu |
| North Carolina | Spanish | Hmong | Vietnamese | Chinese (unspec.) | Arabic |
| North Dakota | — | — | — | — | — |
| Ohio | Spanish | Somali | Arabic | Pennsylvania Dutch | Japanese |
| Oklahoma | Spanish | Cherokee | Native American | Vietnamese | Choctaw |
| Oregon | Spanish | Russian | Vietnamese | Hmong | Ukrainian |
| Pennsylvania | Spanish | Vietnamese | Cambodian | Russian | Korean |
| Rhode Island | Spanish | Portuguese | Haitian Creole | Cambodian | Lao |
| South Carolina | Spanish | Vietnamese | Russian | Japanese | Korean |
| South Dakota | Lakota | German | Spanish | Dakota | Hutterite |
| Tennessee | Spanish | Vietnamese | Kurdish | Arabic | Japanese |
| Texas | Spanish | Vietnamese | Cantonese | Korean | Lao |
| Utah | Spanish | Navajo | Vietnamese | Lao | Portuguese |
| Vermont | Serbo-Croatian | Vietnamese | Spanish | Chinese (unspec.) | French |
| Virginia | Spanish | Vietnamese | Korean | Arabic | Tagalog |
| Washington | Spanish | Russian | Vietnamese | Ukrainian | Cambodian |
| West Virginia | Spanish | Arabic | Japanese | Russian | Korean |
| Wisconsin | Spanish | Hmong | Lao | Russian | Albanian |
| Wyoming | Spanish | Vietnamese | Russian | — | — |

*Note.* A dash (—) indicates that data were either missing or not available from the state. From Kindler (2002, Table 3). Reprinted with permission from the National Clearinghouse for English Language Acquisition and Language Instruction Educational Programs.

TABLE 1.4. Student and LEP Student Growth, by State

| State | Student enrollment growth from 1990–1991 to 1999–2000 | LEP student enrollment growth from 1990–1991 to 2000–2001 | Ranking in terms of % growth from 1990–1991 to 2000–2001 |
|---|---|---|---|
| Alabama[a] | 1.50% | 590.10% | 3 |
| Alaska | 13.00% | 71.70% | 32 |
| Arizona | 27.50% | 107.90% | 25 |
| Arkansas | −1.20% | 430.00% | 7 |
| California | 12.40% | 71.80% | 31 |
| Colorado | 18.50% | 299.90% | 12 |
| Connecticut[a] | 4.50% | 18.80% | 44 |
| Delaware | −5.80% | 55.40% | 34 |
| District of Columbia | −21.90% | 51.50% | 35 |
| Florida | 19.80% | 280.70% | 14 |
| Georgia | 15.00% | 392.30% | 9 |
| Hawaii | −8.10% | 41.90% | 40 |
| Idaho | 27.70% | 415.50% | 8 |
| Illinois | −4.40% | 96.60% | 27 |
| Indiana | 3.80% | 226.90% | 20 |
| Iowa | −4.90% | 180.90% | 21 |
| Kansas | 1.50% | 325.80% | 11 |
| Kentucky | 71.50% | 351.30% | 10 |
| Louisiana | −16.60% | −2.60% | 50 |
| Maine | −6.60% | 50.80% | 36 |
| Maryland | 3.30% | 93.30% | 28 |
| Massachusetts | 1.90% | 12.50% | 47 |
| Michigan | 7.90% | 33.00% | 42 |
| Minnesota | 4.20% | 284.90% | 13 |
| Mississippi | −7.70% | 11.20% | 48 |
| Missouri | 0.50% | 260.00% | 19 |
| Montana | −2.20% | −36.10% | 51 |
| Nebraska | −5.10% | 896.10% | 1 |
| Nevada | 66.30% | 445.20% | 5 |
| New Hampshire | 60.70% | 272.10% | 17 |
| New Jersey | 2.20% | 15.50% | 46 |
| New Mexico | 3.30% | 30.50% | 43 |
| New York | −5.00% | 44.80% | 38 |
| North Carolina | 12.80% | 808.60% | 2 |
| North Dakota | −11.20% | 15.80% | 45 |
| Ohio | −7.20% | 97.50% | 26 |
| Oklahoma | 10.00% | 266.00% | 18 |
| Oregon | 6.30% | 480.20% | 4 |
| Pennsylvania[c] | −11.30% | 43.50% | 39 |
| Rhode Island | −2.00% | 58.90% | 33 |
| South Carolina[b] | −5.10% | 280.40% | 16 |
| South Dakota | −7.10% | 48.10% | 37 |
| Tennessee | 11.90% | 443.00% | 6 |
| Texas | 15.90% | 79.10% | 30 |
| Utah | 9.70% | 121.60% | 24 |
| Vermont | 7.00% | 143.80% | 22 |
| Virginia[d] | 5.00% | 38.10% | 41 |
| Washington | 11.10% | 137.50% | 23 |
| West Virginia | −13.20% | 280.60% | 15 |
| Wisconsin | −5.20% | 89.30% | 29 |
| Wyoming | −5.20% | −0.80% | 49 |

*Note.* Data from National Clearinghouse for English Language Acquisition and Language Instruction Educational Programs (2000a).
[a] Growth is from 1990 to 1991; [b] Growth is from 1991 to 1992; [c] Growth is from 1994 to 1995; [d] Growth is from 1995 to 1996.

data for five states listed in this table come from different time periods; these states are noted in the table.

Table 1.4 clearly demonstrates that the LEP student population increased dramatically during the 1990s. With the exception of Louisiana and Montana, every state and the District of Columbia experienced growth in their LEP school-age population. Simultaneously, 17 states incurred a decrease in their overall student enrollment. In 15 of these 17 states, however, the LEP student population increased. The top 10 states that evidenced the greatest percent growth were Nebraska (896.1%), North Carolina (808.6%), Alabama (590.1%), Oregon (480.2%), Nevada (445.2%), Arkansas (430%), Idaho (415.5%), Georgia (392.2%), Kentucky (351.3%), and Kansas (325.8%). Nine states experienced a 201–300% increase in LEP student population during the time span examined; four states reported a 100–200% increase. The LEP student population more than doubled in 23 states. Moreover, another 8 states and the District of Columbia evidenced a 51–99% growth.

## School Level

A study of the number of LEP students in U.S. public schools has been conducted by the National Center for Educational Statistics (NCES, 1997a). The NCES reported that LEP students were enrolled in 46.3% of schools during the 1993–1994 school year. The six states that had the highest percentage of schools with these students were Hawaii (96.5%), California (90.5%), Arizona (87.5%), Texas (77.1%), New Mexico (77.1%), and Nevada (71.2%; National Center for Educational Statistics, 1997a). The NCES (1997a) also found that seven states—New York (69.1%), Florida (66.5%), Idaho (63.5%), New Jersey (62.9%), Delaware (62.5%), Washington (62.1%), and Utah (61.5%)—had LEP students in 60–70% of their schools during 1993–1994. Five states had LEP students in 50–60% of their schools, and an additional six states had LEP students in 40–50%.

## Classroom Level

The NCES (2002) also conducted a study investigating the number and percent of teachers in U.S. public schools who taught LEP students during the 1999–2000 academic year. Table 1.5 reports the results of their study on national and state levels. As noted in this table, 41.2% of public school teachers taught LEP students during the 1999–2000 academic year. Over half of the teachers in 12 states had instructed LEP students. The top five states with the highest percentage of their teachers instructing LEP students were California (75.2%), Arizona (67.8%), Nevada (67.5%), Hawaii (66.2%), and New Mexico (64.7%).

## SUMMARY

This chapter has highlighted four critical factors that school-based practitioners should recognize and understand in relation to the LEP student population in the United States:

First, it is important for school-based practitioners to understand how students are identified as LEP in their respective states in order to review, evaluate, and incorporate this information into their reporting and decision-making processes.

TABLE 1.5. Percentage of Public School Teachers Who Taught LEP Students, by State, 1999–2000

| State | Total number of public school teachers | Taught LEP students |
|---|---|---|
| 50 states and DC | 2,984,781 | 41.2 |
| Alabama | 50,605 | 19.8 |
| Alaska | 8,248 | 54.3 |
| Arizona | 46,023 | 67.8 |
| Arkansas | 30,410 | 29.9 |
| California | 276,677 | 75.2 |
| Colorado | 41,327 | 53.2 |
| Connecticut | 41,971 | 44.0 |
| Delaware | 7,422 | 44.1 |
| District of Columbia | 5,512 | 36.1 |
| Florida | 127,879 | 50.9 |
| Georgia | 86,879 | 35.2 |
| Hawaii | 12,032 | 66.2 |
| Idaho | 14,447 | 49.6 |
| Illinois | 136,938 | 37.1 |
| Indiana | 61,184 | 29.0 |
| Iowa | 38,116 | 24.7 |
| Kansas | 33,968 | 24.8 |
| Kentucky | 42,879 | 19.6 |
| Louisiana | 50,642 | 16.4 |
| Maine | 17,536 | 15.3 |
| Maryland | 54,583 | 37.4 |
| Massachusetts | 77,281 | 41.2 |
| Michigan | 98,082 | 26.1 |
| Minnesota | 57,534 | 45.5 |
| Mississippi | 33,060 | 15.5 |
| Missouri | 64,094 | 22.6 |
| Montana | 11,937 | 16.8 |
| Nebraska | 23,119 | 33.9 |
| Nevada | 17,245 | 67.5 |
| New Hampshire | 14,985 | 32.2 |
| New Jersey | 97,878 | 43.3 |
| New Mexico | 21,167 | 64.7 |
| New York | 208,313 | 43.4 |
| North Carolina | 85,235 | 46.6 |
| North Dakota | 9,252 | 17.2 |
| Ohio | 123,129 | 20.5 |
| Oklahoma | 45,830 | 32.9 |
| Oregon | 28,584 | 61.5 |
| Pennsylvania | 126,471 | 24.7 |
| Rhode Island | 11,564 | 37.0 |
| South Carolina | 43,721 | 29.3 |
| South Dakota | 11,708 | 20.5 |
| Tennessee | 58,296 | 22.3 |
| Texas | 265,247 | 55.7 |
| Utah | 23,346 | 58.0 |
| Vermont | 9,186 | 24.1 |
| Virginia | 80,987 | 29.9 |
| Washington | 54,816 | 57.6 |
| West Virginia | 22,571 | 10.4 |
| Wisconsin | 67,015 | 32.6 |
| Wyoming | 7,848 | 18.9 |

*Note.* Both full-time and part-time teachers are included. These estimates apply to teachers in traditional public schools (i.e., all public schools in the United States except public charter schools). Detail may not add to totals because of rounding. From National Center for Educational Statistics (2002, Table 1.19, pp. 43–44).

Second, practitioners can expect to find that the LEP student population will vary considerably in terms of native- and English-language abilities (i.e., oral, listening, reading, and writing skills). In addition, determining if the LEP student is a simultaneous versus sequential language learner will provide information about the extent to which the English language has been developed as well as the need for dual-language instructional services.

Third, practitioners need to recognize that the LEP student population in the United States is extremely heterogeneous. Considerable variability exists within the LEP population with regard to the native languages spoken. Although there are over 400 different languages spoken in the United States, Spanish-speaking students constitute 77% of the LEP school-age population. Spanish is the most common language, other than English, in 41 of the 48 states reporting this information. School-based practitioners should also be aware, however, of the other low-incidence language groups that exist in their respective state.

Fourth, the data presented in this chapter indicate that the LEP school-age population doubled during the 1990s and continues to increase rapidly. Nearly every state evidenced growth in their LEP student population. One in every 12.5 students enrolled in U.S. public schools has LEP; 1 in every 10 elementary-age students (prekindergarten to sixth grade) has LEP. Nearly one in two American schools has LEP students on their campus. Two in five teachers taught LEP pupils during the 1999–2000 school year.

Given these statistics and demographic trends, school-based practitioners can realistically expect to assess and intervene with LEP students. It is likely that many practitioners already have assessed LEP pupils but did not know enough about these issues to be as effective as possible. If school psychologists and other personnel have not been trained to incorporate linguistic and cultural factors into their work, the possibility of misdiagnosis is greatly increased. This issue is discussed in the following chapter.

# 2

# Disproportionate Representation of Diverse Students in Special Education

## *Understanding the Complex Puzzle*

The assessment and placement process of ethnic minority as well as culturally and linguistically diverse schoolchildren for special education services has been controversial for more than 30 years. This controversy began in 1968, when Dunn first noted that there was a disproportionate number of culturally diverse children identified as "mentally retarded." Beginning in the early 1970s, litigation (*Diana v. California*, 1970; *Larry P. v. Riles*, 1972, 1974, 1979, 1986) pertaining to two cases alleging the inappropriate placement of culturally and/or linguistically diverse children in special education programs brought this issue to the national forefront. The impact of these two cases was clearly evident in Public Law 94-142, the Education for All Handicapped Children Act of 1975. This law required that students be assessed in their native language when feasible and in a nondiscriminatory manner. Subsequent revisions of this law—Individuals with Disabilities Education Act (IDEA) 1990 and 1997—continue to mandate these safeguards. Additional safeguards pertaining to culturally and linguistically diverse students were included in the 1997 reauthorization of IDEA.

Despite these litigation and legislation efforts, disproportionate representation of ethnically and linguistically diverse students in special education continues to exist. Moreover, this representation has been noted to occur in the disability categories of mental retardation (MR), learning disabled (LD), and seriously emotionally disturbed (SED). The federal government acknowledges the disproportionality problem:

This chapter is by Salvador Hector Ochoa.

The U.S. Office of Special Education Programs (OSEP) and the U.S. Office of Civil Rights (OCR) view the issue of disproportionate placement as an ongoing national problem that varies from district to district, from state to state and from region to region. . . . Congress has made the issue of disproportionate representation of minorities in special education a national priority that must be addressed decisively. (Daugherty, 1999, p. 16)

Given that disproportionate representation continues to be an unresolved problem, it is important for school-based practitioners to understand its critical components. This chapter examines four areas that illuminate the phenomenon of disproportionate representation: (1) a review of studies across approximately 20 years to examine trends and illustrate the extent of the problem; (2) the methodological and conceptual issues that must be considered when examining this issue; (3) the potential factors that help to explain why this problem continues; and (4) solutions that have been recommended to address this matter, along with policy recommendations.

The discussion of potential factors that contribute to overrepresentation will help psychologists and other school personnel understand how sociodemographic factors, school factors that include, but are not limited to, instructional, referral, and assessment practices, as well as other external factors have a bearing on the problem of disproportionality. As previously noted, this is not to say that only these factors in general education and in the referral-assessment-placement process have a bearing on disproportionate representation. However, factors in these areas are ones on which school-based practitioners and educators can have a direct influence on a day-to-day basis via their professional practices. In other words, these are areas in which school-based practitioners and educators can help to resolve a part of the disproportionality problem.

Each of the remaining chapters in this book addresses critical instructional, referral, and/or assessment issues and practices that hopefully will result in more accurate diagnosis of culturally and linguistically diverse students who are referred for special education. A review of the potential solutions will help practitioners and educators recognize that there are additional solutions that have been recommended and that must occur in order to effectively address the problem of disproportionality; furthermore, school-based practitioners can play a critical role in some of the recommended solutions. Policy recommendations are also provided; several of these policies involve the creation of guidelines that would have significant bearing on school psychology practices pertaining to culturally and linguistically diverse pupils.

## THE EXTENT OF THE PROBLEM ACROSS 20 YEARS

### Ethnic Diversity

The primary source that has been used to document and demonstrate the extent of disproportionate representation has been the U.S. Office of Civil Rights (OCR) Surveys of Elementary and Secondary Schools. OCR surveys are conducted every 2 years. The first thorough examination of this issue was conducted by the National Academy of Sciences' Panel on Selection and Placement of Students in Programs for the Mentally Retarded, whose results were reported in a book by Heller, Holtzman, and Messick in 1982. As a member of this panel, Finn (1982) analyzed data from the 1978 OCR survey and reported that the representation of African Americans in classrooms for the educable mentally retarded (EMR) were "noticeably higher" on a national scale (p. 367). Hispanics were not identified disproportionately as EMR on a national level, but they were in states (Arizona, Colorado, New Mexico, and Texas) with large Hispanic populations. Moreover, Finn noted that disproportionate numbers of Hispanics were labeled EMR in school districts that had high concentration of Hispanics.

Chinn and Hughes (1987) conducted an analysis of the 1978–1984 OCR survey data on a national scale (they did not examine OCR data on a state level) and reported that African Americans were disproportionately represented in the SED and EMR categories for 1978, 1980, 1982, and 1984. Hispanics were disproportionately identified as LD when the 1980, 1982, and 1984 OCR survey data were analyzed.

Harry (1994) reviewed the 1986 and 1990 OCR survey data on both a national level and by state, and found that African Americans were overidentified as SED, trainable mentally retarded (TMR), and EMR at the national as well as at state levels. Hispanics were disproportionately identified as TMR on a national scale in the 1990 OCR data set. Harry also noted that in the 1986 OCR survey data, Hispanics were overidentified in "states where they represented a larger proportion of the school population. . . . [F]or example, overrepresentation was evident in Arizona, where Hispanics accounted for 24 percent of the total enrollment, 31 percent of EMR, and 30 percent of TMR classes . . . " (p. 18).

The overrepresentation of culturally diverse pupils in special education was only investigated by analyzing OCR survey data from the 1970s to the 1990s because states were not required to collect and report race/ethnicity information on pupils who were identified as having a disability. In the reauthorization of IDEA in 1997 (Public Law 105-17), Congress required states to:

> (a) report, annually, the extent of minority representation by disability category; (b) determine if significant disproportionality exists, and (c) if observed, review and revise policies, practices, and procedures in identification or placement to ensure that minority children are not inappropriately identified or served in more restrictive settings. (Oswald, Coutinho, Best, & Singh, 1999, p. 196)

The *Twenty-Second Annual Report to Congress on the Implementation of the Individual with Disabilities Education Act* (Office of Special Education and Rehabilitation Services, 2000) did include information on race/ethnicity, as required by Public Law 105-17. Data obtained from this report were analyzed by the National Research Council's (NRC, 2002) Committee of Minority Representation in Special Education and Parrish (2002). The NRC (2002) committee reported that on a national level, African American students have a 135% and 59% greater probability, when compared to white pupils, of being identified as MR and ED (emotional disturbance), respectively. Similarly, Parrish reported that on a national scale, compared to white students, African American students have a 188% greater probability of being identified as MR and a 92% greater probability of being identified as ED. The NRC (2002) committee found that in comparison to white pupils on a national level, Native Americans/Alaskan Natives have a 24% greater probability of being identified as LD and a 12% greater probability of being labeled as ED. Parrish (2002) found that in comparison to white pupils on a national level, Native Americans/ Alaskan Natives have a 50%, 31%, and 24% greater probability of being labeled as LD, MR, and ED, respectively. Nationally, Hispanics had a 13% lower probability of being identified as MR and a 7% greater probability of being labeled LD when compared to whites students (National Research Council, 2002). Parrish (2002) reported that on a national scale, Hispanics had a 23% lesser probability of being identified as MR and a 17% greater probability of being labeled LD when compared to white students.

*Variability across States*

It is important to note that both the NRC (2002) committee and Parrish (2002) reported that there is considerable variability across states with respect to ethnic representation across different categories. For example, the NRC committee reported that Hispanics in Massachusetts and Hawaii had a 239% percent and 151% percent greater probability, respectively, of being identified as MR when compared to whites in each of these states. These percentages are in the opposite direction from the percentage reported by the NRC for Hispanics on a national level noted above.

Parrish (2002) found that Hispanics, African Americans, Asian/Pacific Islanders, and Native Americans were more likely to be labeled MR in states that had the largest ethnic populations. Parrish conducted an analysis of the MR representation in the 10 states with the highest and lowest proportion of students from each major ethnic group and found that

> for black children, the risk of being designated mentally retarded (in comparison to whites) ranged from 3.59 in the ten states in which their proportion is the highest to 1.77 in the ten states where the proportion is the lowest. . . . For Hispanic children, the odds are more than three times as great in ten states with the highest percentage of Hispanics (1.55 vs. 0.42) as in states with the lowest percentage of Hispanics. (p. 24)

This means that Hispanic children have a 55% greater probability of being identified as MR when compared to whites in the 10 states with the highest proportion of Hispanics. However, Hispanics have a 58% lesser probability of being identified as MR when compared to whites in the 10 states with the lowest proportion of Hispanics.

Similarly, Parrish (2002) found these same trends in MR classifications for both Native Americans and Asian/Pacific Islanders. Native Americans had a 75% greater probability of being identified as MR when compared to whites in the 10 states in which they constituted the highest proportions. However, they had only a 7% greater probability of being identified as MR when compared to whites in the 10 states in which they constituted the lowest proportions. Parrish reported that Asian/Pacific Islanders had a 14% greater probability of being identified as MR when compared to whites in the 10 states that have the largest proportions of Asian/Pacific Islander, whereas they have a 44% lesser probability of being labeled MR when compared to whites in the 10 states in which they constituted the lowest proportions. These statistics clearly illustrate that data obtained on a national level can mask disproportion that exists within and across states.

*Infants, Toddlers, and Preschoolers*

Interestingly, the *Twenty-Second Annual Report to Congress on the Implementation of the Individuals with Disabilities Education Act* (Office of Special Education and Rehabilitation Services, 2000) found different trends when examining the racial/ethnic characteristics of infants, toddlers, and preschoolers served under Part C of IDEA. Early intervention services are critical, given that research has shown their positive impact (National Research Council, 2002). School districts are required to undertake activities to help identify these youngsters (e.g., Child Find) and provide these services to them. The data in this report indicate that Hispanics are being underserved. Although Hispanics account for 18.2% of the national population from birth to 2 years of age, only 14.9% of infants and toddlers served under Part C of IDEA are Hispanic. Additionally, whereas

Hispanics account for 17.2% of preschoolers (ages 3–5) nationally, only 12% of preschoolers served under Part C of IDEA are Hispanic. Contrastingly, this report noted that "Black students' representation in the . . . developmental delay categor[y] was more than twice their national population estimates" (p. II-26).

### Underrepresentation in Programs for the Gifted

It should be noted that although this chapter focuses on disproportionate representation of culturally diverse students in special education, it is important to recognize that they have been underrepresented on the other end of the exceptionality continuum: gifted students. Based on analysis of the 1992 OCR Elementary and Secondary School Civil Rights Compliance Report, Ford (1998) reported that Hispanics and African Americans were underrepresented in gifted education by 42% and 41%, respectively. The NRC (2002) committee examined ethnic representation in gifted programs by analyzing the 1998 OCR data and found that in comparison to white pupils on a national level, Asian/Pacific Islanders have a 34% greater probability of being placed in gifted education programs. The NRC committee reported that on a national level, there is lesser probability of being identified as gifted compared with whites for Native Americans/Alaskan Natives (35%), Hispanics (52%), and African Americans (59%).

### Least-Restrictive Environment Placement Issues

Another important issue pertaining to minorities in special education that has received little attention is the need to ensure their placement in the least restrictive environment. Fierros and Conroy's (2002) research concluded that "special education students from minority racial groups [Hispanics and African Americans] are more likely than whites to be placed in restrictive educational settings" (p. 40). They conclude that on national and state levels, their "research suggests . . . widespread violations of IDEA's least restrictive environment requirements" (p. 42). Parrish (2002) found that in California, Native American, Hispanic, African American, and Asian/Pacific Islander special education students were placed in self-contained classrooms to a greater extent than was warranted based on their identified needs; an 8–9% overassignment for each of these ethnic groups occurred.

## Linguistic Diversity

Whereas substantial data have been collected to document ethnic disproportionate representation of ethnic groups in special education, very little research has been conducted with culturally diverse students who are not English proficient. Language status is a factor that has received little attention in the special education literature on disproportionality. Language status cuts across all ethnic groups—Hispanics, African Americans, Native Americans, Asian/Pacific Islander, and whites. (The latter group could include recent immigrants from Eastern Europe.) No research is available that simultaneously examines the influence of language and ethnic status on special education representation. The research question remains uninvestigated: *Does special education representation vary for ethnically diverse students who are, and are not, proficient in English?*

The limited research that has examined LEP students' representation in special education on a national level has lumped together all different LEP language subgroups. Macias's (1998) survey of state education agencies found that 5.9% and 8.2% of LEP students were enrolled in special education programs during the 1994–1995 and 1995–1996 academic years, respectively. Macias's survey also noted that in 1996–1997, LEP students constituted 7.4% of the student population in the United States and its territories. During this same time period, 7.6% of LEP students were enrolled in special education programs.

The *Twenty-Third Annual Report to Congress on the Implementation of the Individuals with Disabilities Education Act* (Office of Special Education and Rehabilitation Services, 2001) also provides information about the representation of LEP students in the disability areas of MR, LD, and ED. This report cites the following figures obtained from the U.S. Department of Education's (1999b) 1997 Elementary and Secondary School Civil Rights Compliance reports: "LEP students represented 5.5 percent of the students identified as having LD, they represented just 3.7 percent of students identified with MR and 1.9 percent of students identified as having emotional disturbance" (pp. II-32–33).

Texas is one of the very few states that collects information on the number of LEP students that are in special education. In 2003–2004, LEP students comprised 15.3% of the school-age pupils in Texas; during this same academic year, LEP students comprised 14.4% of all special education students (Gonzalez, 2004; Texas Education Agency, 2004; T. Zhang, personal communication, September 2004). Thus, when examining the data on a state level, LEP students do not appear to be disproportionately represented in special education in Texas. A different picture emerges, however, when LEP students representation is examined by district level.

The Texas Education Agency (TEA) investigates disproportional representation of LEP students in special education on a district level. (This process is explained in detail later in this chapter.) This analysis is conducted for school districts that have at least 10 LEP students. The TEA compares each district's overall enrollment of LEP students with their enrollment of LEP special education students. Percentages for both of these enrollments are then compared to one another in order to obtain a "difference score" for each school district. A low score indicates that there is little or no difference between the district's percentage of LEP students in special education and their percentage in the district's overall representation. The larger the difference score, the greater the discrepancy between the district's percentage of LEP students in special education and the district's overall percentage of LEP student enrollment. For the 2000–2001 academic year, the TEA obtained difference scores for 752 school districts and found that 36 out of these 752 school districts (5%) were assigned the high-risk level (i.e., level 4) for LEP special education representation (P. Baker, personal communication, October 4, 2002). School districts that were assigned this level of risk evidenced difference scores greater than 18. Moreover, 114 school districts (15%) were assigned the second highest risk level (i.e., level 3) because their difference scores ranged from 3.6 to 18 (P. Baker, personal communication, October 4, 2002). Approximately 45% ($n = 434$) of the school districts in Texas that were rated did not evidence disproportionate representation of LEP students in special education (P. Baker, personal communication, October 4, 2002). These data clearly indicate that LEP students are disproportionately represented in special education in some but not all school districts in Texas, suggesting a considerable level of variability among districts within a state.

Disproportionate representation of LEP students in special education was also noted on a district level in a study conducted by Artiles, Rueda, Salazar, and Higareda (2002). These researchers examined LEP representation in the MR and speech and language disorder disabilities categories in 11 urban school districts in California that had significant number of students who were second-language learners, Hispanic, and poor. In comparison to pupils who were English proficient, LEP students had a greater probability of being identified for special education services in the elementary (27%) and secondary (91%) levels. In particular, the researchers noted that LEP students had a 225% greater probability of being labeled MR at the secondary level. They also noted that disproportionate representation of LEP students in special education was not evident in kindergarten through fourth grade. Disproportionate representation of pupils with LEP began in 5th grade. Artiles et al.'s (2002) findings are consistent with those of Parrish (2002) and Finn (1982): All found that disproportionate representation frequently occurs in districts or states that have high minority enrollments.

## Summary

Although it is important to acknowledge that there are limitations to the data on disproportionate representation in special education (discussed in the next section), a review of the data across a 20-year time span provides empirical support for the contention that this disproportionality continues to exist for both ethnically and linguistically diverse students. Three important groups have reached similar conclusions about the disproportionate representation of ethnically diverse students in special education. First, President Bush's Commission on Excellence in Special Education Report, *A New Era: Revitalizing Special Education for Children and their Families* (President's Commission, 2002), stated: "A particularly disturbing finding is that children of minority status are over-represented in some categories of special education. . . . The magnitude of the overrepresentation problem varied across state and local education agencies within all high-incidence categories" (p. 26). Second, the NRC's (2002) Committee on Minority Representation in Special Education's Executive Summary states: "The higher representation of minority students occurs in high-incidence disabilities categories of mild mental retardation (MMR), emotional disturbance (ED), and to a lesser extent learning disabilities (LD), categories" (p. 1). Third, the *Executive Summary—Conference on Minority Issues in Special Education*, written by the Civil Rights Project (2000) at Harvard University, states the following:

> Historically, special education has too often been a place—a place to segregate minorities and students with disabilities. . . . To the extent that minority students are misclassified, segregated, or inadequately served, special education can contribute to a denial of equality of opportunity, with devastating results in communities throughout the nation. (p. 1)

The research suggests that it is important to examine the disproportionate representation data on various levels. At times, disproportionate representation might not be evident at a national level but exists at either or both the state and district levels. The limited research on least-restrictive environment placement indicates that when compared to white students, minority pupils are placed in more restrictive educational settings within special education.

## METHODOLOGICAL AND CONCEPTUAL ISSUES

There are several methodological and conceptual issues to consider when examining the problem of disproportional representation. These issues include (1) use of different methods with which to calculate representation in special education; (2) the methodological limitations of the OCR survey data; (3) different eligibility criteria used by states to qualify a child in a given disability category; and (4) different degrees of difference used by states to constitute disproportionate representation. These factors need to be acknowledged when interpreting data on disproportionate representation. The degree to which these factors influence the picture of disproportionality is not known. Thus, these issues must be addressed in order to identify and rectify the extent of the disproportionality problem.

## Use of Different Calculation Methods

Three different methods have been used in the research literature on disproportionate representation: the risk index, odds ratio, and composition index (Losen & Orfield, 2002; National Research Council, 2002). All three of these methods were used in the literature discussed in the previous section.

### Risk Index

The risk index is obtained by dividing the number of pupils from a given ethnic background who are identified as having a particular type of disability by the total number of pupils who exist in a given population. The given population can be a school district, a state, or the nation. For example, there are 500 Hispanics in District A. Of these, 11 have been identified as MR. Thus, we would divide 11 by 500 to obtain a risk index of 2.2. This means that 2.2% of all Hispanics in District A are identified as MR.

### Odds Ratio

The odds ratio is obtained by using the risk index of an ethnic minority group as the nominator and the risk index of whites as the denominator in the division equation for the same disability category. For example, in the same District A mentioned in the previous paragraph, there are 1,000 white students of which 10 have been identified as MR. Thus a risk index of 1.0 is obtained for this group in District A by dividing 10 by 1000. The odds ratio is obtained by dividing the risk index for Hispanics with MR in District A (2.2) by the risk index for whites with MR in District A (1). The odds ratio is 2.2. This means that, in comparison to whites, Hispanic students have a 220% greater probability—or are slightly more than twice as likely—of being identified as MR in District A. In this example, the risk index for Hispanics is larger than it is for whites. When the risk index for a particular ethnic group is greater than it is for whites, this ethnic group will have a greater probability of being identified as MR. If, however, the risk index for a particular ethnic group is less than it is for whites, it means that this ethnic group has a lesser probability of being identified.

### Composition Index

"The composition index is calculated by dividing the number of students of a given racial or ethnic group enrolled in a particular category by the total number of students . . . enrolled in that same disability category" (National Research Council, 2002, p. 43). For example, in the same District A mentioned above, we have the following distribution of students identified as MR: 11 Hispanics, 14 African Americans, and 10 whites. Thus, there are a total of 35 students who are identified as MR in District A. The MR composition index for Hispanics (11/35) is 31.42%, for African Americans (14/35), 40%, and for whites (10/35), 28.58%. The composition indexes for all examined ethnic groups, when added together, should equal 100%. The composition index for each ethnic group is usually compared to the group's respective percentage in the total student population.

In District A, for example, there is a total of 2,000 students, of which 500 are Hispanic, 500 are African American and 1,000 are white. Thus, District A is comprised of 25% Hispanic, 25% African American, and 50% white students. In this scenario, the Hispanic MR composition index of 31.42% is compared with the percent of total Hispanics in District A (25%); there is a +6.42% difference. The African American comparison would be 40% (MR composition index) versus 25% (percent of total African American enrollment), resulting in a +15% difference. The difference between the white MR composition index and the percent of total white enrollment is −21.42%.

Given that these three different indices are used in the disproportionate representation research, it is important to understand what each means to reduce confusion. Knowing which of the indices is used by their respective state education agency will enable psychologists and educators to accurately interpret the disproportionate representation data from their state and, if applicable, school district. As is noted below, many states used the composition index to determine the existence of disproportionality.

## Methodological Limitations of the OCR Survey Data

Several researchers have noted limitations in the OCR survey data sets used to examine the disproportionality problem. Finn (1982) reported that the 1978 OCR survey was not a representative sample on a national scale. This OCR data set consisted of the 50 largest school districts and a sample of other districts. MacMillian and Reschly (1998) noted that "the methods for selecting districts has varied over the different surveys, thereby comprising comparison results" (p. 17). Harry (1994) reported that the 1990 OCR survey only reported national data and failed to include state data. Harry (1994) states that this omission is a problem because there is much variance across states; however, she concludes:

> These flaws suggest that some caution must be exercised in using the OCR data. Nevertheless, the data provide a comprehensive national picture that is unavailable elsewhere. Further, the bi-annual summaries for 1978 to 1990 consistently display evidence of minority disproportionate representation. . . . (p. 10)

## Different Eligibility Criteria Used by States to Qualify Students for Special Education

Researchers (Finn, 1982; Harry, 1994; National Research Council, 2002; Parrish, 2002) examining the disproportionality problem have also found that there is much variance by state. What causes this variability to occur? One possible explanation that has not been sufficiently addressed is the impact of different criteria used across states to qualify a child for a particular disability category (MacMillian & Reschly, 1998). For example, some states use a discrepancy method to qualify a student as LD. There must be a significant discrepancy between the child's intellectual functioning and his or her academic achievement in order to meet eligibility criteria as LD. Schrag (2000)

examined how each state defined "significant discrepancy" and found that there was much variance across states and that some states used more than one discrepancy criterion. Twenty-two
states use a standard score comparison, whereas 17 use a regression formula. Moreover, the
amount of the discrepancy needed to qualify as LD varies by states. Texas requires a 16-point discrepancy. In Alabama, Georgia, and New Mexico, the amount of discrepancy needed varies
depending on the child's age. Because of the varying discrepancy amounts needed, it is conceiv-
able that a student could be classified as LD in one state, relocate to another, then not be classified as LD. Thus, the number of students identified as LD in a given state can vary by the size of
the discrepancy required under state regulations. Moreover, states such as Louisiana require a
different type of discrepancy (between-subject discrepancy). MacMillian and Reschly (1998) note
that these varying criteria are problematic when interpreting overrepresentation data:

> Overrepresentation data, however, do not make adjustments for such difference—if a child is called
> LD, the data treat all such cases *as though they represented the same psychological profile.* Clearly this
> is not the case. . . . When the data are aggregated nationally, such variations are obscured and the
> results of overrepresentation data rendered hopelessly uninterpretable when considered by specific
> categories. (p. 21)

## Varying Degrees of Difference Used by States to Constitute Disproportionality

States vary as to the criteria they use to determine a disproportional level. Markowitz (1996b,
2002), from the National Association of State Directors of Special Education, examined the 29
states that have operationally defined what constitutes disproportionality. The following criteria
are used by states: "percentage point discrepancy" ($n = 10$), chi-square tests ($n = 5$), $z$-scores ($n = 3$), confidence interval bands ($n = 1$), odds ratio ($n = 3$), equity index ($n = 1$), or other state-
developed formulas ($n = 1$). Some states employ more than one method.

A few examples of how different states operationally define disproportionality helps to illustrate the variability across states. In Arkansas, disproportionality exists "if the difference between
percentage of students from a racial/ethnic group in the general student population and the percentage of students receiving special education services who are from that group is greater than
8.3%" (Markowitz, 1996b, p. 7). The percentage difference required to constitute disproportionality varies from as low as 3% in Indiana to 10% in North Carolina (Markowitz, 2002).

In New Mexico, two figures are obtained. First, the difference between the percentage of
pupils from a particular ethnic group in special education by disability category and the percentage of students from a given ethnic background in the general school-age population in the district is calculated. "If the percentage of students with disabilities in a given racial/ethnic category
is five percent above or below the percentage of that racial/ethnic group in the district, it is considered to be disproportional" (Markowitz, 1996b, p. 15). Second, an equity index is calculated for
each disability category. "This index is calculated by dividing the percentage of students with disabilities in a given racial/ethnic group by the percentage in that racial/ethnic group" (Markowitz,
1996b, p. 15). An equity index that is greater than or equal to 1.5 constitutes significant
disproportionality. Pennsylvania also uses two figures to ascertain the existence of disproportionality. The first is similar to the 5% difference used in New Mexico. The second measure is
a $z$-test of statistical significance of a proportion. This statistical technique is used in order to

determine if the difference between the two percentages (% of ethnic group in special education vs. % of ethnic group in the school district) is statistically significant. School districts that achieve a $z$-score of 1.65 or higher are considered to have disproportionate representation.

The TEA appears to be the only state agency that examines disproportionality by comparing district characteristics across the state. Disproportionate representation is examined with respect to ethnic status (Hispanic, African American, white), low socioeconomic status, LEP status, and overall special education enrollment. In particular, the state examines disproportionate representation of African Americans labeled MR and LEP students identified as speech and language disordered. In order to accomplish this task, a district-level composition index is obtained for each of the factors. Each of these special education factor composition indices is compared with its respective total district composition index, and a "difference score" is obtained by subtracting one index from the other. For example in Texas District B, 12% of LEP students are in special education (i.e., special education LEP status composition index), compared with 3% of LEP students in the total student population (i.e., general education LEP status composition index); the resulting difference score is +9%. The TEA then compiles all school districts' LEP status difference scores. (There are over 1,100 districts in Texas.) The median LEP status difference score is thereby obtained for the state and serves as the benchmark from which to determine if a particular district has disproportionate levels of LEP students in special education. The greater the distance between a particular district's LEP difference score with the state's median difference score, the greater the disproportionality (over or under) level assigned. The TEA uses a 5-point scale (0–4) to assign a risk level: A score of zero indicates that no disproportionate representation of LEP students exists. Districts that are assigned a risk factor of 3 or 4 on LEP status will have to address their disproportional LEP representation during the state's special education monitoring compliance visit. This same process is used to determine disproportionate representation for each of the following factors: ethnicity, low socioeconomic status, and overall special education enrollment, African Americans labeled as MR, and LEP students identified as speech and language disordered.

Coutinho and Oswald (2000) note that "although estimates of the extent of disproportionality have varied substantially, at least in part because of differences in definition and method, the fact of disproportionate representation of minority school children in special education is no longer in dispute" (p. 138). Based on the varying criteria for disproportionality across states, the question that still needs to be asked is what constitutes proportionality (Kauffman, Hallahan, & Ford, 1998) or disproportionality? Recognizing that states use different criteria to determine disproportionality is important because the criteria impact the number of school districts in a given state that will evidence disproportionality. Thus, caution should be exercised when comparing the percentage of school districts that evidences disproportionality in one state versus the percentage in another, because the obtained data can be greatly influenced by the criteria used. One state might appear to have significant problems with disproportionality if they use less stringent criteria.

Recognizing that states use different criteria for determining disproportionality is also important from a practical perspective. State education agencies can require school districts that have disproportionate representation to submit a corrective action plan (CAP) to address this problem. The number of school districts in a given state that submit CAPs will vary depending on the criteria set forth by that state.

School-based practitioners need to be aware of how disproportionate representation is operationally defined in their respective state and, if applicable, school district. Those employed in school districts that evidence disproportionate representation need to critically review the reasons for this problem. The following section provides a review of factors that need to be considered during this review.

## POTENTIAL FACTORS THAT ARE ASSOCIATED WITH, OR INFLUENCE, DISPROPORTIONALITY

Several potential factors are believed to be associated with and/or to influence disproportionality (see Harry, 1994; Artiles & Trent, 1994): (1) a deficit view/philosophy about culturally diverse students; (2) the sociological and economic characteristics of culturally diverse families and communities; (3) systemic school bias occurring in instruction, referral, and assessment; (4) school accountability requirements; (5) funding formulas; and (6) the ambiguity in how different disability categories are defined and constructed (Harry, 1994). Harry's (1994) thorough review of "explanations" for disproportionality concludes the following:

> This report has attempted to show that there is no single reason for this continuing problem.... [T]his report finds that the disproportionate placement of minority students in special education programs is a problem, by virtue of many gross educational and social inequities, whose strands combine into a complex and mutually inextricable force to place poor, and, in particular, poor minority students at a disadvantage. This disadvantage too often leads to failure, inappropriate assessment, the designation of a disability, and placement in stigmatizing, ineffective programs. (p. 65)

Examining these potential factors is critical in order to ascertain what changes need to take place to address the problem of disproportionality.

### Deficit View/Philosophy of Culturally Diverse Pupils

In the disproportionality context, Artiles and Trent (1994) state that "disability and cultural difference" have been "implicitly equated" (p. 424). Artiles (1998) further states:

> Indeed, we cannot and should not ignore the fact that the disproportionate representation debated is imbedded in our historically contested discourse about cultural differences. The question is, are we willing to acknowledge in our discussions about disproportionate representation that our views of cultural differences have been based on deficit thinking? (p. 33)

How we view cultural diversity has a significant impact on our expectations about the performance of ethnic minority schoolchildren and on how we frame student failure. For example, if a school psychologist believes students who are not exposed to English are at a higher risk for reading problems, then there may be a bias to "find" reading problems.

### Sociodemographic Characteristics of Culturally Diverse Families and Communities

Several researchers (MacMillian & Reschly, 1998; Wagner, as cited in Daniels, 1998) have suggested that poverty, rather than ethnicity, is the critical variable that needs to be examined in the disproportionality discussion. MacMillian and Reschly (1998) state that ethnicity and social class are not separated out in the OCR data sets. Moreover, they argue that social class, not ethnicity, is critical: "We are willing to wage that in such a matrix, the intercorrelation between ethnicity and social class would be moderately high and that social class, not ethnicity, would explain more variance in the rates of detection for these high-incidence disabilities, particularly MMR" (p. 20). MacMillian and Reschly (1998) state that if only ethnicity is examined, "interpretations tend to emphasize 'the figment of the pigment' " (p. 20).

The NRC (2002) Committee on Minority Representation in Special Education noted that many culturally diverse students are poor. They reviewed many of the risk factors usually found in families and communities that are poor, such as being exposed to "harmful toxins" (p. 4). The NRC committee stated that: "Poor children are also more likely to be born with low birth weight, to have poorer nutrition, and to have home and child care environments that are less supportive of early cognitive and emotional development than their majority counterparts" (p. 4). Furthermore, there are ethnic differences in the development of school readiness skills, as measured upon entering the public schools. The NRC (2002) Committee's review of empirical research clearly provides support for the use of early intervention methods with children who live in conditions that place them at risk.

The NRC (2002) Committee also stated that "while the committee considers the importance of early experiences to be incontrovertible, it is only one piece of the puzzle" (p. 167). This line of argument is labeled the "differential susceptibility" hypothesis (Oswald, Coutinho, & Best, 2002): "If this overrepresentation is a function of genuinely higher disability rates among students of color, national and local responses must address the social conditions that are risk factors for disability" (p. 2). Oswald et al.'s (1999) study simultaneously examined the influence of both demographic variables and ethnicity on special education placement of African Americans in the SED and MMR categories in 4,454 school districts included in the 1992 OCR data survey. Demographic data for each district were obtained from the National Center for Educational Statistics (NCES) (1992) Data Center Common Core of Data. Information on the following six demographic variables were collected: "median value housing," "median income for households with children," "percentage of children below poverty level," "percentage of children enrolled in school who are at-risk," "percentage of adults in the community who have 12th-grade education or less and no diploma," and "percentage of children who are Limited English proficient" (p. 197). Oswald et al. (1999) reported that "demographic variables were found to be significant predictors of identification of students as MMR or SED; however, after the effects of these variables were accounted for, the likelihood of being identified as MMR or SED was still significantly influenced by ethnicity" (p. 203).

Oswald et al. (2002) conducted another similar study to the one previously mentioned. In this study the researchers used the 1994 OCR data set and the NCES's 1993 data set to examine nine sociodemographic variables in relation to Hispanics, African Americans, and Native Americans. The same six variables used in the Oswald et al. 1999 study were used in this study, plus "per pupil expenditure," "student–teacher ratio," and "percent of enrolled children who are non-White." Oswald et al. (2002) report that their

> findings indicate that, even after accounting for the effects of district socio-demographic characteristics, students' gender and ethnicity are important in determining the likelihood of identification. In addition, . . . the impact of socio-demographic factors is different for each of the various gender/ethnicity groups. (p. 7)

With regard to the variable of poverty, Oswald et al. (2002) state that the data "can be viewed as supporting differential susceptibility for SED and LD among Black and Hispanic students. The MR data, however, appear to support a hypothesis of systemic bias" (p. 8). (Systemic bias is discussed in the next section.) Moreover, Oswald et al. (2002) state:

> In spite of the importance of sociodemographic factors, however, child gender and ethnicity also contribute to the likelihood of identification in important ways. This finding, along with the patterns observed in some of the sociodemographic variables, lend support to the systemic bias hypothesis. (p. 11)

## Systemic School Bias

Several researchers (Losen & Orfield, 2002; Parrish, 2002) have asserted that poverty and its associated risk factors cannot completely account for minority disproportionate representation in special education. Losen and Orfield (2002) state:

> The theory that poverty and socioeconomic factors can explain all or most of the observed racial disparities fails to account for the extreme differences between black overrepresentation and Hispanic underrepresentation, differences that are even more significant in many states than disparities between blacks and whites. . . . Yet Hispanics, like blacks, are at a greater risk than whites for poverty, exposure to environmental toxins in impoverished neighborhoods, and low-level achievement in math and reading. Thus, the high variations in identification rates among minority groups with similar levels of poverty and academic failure cast serious doubts on assertions by some researchers that it is primarily poverty and not bias that creates these deep racial disparities. (pp. xxiv–xxv)

Given that some question the validity of, or the extent of, the differential susceptibility hypothesis, others have claimed that the disproportionate representation is partially influenced by systemic bias that occurs within schools. The systemic bias hypothesis contends that there are factors in schools that place culturally diverse students at risk for being identified as disabled. Oswald et al. (2000) state that "if . . . the [disproportionality] problem arises from system bias and discrimination within the public school system, aggressive efforts are required to correct attitudes and behavior associated with special education identification of minority school children" (p. 2). Three critical factors in this area have been noted in the literature: instructional issues, referral procedures, and assessment practices. Given the importance of these factors, each is reviewed here.

### Instructional Factors

School quality varies considerably across the United States. Many minority children are educated in schools that are in low-income areas that do not have the same per-pupil expenditures as those in higher socioeconomic communities (National Research Council, 2002). Teachers in low-income area schools typically do not have the same level of teaching experience and training and are often paid less than teachers in higher socioeconomic area schools (U.S. Department of Education, 2001). Furthermore, there is a greater number of uncertified teachers in schools with low-income pupils (U.S. Department of Education, 2001). Moreover, a significant number of LEP students are not taught by certified bilingual education teachers (Kindler, 2002; Urban Teacher Collaborative, 2000). Heubert (2002) states that minority and LEP students are often not taught the skills and content that are required by state-mandated tests. Failure to be exposed to the standard curriculum places these children at risk for failure.

The importance and impact of instructional factors on eligibility for special education is best noted by changes in IDEA 1997 (Public Law 105-17): "In making a determination of eligibility under paragraph 4(A), a child shall not be determined to be a child with a disability if the determinant factor for such determination is lack of instruction in reading or math or limited English proficiency" (sec 614 [b] [5]). Kovaleski and Prasse (1999) state:

> The authors of IDEA '97 believed that students were being incorrectly identified as having a disability (typically learning disability) because they displayed academic difficulties that were a direct result of ineffective instruction or the lack of opportunity to receive effective instruction. To prevent these students from being over-identified, the "lack of instruction" requirement was added to the law. (p. 24)

The lack of effective instruction has been cited as one reason why culturally and linguistically diverse students do not experience academic success (Cummins, 1983). In schools, these children are identified as LEP if they do not possess adequate English-language skills. Several instructional programs are available to LEP children in the United States. (These programs are described briefly here and discussed in detail in Chapter 4.) One such program involves immersion, which is also referred to as the "sink or swim" method. In this program, LEP students are placed in classrooms with monolingual English-speaking students and where instruction is provided only in English.

Other instructional programs available to LEP students include the following four types of bilingual education: English as a second language (ESL), transitional/early-exit, maintenance/late-exit, and two-way/dual. These types of bilingual education vary in the length of time they offer instruction in the child's native language. ESL programs do not offer any instruction in the child's native language. Instead, teachers in ESL settings utilize teaching strategies to facilitate the learning process in English. Transitional or early-exit programs offer instruction in the child's native language for approximately 2–3 years, and maintenance or late-exit programs offer instruction in the child's native language for approximately 5–6 years. It should be noted that children in both transitional and maintenance programs also receive instruction in English. Two-way or dual bilingual programs are comprised of approximately an equal percent of LEP students and monolingual English-speaking students. In this program, instruction in both English and the other language is approximately equal.

Research has clearly demonstrated that these different types of program options for LEP students vary in their effectiveness. Studies have found that maintenance programs (Ramirez, 1992; Thomas & Collier, 1996, 1997, 2002) and dual bilingual programs (Thomas & Collier, 1996, 1997, 2002) are effective. However, these two instructional program options are the least used and/or are often not available to LEP students. The other three instructional programs (immersion, ESL, transitional) are used most frequently with LEP students, but these programs have been shown to be less effective than maintenance and/or dual/two-way programs (Ramirez, 1992; Thomas & Collier, 1996, 1997, 2002). Given these findings, it is important to note that the NRC's (2002) Committee on Minority Representation in Special Education states: "We reiterate that special education should not be considered unless there are effective general education programs" (p. 302). Bilingual education is part of general education; the effectiveness of some types of bilingual education programs has been questioned. (This issue is addressed in Chapter 4.)

Other research has documented the impact of not receiving bilingual education services. Finn (1982), who used the 1978 OCR survey data, reported that "districts with the highest disproportion levels have the smallest proportion of students in bilingual programs. It is possible that Hispanic students with poor English proficiency are misclassified as EMR when bilingual program are not available" (p. 372). Figueroa, Fradd, and Correa's (1989) summary of key findings of two federally funded Hispanic Handicapped Minority Research Institutes that examined special education issues stated: "Few children receive primary language support before special education, even fewer during special education" (p. 176). Artiles et al. (2002) found that LEP students who were taught in immersion instructional settings (i.e., English only) were "almost 3 times more likely than English language learners placed in bilingual education" to be placed in special education (p. 129).

The implications of these research findings, along with the requirements for effective instruction in IDEA (1997) are profound. Holtzman (1982), who chaired the National Academy Panel, stated that one of "two key issues . . . at the heart of the debate about disproportion" is the following:

> Disproportion is a problem when children receive low-quality instruction. This problem may arise in the regular classroom, where opportunities for academic success may be restricted or in the special education classroom, where a child's educational progress may falter due to lowered or inappropriate expectations and goals. (p. xi)

Based on this research, we might conclude that the academic difficulties and/or underachievement of some LEP students could be pedagogically induced. In these situations, identifying these LEP students as learning disabled is problematic. Moreover, the extent to which this research should be considered when complying with the "lack of instruction requirement" or "limited English proficiency" determination factors set forth in 1997 is an important factor that needs to be addressed.

## Referral Procedures

Bias in the referral process has been noted to influence disproportionality (Artiles & Trent, 1994). This bias can be manifested in two ways: (1) in terms of who gets referred, and (2) lack of prereferral interventions. Reynolds and Kaiser (1990) note that "there is evidence that persons are not always referred for services on the basis of impartial objective rationales" (p. 646). Fuchs (1991) states that referrals to special education "may be arbitrary, if not biased" on the basis of gender and minority status (p. 243). The NRC's (2002) review of research in this area found that although bias occurs in scenario-type research, the generalizability of the findings to actual real-life cases is "not clear" (p. 358).

There is evidence to suggest that a lack of prereferral interventions exists. Jean Peelen of the OCR (as cited in Markowitz, 1996a) made the following statement in September of 1995 when addressing the Project Forum's Policy Forum on Disproportionate Representation:

> What is OCR finding? There are problems related to interventions, particularly interventions implemented haphazardly and inconsistently across schools in the same district. When inconsistent interventions are combined with a high referral rate to special education for minority students, this may be

a violation of Title VI. Sometimes we see school districts where the pre-referral programs are good in schools with a high concentration of non-minority students and poor in schools with a high concentration of minority students. The OCR would probably find these districts in violation of Title VI. (p. 4)

Additionally, one of the findings noted in Figueroa et al.'s (1989) summary of the Hispanic Institutes' examination of special education issues was that "prereferral modifications of the regular program [were] rare" (p. 176). Moreover, when prereferral modifications were implemented, they were of "poor quality" (National Research Council, 2002, p. 302).

A critical area in relation to the referral process is to ascertain why linguistically diverse children are referred. Ochoa, Robles-Piña, Garcia, and Bruenig's (1999) study investigated reasons why linguistically diverse children are referred and found that nearly half of the 17 most common reasons for referral could be explained by, or were associated with, language or cultural factors. One important finding noted in Figueroa et al.'s (1989) summary of the Hispanic Institutes' examination of Hispanic representation in special education was the following: "The behaviors that trigger teacher referral suggest that English-language–acquisition stages and their interaction with English-only programs are being confused for handicapping condition" (p. 176). These findings suggest that school personnel's lack of knowledge about cultural factors and second-language acquisition might be a contributing factor. Ortiz (1990) found that when prereferral teams are trained on culture and language issues, the number of referrals of culturally and linguistically diverse students to special education is substantially reduced. Ortiz's study revealed that approximately 70% of the students being reviewed by these trained prereferral teams were not referred to special education.

## Assessment Practices

Several factors associated with the assessment process merit attention when reviewing the problem of disproportionality: (1) inadequately trained examiners, (2) inappropriate assessment practices, and (3) failure to comply with federal and/or state guidelines. Each of these factors can influence the eligibility decision of culturally and linguistically diverse students being considered for special education.

Research clearly indicates that many school psychologists are not trained to assess culturally and linguistically diverse pupils. Ochoa, Rivera, and Ford (1997) surveyed school psychologists in eight states (Arizona, California, Colorado, Florida, New Jersey, New Mexico, New York, Texas) with large Hispanic populations to determine how school psychologists assessed culturally and linguistically diverse students for learning disabilities and mental retardation. They found that 83% of the school psychologists self-reported that they were less than adequately trained by their university program to conduct bilingual assessment. It should be noted that these school psychologists indicated that they had actually conducted assessment of LEP students. Additionally, 56% of the school psychologists also self-reported that they were less than adequately trained to interpret the assessment results of bilingual and/or LEP students. Ochoa, Rivera, and Ford (1997) concluded the following:

These figures raise serious questions about the validity of test results when LEP students are assessed. The implications of these findings regarding the eligibility decisions of culturally and linguistically diverse students [are] frightening. The field of school psychology must ask itself whether the lack of adequate training by approximately 80% of school psychologists conducting bilingual psychoeducational assessment has any bearing on the overrepresentation of minority children in special education. (p. 341)

Moreover, Ochoa, Morales, and Hernandez (1997) found that misdiagnosis/overidentification of bilingual and LEP students was the fourth most frequently cited concern of school psychologists in the area of bilingual assessment.

A lack of adequately trained school psychologists has also been documented of assessments intended to ascertain if a student has a serious emotional disturbance (SED). Amado, Sines, and Garza (1999) and Ochoa, Garza, and Amado (1999) found that approximately 70% of school psychologists self-reported they were less than adequately prepared by their university training programs to conduct emotional/behavioral assessments with Hispanics and African Americans, respectively. Moreover, approximately 40% of the school psychologists in both studies reported they had not received inservice training after graduation, whereas approximately 50–60% indicated they had. These data clearly indicate that a significant number of examiners who assess Hispanics and African Americans for serious emotional disturbance do not have sufficient or appropriate training to do so.

Given these data, it is not surprising to note that the testing practices used to assess culturally and linguistically diverse students have come under intense scrutiny and criticism. Questionable assessment practices with culturally and linguistically diverse students include the use of untrained interpreters, insufficient or inadequate language proficiency testing, and intellectual and academic assessments conducted only in English. Because of the lack of bilingual examiners (Nuttall, 1987; Rosenfield & Esquivel, 1985), school psychologists often have to resort to using interpreters to assess culturally and linguistically diverse youngsters. Ochoa, Gonzalez, Galarza, and Guillemard's (1996) research on interpreter usage found that approximately 75% of school psychologists have used interpreters to assess bilingual and/or LEP students. They also found that

> Seventy-seven percent of the school psychologists who reported using interpreters had received no or very little training to do so. Only 37% of the school psychologists reported that their interpreter had received training. In only 7% of the cases were both school psychologists and interpreters trained in the interpretation process. (p. 19)

Thus, this research indicates that the use of untrained interpreters is common practice. Figueroa (1990a) contends that the use of untrained interpreters calls into question the validity of obtained assessment results. Moreover, the data presented here clearly indicate that Standard 9.11 of the 1999 *Standards for Educational and Psychological Testing*, which was created by the collaborative efforts of the American Educational Research Association, the American Psychological Association, and the National Council of Measurement in Education, is frequently violated or not observed or implemented. Standard 9.11 states: "When an interpreter is used in testing, the interpreter should be fluent in both the language of the test and the examinee's native language, should have expertise in translating, and should have a basic understanding of the assessment process" (p. 100).

A critical factor that must be considered when culturally and linguistically diverse students are being assessed for special education—and, in particular, for learning disabilities and mental retardation—is their language proficiency in both English and their native language. IDEA

(1997) legally requires that students be assessed in their dominant language; professional standards demand that it should be done. Standards 9.3 and 9.10 of the *Standards for Educational and Psychological Testing* (1999) emphasize the importance of language proficiency:

> 9.3 When testing an examinee proficient in two or more languages for which the test is available, the examinee's relative language proficiencies should be determined. The test generally should be administered in the test taker's most proficient language, unless proficiency in the less proficient language is part of the assessment.

> 9.10 Inferences about test takers' general language proficiency should be based on tests that measure a range of language features, and not a single skill. (pp. 97–100)

Moreover, the National Association of School Psychologists' (1997) *Standards for the Provision of Psychological Services* states: "Communications are held and assessments are conducted in the client's dominant spoken language or alternative communication system. All student information is interpreted in the context of the student's sociocultural background and the setting in which she/he is functioning" (p. 62).

There is research to support the contention that the standards have not always been followed when culturally and linguistically diverse students have been assessed for special education services. Figueroa et al.'s (1989) summary of the Hispanic Institutes' examination of Hispanic representation in special education noted two key findings with regard to language proficiency testing and language factors, in general:

> Language proficiency is not seriously taken into account in special education assessment. . . . English-language problems that are typically characteristic of second-language learners (poor comprehension, limited vocabulary, grammar, and syntax errors, and problems with English articulation) are misinterpreted as handicaps. (p. 176)

More recently, Ochoa, Galarza, and Gonzalez (1996) examined language proficiency assessment practices of school psychologists who assess culturally and linguistically diverse learners. They found that many school psychologists do not use best practices in this area. Without adequate and sufficient language proficiency assessment, school psychologists will not be able to ascertain in which language(s) they should proceed when conducting intellectual and academic assessment. Moreover, Ochoa, Galarza, and Gonzalez (1996) note that "the inclusion of appropriate language proficiency assessment will prevent school psychologists from negating the significance that language has on the educational status of bilingual and LEP students" (p. 33).

Test bias (Valdés & Figueroa, 1996) and inappropriate assessment practices when assessing academic achievement and intelligence have also been problematic (Figueroa et al., 1989). Inappropriate assessment practices have been consistently observed since the *Diana v. California* case in 1970 (see Chapter 3). Figueroa's (1984, as cited in Harry, 1994) study noted that school districts were still failing to comply with appropriate assessment requirements set forth in *Diana v. California*. Another important finding noted in Figueroa et al.'s (1989) summary of the Hispanic Institutes' examination of Hispanic representation in special education was that "testing is done primarily in English, often increasing the likelihood of establishing an achievement or intelligence discrepancy" (p. 176). Ochoa, Powell, and Robles-Piña's (1996) study of how school psychologists assess the intellectual functioning and academic achievement of bilingual or LEP students also found that examiners utilize some inappropriate assessment practices, such as translating measures in English to Spanish and intermixing two languages during administration of a particular test that resulted in violating standardized test administration procedures.

## Noncompliance with State and/or Federal Guidelines

One area that has not received much attention in the disproportionality debate is noncompliance with state and federal guidelines. As noted previously, federal guidelines requiring that culturally and linguistically diverse students be assessed in their native language have been in place for more than 25 years. A review of data indicates that this assessment safeguard is not always practiced.

Another safeguard that was included in Public Law 94-142 and still remains in IDEA 1997 is the exclusionary clause. According to this clause, a student should not be considered learning disabled if the "discrepancy between ability and achievement is primarily the result of environmental, cultural, or economic disadvantage" (U.S. Department of Education, 1977, p. 65083). However, there is very limited information or research about how this federal requirement is to be implemented. Esquivel (1988) states that "legal requirements often stipulate what needs to be done, yet fail to specify how the task should be accomplished" (p. 115). The impact or influence of the exclusionary clause has not been part of the disproportionality debate. How can noncompliance with the exclusionary clause impact disproportionate representation of minorities in special education?

Ochoa, Rivera, and Powell (1997) examined how school psychologists comply with the exclusionary clause in relation to bilingual or LEP students. They conclude:

> The results of this study indicate that a number of critical factors are considered by some school psychologists to comply with the exclusionary clause when assessing bilingual and LEP students. The extent to which many of these factors are used, however, appears to be low. Moreover, many additional factors are completely overlooked by school psychologists. (p. 163)

Reviewing the extent to which language instruction and language acquisition factors were considered when complying with the exclusionary clause, Ochoa, Rivera, and Powell (1997) note:

> These findings are especially disheartening because it shows that the majority of school psychologists fail to recognize the significance of language in the educational status of LEP and bilingual students. It is especially important that language-related factors be addressed if the severe discrepancy between intelligence and achievement is in the areas of oral expression, listening comprehension, written expression, spelling, basic reading skills, and reading comprehension. (p. 165)

Another critical factor that needs to enter this discussion is the inaccurate identification of children as having a disability when they fail to meet federal or state guidelines (MacMillian & Reschly, 1998). Based on their review of the literature, MacMillian and Reschly (1998) state:

> Thus, since 1978, when P.L. 94-142 was to be fully implemented, there has been consistent evidence that between 52% and 70% of children identified by the schools as LD do not meet the standards as conceptualized in federal and state definitions of the disability category. These are startling figures

when one considers that the research has been conducted in different states, at different times, and with different strategies for selecting the samples of students with LD. How are we to interpret the overrepresentation data when over half the children classified as LD by the schools do not meet the criteria? (p. 22)

When one reviews this research on the assessment process collectively, one can find support for the conclusion reached by the Civil Rights Project (2000) at Harvard University. The project's executive summary states: "The special education evaluation process is often described as a set of discrete decisions based on scientific analysis and assessment. In reality, the evaluative decisions are more subjective, with many interdependent variables including school politics and cultural bias" (p. 2).

## School Accountability

School accountability, a subject that has received much attention in the media, is usually associated with higher educational standards. This accountability is typically measured via state competency-based testing. Schools are often rated on the collective performance of their students on their respective state competency-based test. Until recently, schools had the option of exempting students who were identified as disabled from taking this test. Thus, in order to improve the rating/ranking a school could earn, school personnel could be influenced to place more children in special education to prevent these students from lowering the school's overall results (Heubert, 2002; Project Forum, 1995).

The use of state competency-based testing is problematic when used as criteria for promotion and graduation. As previously noted, Heubert (2002) states that minorities and LEP students are among the most likely candidates *not* to receive instruction covering the full content and skills that are measured on states' competency-based measures. When this omission occurs, minority students and second-language learners are at risk for failure. If the LEP and culturally diverse pupils who fail these high-stake tests are educated in schools that are located in low socioeconomic communities, general education might not be able to meet their needs. In these situations, special education may become a preferred, or only, alternative to "save" the child. As Parrish (2002) notes, this practice, however, does not solve—and perhaps even exacerbates—the problem:

> Pressure to place more students in special education may also be increased by the recent emphasis on education accountability. If higher minority districts are held to higher standards of performance without the supplemental resources needed to achieve them, minority children may increasingly be found to need remediation, and without alternatives it may become even more likely in the future that these services will be provided through special education. This is unlikely to be the best way to assist many of these children and will continue to drive minority overrepresentation. (p. 21)

## Ambiguity of Disability Definitions and Constructs

Much has been made of problems with how mild disability categories have been defined and constructed (Artiles & Trent, 1994; Harry, 1994; MacMillian & Reschly, 1998; Ysseldyke, Algozzine,

& Thurlow, 1992). Mild disability categories include learning disabilities (LD), mild mental retardation (MMR), serious emotional disturbance (SED), and speech impaired (SI) (Harry, 1994). As noted in the methodological and conceptual issue section of this chapter, states use different criteria for determining a learning disability. Harry (1994) also notes that there is a subjective component to classifying students with mild disabilities:

> The subjective and shifting nature of the mild disability classification systems (EMR, LD, SED, SI) seriously calls into question the validity of these labels for all students, but particularly for the poor and minorities, whose life experiences, early education, language and behavioral styles make them more vulnerable to inappropriate judgments, than are their white and middle class peers. (pp. 31–32)

It should be noted that the areas of disproportionate representation noted in the first section of this chapter were in these mild disability categories. Moreover, "it is important to note that ethnic proportions in clearly biologically determined disability categories (e.g., blind, deaf, orthopedic disability) and those cases of mental retardation considered severe and profound do not yield dramatic deviations from proportions one would expect" (MacMillian & Reschly, 1998, p. 16).

## RECOMMENDED SOLUTIONS

Recommendations to address the disproportionality problem have been made by many researchers and national associations (Artiles, 1998; Artiles & Trent, 1994; Harry, 1994; Kea & Utley, 1998; National Association of State Directors of Special Education's Project Forum, 1995; National Research Council, 2002; Serna, Forness, & Nielsen, 1998; Valles, 1998). Most of these recommendations can be grouped into the following five areas: (1) teacher training at both the preservice and inservice levels; (2) improvement in early intervention/prereferral activities; (3) additional research; (4) activities that need to be undertaken by OCR; and (5) factors that should be considered by the profession.

### Teacher Training

In 1993 and 1994, Project Forum at the National Association of State Directors of Special Education Convention held three different activities that solicited input from different stakeholders, examined state efforts, and reviewed the research about the disproportionality problem. From these three activities, Project Forum compiled a list of 35 recommendations to help address disproportionality. In 1994, Project Forum invited 24 individuals from advocacy groups, universities, school districts, professional organizations, state education departments, and OCR to select 10 of the 35 recommendations that they believed "would be most likely to correct disproportionate representation" (Project Forum, 1995, p. 60). The same individuals then ranked the top 10 recommendations that emerged. The second most-often endorsed recommendation was: "Training should be provided to address the diverse learning strengths and needs of an increasing heterogeneous student population" (p. 17). Other researchers have also recommended teacher training as an important factor in addressing disproportionality. Recommended training topics included: (1)

multicultural education information (Artiles & Trent, 1994; Harry, 1994; Project Forum, 1995; Valles, 1998), (2) information on bilingual education or second-language acquisition issues (Harry, 1994; Project Forum, 1995; Valles, 1998), (3) "culturally responsive instruction" (Kea & Utley, 1998, p. 44; see also National Research Council, 2002, p. 373), (4) home–school collaboration (Project Forum, 1995), (5) behavioral management (National Research Council, 2002), and (6) "effective intervention strategies" (National Research Council, 2002, p. 373).

## Early Intervention/Prereferral Intervention

Prereferral intervention was endorsed most often and ranked as the most recommended remedy to address disproportionality by the 24 individuals surveyed by Project Forum (79% of the individuals endorsed this recommendation; Project Forum, 1995). Serna et al. (1998) also emphasize the importance of implementing empirically supported prereferral interventions. Along these same lines, the NRC (2002) Committee on Minority Representation in Special Education recommends that intervention should begin once problems are noted. Thus, the committee recommends that "universal screening programs" be in place to provide interventions to pupils who are in need of such services (p. 366).

## Research

There are many unanswered questions and unresolved issues about the disproportionality problem. Two critical lines of research have been recommended: (1) to further examine and clarify the differential susceptibility hypothesis versus the systemic bias hypothesis, which have been proffered explain the disproportionate representation of minorities in special education (Coutinho & Oswald, 2000); (2) to "emphasize the interplay between the ecological and cultural factors of children's development and learning processes" (Artiles & Trent, 1994, p. 427). Other research agendas are listed in the policy recommendations section.

## OCR Activities and Data Collection

The OCR performs many important activities with regard to the disproportionality problem. Historically, the office has conducted biannual surveys to collect data on racial/ethnic representation. Harry (1994) states that the OCR should continue to conduct its surveys but recommends that state-level data be collected and that the biannual OCR surveys should include information about whether the children are LEP or monolingual English speakers. The NRC (2002) recommends that state- and district-level data be collected. As noted, there is much evidence to suggest that there is great variability in the disproportionality problem across states. The NRC also recommends that data on LEP status be obtained, and Harry also recommends that information about the children's placement in special education be collected.

In addition to collecting data, the OCR conducts compliance reviews and complaint investigations concerning disproportionate representation in special education (Glennon, 2002). Glennon (2002) states that the OCR should increase the number of compliance visits conducted on an annual basis; moreover, Glennon recommends that compliance visits check for variables that have been associated with disproportion representation.

## Critical Issues in the Field of Special Education

There are several critical issues to consider in the field of special education with regard to the disproportionality problem. One issue is how to identify children for special education services. Presently, states identify children for these services by ascertaining if they meet state-specified criteria for a typical disability category. Harry (1994) and Project Forum (1995) advocate replacing this system with a noncategorical one that would stress examining "the identification of student needs and the provisions of services to address those needs" (Project Forum, 1995, p. 18). Another issue that the field of special education should continue to refine is that of defining/clarifying the mild disabilities categories (Artiles & Trent, 1994). Moreover, the field should also determine what constitutes disproportionality (Project Forum, 1995).

## WHERE DO WE GO FROM HERE?: POLICY RECOMMENDATIONS

This section provides policy recommendations that address the disproportional representation of culturally diverse students in special education. Some of these recommendations are based on the recommendations provided in the section on recommended solutions. Additionally, some of these recommendations have been proposed by the NRC (2002). Other recommendations have been included based on the proposed influences of disproportionality reviewed in this chapter. This list is not intended as exhaustive but rather represents critical areas that need to be undertaken if the disproportionality problem is to be understood and addressed.

1. The NRC (2002) recommends that the current "wait-to-fail" assessment model be replaced with a "universal screening program" that results in "early intervention" (pp. 365, 366). In particular, the NRC (2002) states that intervention should be undertaken when students evidence difficulty in reading. The NRC (2002) provides empirical support that early intervention efforts result in positive gains for culturally diverse children who are poor.

2. Federally funded special education research institutes should be established in order to investigate the systemic bias versus the susceptibility bias research agenda recommended by Coutinho and Oswald (2000). This information can provide critical information about the potential causes for disproportional representation.

3. Along similar lines, the NRC (2002) recommends that a panel be "convened to design the collection of a nationally representative longitudinal data that would allow for a more informed study of minority disproportion in special education" (p. 380). In particular, the NRC recommends that that some factors that need to be included in the data collection procedures include "how long the family has lived in the United States; birth country of students, their parents, and their grandparents; language proficiency (in both English and native language; education levels of parents; level of acculturation; and experiences with literacy [artifacts] and practices" (p. 380). Harry (1994) also recommended that the OCR collect language status information. Language status and the above variables recommended by the NRC apply to many different ethnic groups. Data collection on these variables will help to illustrate if there are significant between-group ethnic differences (e.g., Hispanics vs. African Americans) as well as within-group ethnic variability (e.g., Mexican American vs. Cuban American vs. Puerto Rican). Moreover, it would help to see if there

are differences within particular subgroups (e.g., nearly two in five Hispanics in 2000 were born outside the United States (Thierren & Ramirez, 2000), making the examination of first- vs. second-generation children important).

These data would help us understand the extent to which each of these variables, or their combination, influences disproportionate representation of different minority groups as well as within particular ethnic groups (e.g., Hispanics). This information would allow us to conduct analyses of language status by race/ethnicity, thereby clarifying whether language status is a critical factor in disproportionate representation for some or all racial/ethnic groups.

4. Both the OCR's and the Office of Special Education's (OSEP) annual report to Congress on the implementation of IDEA data sources should include information in addition to what is proposed by Harry (1994) and the NRC (2002) pertaining to language status. This information would include (1) the availability of dual-language instruction prior to referral; (2) parent denial of bilingual education services; and (3) type of bilingual education offered. As noted earlier in this chapter, two of these instructional situations (the availability of dual-language instruction prior to referral and parent denial of bilingual education) can have a significant bearing on second-language learners' academic outcomes and possible placement in special education. These recommendations would expand the research conducted by Artiles et al. (2002) in this area to a national level and would include different disabilities categories (e.g., LD). Research in this area is critical, given that IDEA 1997 clearly specifies that LEP and lack of instruction cannot be determining reasons for qualifying a child for special education services.

5. National guidelines need to be developed to help school personnel comply with determining that LEP is not a factor in eligibility for special services, as outlined in IDEA 1997. These guidelines will also provide a framework for the OCR to use when conducting monitoring activities.

6. National guidelines need to be developed to help school personnel comply with the "lack of instruction" requirements in IDEA 1997. These guidelines will also provide a framework for the OCR to use when conducting monitoring activities.

7. National guidelines should be developed to help school personnel comply with the exclusionary clause provision in IDEA 1997. This clause is a significant safety net that can reduce the disproportionality problem if multidisciplinary decision-making school committees understand how to implement it in their school settings. These guidelines will also provide a framework for the OCR to use when conducting monitoring activities.

8. Given the scarcity of bilingual school psychologists and the simultaneous increase in the LEP student population in the United States, national guidelines should be developed concerning the use of interpreters in assessment with students who speak low-incidence languages. Once formulated, training in this area should be provided to relevant school personnel. Federally funded research needs to examine if the use of either trained or untrained interpreters has a bearing on the disproportionality problem.

9. Given the shortage of school psychologists who are adequately prepared to assess culturally and linguistically diverse pupils for special education, state certification boards should consider requiring a separate licensing credential in the area of bilingual assessment with Spanish-speaking students. This bilingual examiner credential should require dual-language competency as well as a knowledge base of cultural and linguistic factors. Such an examiner would better ensure that children are assessed in their native language when appropriate and necessary. In this

manner, the legal safeguards of the *Diana v. California* case and IDEA 1997 will be implemented effectively.

10. Federally provided special education research funds should be allocated to develop and evaluate assessment models/methods for use with culturally and linguistically diverse students. Moreover, significant priority for funding should be given to investigate psychometric test bias with culturally and linguistically diverse populations.

11. As recommended by Artiles and Trent (1994) and Harry (1994), clarification of the mild disabilities constructs needs to be undertaken, particularly the LD category. The special education profession should advocate for uniform national criteria. Refinement of the LD construct should incorporate theoretical and empirical research in the field.

12. A uniform national standard of what constitutes disproportionality needs to be determined. This standard will allow for comparisons across states and will help to clarify the extent of the disproportionality problem.

13. Federally funded research should be allocated to develop and evaluate empirically supported interventions as well as to develop prereferral models that address issues of culture and language (National Research Council, 2002).

14. State monitoring components in special education should investigate the degree to which state guidelines for eligibility in the mild disabilities categories are followed in schools. This information should be analyzed by both race/ethnicity and language levels.

Implementation of these policy recommendations would help provide a better understanding of, and increase the probability of addressing, the disproportionality problem from both a theoretical and an applied perspective. Improvements on both of these fronts are critically needed.

## SUMMARY

Disproportionate representation of culturally diverse and linguistically diverse pupils in special education continues to exist. Many factors contribute to disproportionate representation. The research reviewed in this chapter provides support for both the differential susceptibility hypothesis and the systemic school bias hypothesis. This review suggests that practices associated with school systemic variables (bilingual and general education instructional practices; referral practices; inadequately trained school psychologists; use of untrained interpreters; insufficient or inadequate assessment practices pertaining to language proficiency, academic achievement, and intelligence; and noncompliance with state and/or federal guidelines [e.g., exclusionary clause]) need to be addressed and improved by school-based practitioners and educators to reduce the mislabeling of second-language learners. The remaining chapters of this book address these factors. It is our hope that once these factors are addressed, professional practices pertaining to assessment procedures and eligibility decisions will be improved. The assessment of second-language learners is extremely controversial, complex, and difficult and involves far more factors than which tests should be administered.

It is important that practitioners work collaboratively with other educators in general education to address the influence of systemic school factors on disproportionate representation. In short, significant changes need to occur in general education. How general education practices respond to LEP students who are experiencing failure or who are at risk for failure is critical. In these situations, an immediate referral to special education is not acceptable. How general education practices respond to the educational needs of second-language learners is critical. Bilingual education is not a remedial program but rather a part of general education. A referral to special education simply because the LEP student experiences academic failure when there is no bilingual education program available or when the bilingual education program is provided only to a certain elementary grade level is not an acceptable practice. How general education views special education is also important; special education should not be considered a means to "save" a child because he or she is going to drown in a general education program that does not address his or her linguistic needs.

The problems associated with disproportionate representation are complex, as are the potential solutions. Although the focus of this book is to provide both theoretical and practical information to improve practice, it is important to recognize that addressing the disproportionality problem will require further research. Moreover, the development of professional guidelines is needed and would help educators to meet the egalitarian intent of Public Law 105-17. The implementation of the specific policy recommendations would help as well.

# 3
---

# Legal and Ethical Requirements
# for the Assessment of Culturally
# and Linguistically Diverse Students

In these days it is doubtful that any child may reasonably be expected to succeed in life
if he is denied the opportunity of an education. Such an opportunity . . . is a right which
must be made available on equal terms to all.

—*Brown v. Board of Education* (1954)

In its current form the assessment of students who are culturally and linguistically diverse is, at
best, a work in progress and, at worst, a biased and damaging process. Even the most well-
intentioned school-based practitioner may easily overlook key environmental, cultural, and economic factors, language acquisition issues, and acculturation characteristics. In order to minimize
potential harm and maximize assessment and intervention effectiveness, it is essential that school-
based practitioners develop a clear understanding of the legal requirements and ethical guidelines established during the past half century.

## LEGAL REQUIREMENTS

Legal requirements for school-based practice are largely reactionary: Someone somewhere did
something wrong, and now there is a law restricting individuals from doing that same thing again.
When at a later date someone else does something similar but somehow uniquely different, the
law is often altered and expanded to restrict this new type of behavior as well. An understanding
of this overly simplistic, although generally accurate, description of the evolution of legal requirements is fundamental to an appreciation of their purpose as well as their limitations. Legal

This chapter is by Robert L. Rhodes.

42

requirements establish minimal standards of practice. They are not aspirational in nature, nor do they provide a sufficient safeguard to ensure appropriate and accurate assessment of each student, even if followed in a prescriptive fashion.

## THE LETTER OF THE LAW VERSUS THE SPIRIT OF THE LAW

The underlying meaning of the phrase "the letter of the law versus the spirit of the law" is that simple adherence to the legal requirements of a given situation may not yield the result that the law was intended to produce. This failure to capture the "spirit" or intention of the law is perhaps nowhere more evident than in the school-based application of federal and state regulations. On occasion as school psychologists, we have met each legal requirement of a given scenario, only to be wholly dissatisfied with the end result. More often than not, the scenario involved our work with a student who was culturally and linguistically diverse and our own inability to sufficiently address the complexities of the case through a paint-by-numbers legalistic approach.

Recognition that a minimalistic legal approach alone is insufficient should not hinder a pursuit of the spirit of the law, however. Educational law must be used in the manner in which it is intended to be used: as a foundation for practice upon which educators can enthusiastically build. The answer to appropriate and comprehensive assessment of students who are culturally and linguistically diverse is *not* found in the abandonment or circumvention of the law. Instead, the legal rights and privileges that all students have been afforded over the years must be preserved while individually appropriate methods are implemented. When a thorough understanding of the legal requirements of federal and state regulations is combined with unique and innovative approaches to working with culturally and linguistically diverse children and their parents encouraging results are often generated (see Rhodes, 1996).

The purpose of this chapter is to provide school-based practitioners with an overview of consent decrees, case law, and federal law related to the assessment of students who are culturally and linguistically diverse. Associated ethical considerations and guidelines are also discussed. In keeping with the practical nature of this book, specific portions of federal law, ethical guidelines, and professional standards are provided.

## CONSENT DECREES

A "consent decree" is a negotiated agreement between the parties to a lawsuit that resolves the disputed issues and is sanctioned by the court. The plaintiff and defendant in a civil lawsuit often reach such an agreement prior to an official ruling in order to avoid the cost of further litigation. A consent decree is a legally enforceable court order or legal mandate that represents the agreement reached between the two parties. It is often the case in this type of arrangement that the defendant agrees to cease an activity or practice asserted by the government to be illegal. Consent decrees describe the actions that must be taken by one or both of the parties to end the disagreement and are binding only to the parties to the decree. Although consent decrees do not make case law or set legal precedent, they are often very influential in the development of state and federal regulations (Reynolds, 2000). *Diana v. State Board of Education* and *Guadalupe Organization v. Tempe Elementary School District No. 3* are two well-known consent decrees related to students who are culturally and linguistically diverse that have had a significant impact on special education legislation and litigation.

### Diana v. State Board of Education (1970)

*Diana*, named for one of nine plaintiffs in a class-action suit, alleged disproportionate representation of bilingual, Spanish-surnamed students in a program for the mentally retarded. Diana's case is a poignant example of the harmful effects of inappropriate assessment practices and a failure to account for linguistic differences. Diana, a member of a Spanish-speaking household, was assessed and placed in a classroom for students with mental retardation after receiving an IQ score of 30. When she was later reassessed with the same instrument by a bilingual psychologist in both Spanish and English, she received a score that was almost 50 points higher and no longer qualified for special education services. The consent decree in this case mandated the assessment of children in their native language or with sections of tests that do not require knowledge of the English language.

### Guadalupe Organization v. Tempe Elementary School District No. 3 (1972)

The plaintiff's request in this case was to require the local school district to provide all non-English-speaking Mexican American (Hispanic) and Yaqui Indian students with bilingual–bicultural education. Similar to the *Diana* consent decree, provisions set forth in *Guadalupe* mandated the assessment of students in their primary language or through the use of nonverbal measures if the student's primary language was not English. The *Guadalupe* consent decree further specified that IQ tests could not be the sole criteria or primary basis for the diagnosis of mild mental retardation and that adaptive behavior must be assessed outside of the school setting.

## CASE LAW AND THE ASSESSMENT OF CULTURALLY AND LINGUISTICALLY DIVERSE STUDENTS

Civil cases that ultimately result in a formal court ruling establish case law. Similar to consent decrees, case law often serves as a foundation for public law. To understand the origin and purpose of today's public laws regarding the assessment of culturally and linguistically diverse students, it is important to understand the court cases upon which they were built. The following cases, presented in chronological order, provide an example of the sequential progression of legal requirements. From *Brown v. Board of Education* to *Mills v. Board of Education*, the rationale and need for broad-based protection and procedures for students with disabilities, including students with disabilities who were culturally and linguistically diverse, were increasingly established.

### Brown v. Board of Education (1954)

In this landmark case, the court ruled that segregation of students on the basis of race or ethnicity was a direct violation of the 14th Amendment of the U.S. Constitution. The Equal Protection Clause of the 14th Amendment specifies that no state shall "deny any person within its jurisdiction the equal protection of the laws." A separate education for students who were African American was determined to be an unequal education and was viewed as resulting in arbitrary discrimination. The *Brown* ruling opened the door to future litigation and legislation limiting discriminatory practices against students who were viewed as different because of race, ethnicity, culture, language, or disability.

### *Pennsylvania Association for Retarded Citizens v. Commonwealth of Pennsylvania* (1972)

*PARC* was a class-action suit filed on behalf of 13 mentally retarded students. The suit alleged that the denial of attendance of students with mental retardation in the public schools of Pennsylvania was a violation of the equal protection and due process clauses of the 14th Amendment. A U.S. federal court ratified the consent agreement reached between the two parties that disallowed the exclusion of mentally retarded students from the public schools. The court also mandated several provisions that are routinely included in present-day statutes. In accordance with the court ruling, the state of Pennsylvania was required (1) to provide a free, appropriate education to all students, regardless of the nature or extent of their disability; (2) to educate children with disabilities alongside children without disabilities to the extent possible; (3) to conduct an annual census to locate and serve children with disabilities; (4) to cease and desist from applying school exclusion laws; (5) to notify parents before assessing a child to determine the presence of a disability or prior to placement in a special education program; (6) to establish due process procedures; (7) to reevaluate children identified as having a disability on a regular basis; and (8) to pay for private-school tuition if the school refers the student to a private school or cannot reasonably meet the needs of the student in the public school (Reynolds, 2000).

### *Mills v. Board of Education* (1972)

Similar in nature to *PARC*, *Mills* was a class-action suit filed by the parents of students with disabilities against the District of Columbia Board of Education for failure to provide all students with disabilities a public education. The court ruling in this case required that the plaintiffs be provided a free public education, that due process procedures be established, and that students with disabilities receive special education services regardless of the school district's financial capability.

## PUBLIC LAW AND THE ASSESSMENT OF CULTURALLY AND LINGUISTICALLY DIVERSE STUDENTS

The rulings of *PARC* and *Mills* opened a floodgate of litigation and garnered the attention of state departments of education and legislators alike. That same year (1972), the U.S. Congress, prompted by the significance and volume of cases, initiated federal legislation to protect the rights of students with disabilities (Jacob-Timm & Hartshorne, 1998). After extensive debate, the revolutionary and broad-based Education for All Handicapped Children Act (EHA) was signed into law 3 years later.

## Education for All Handicapped Children Act

The EHA (Public Law 94-142; 1975) was the culmination of two decades of consent decrees, court rulings, and parent advocacy. It set into federal law much of what had been established through state and federal courts during the previous 20 years and, as a result, brought about sweeping changes for all children with disabilities. Children who qualified under the newly established categories of disability were guaranteed numerous rights and privileges, including a free and appropriate public education (FAPE), education in the least restrictive environment (LRE), the development of an individualized education program (IEP), and nondiscriminatory assessment procedures to determine eligibility for services.

The nondiscriminatory assessment procedures implemented by EHA are encapsulated in the Act's "Protection in Evaluation Procedures" provisions (PEP; Education for All Handicapped Children's Act, 1975). Donovan and Cross (2002) note that specific features of the PEP provisions were derived verbatim from previous court cases (*Diana*, 1970; *Guadalupe*, 1972; *Mills*, 1972; *PARC*, 1972). Incorporating the agreements and rulings from these cases, the PEP required (1) a comprehensive, individualized evaluation; (2) nondiscriminatory procedures for ethnic and cultural minorities; (3) the evaluation of multiple domains and the use of multiple measures rather than one single measure; and (4) team-based decision making that involved the participation of parents. Donovan and Cross state that the dual purposes of the PEP regulations were to ensure that students who had a true disability were determined to be eligible for special education services, and that those students who had different learning patterns and behaviors because of cultural and language differences, rather than a disability, were not determined to be eligible. It is this very distinction with which we continue to struggle today.

The EHA was amended in 1978 (Public Law 98-773), 1983 (Public Law 98-199), 1986 (Public Laws 99-457 and 99-372), 1988 (Public Law 100-630), and 1990 (Public Law 101-476). The growing number of diverse students, newly established consent decrees and court rulings (see *PASE v. Hannon*, 1980; *Larry P. v. Riles*, 1986; *Daniel R. R. v. Texas Board of Education*, 1989), and continued difficulty differentiating difference from disability resulted in increasingly specific requirements and procedures for the assessment of culturally and linguistically diverse students.

## Individuals with Disabilities Education Act

During the 1990 amendments to the EHA (Public Law 101-476), the law was renamed the Individuals with Disabilities Education Act (IDEA, 1990). The term *handicapped* was replaced with *disabilities* and a greater emphasis was placed on timely and comprehensive multidisciplinary evaluations. Early intervention services were emphasized for children from birth to 2 years of age, and autism and traumatic brain injury were added to the list of eligible disability categories. The PEP regulations were maintained as a guide for nondiscriminatory assessment.

## Individuals with Disabilities Education Act, Revisions of 1997

Although a thorough discussion of the extensive revisions to the IDEA in 1997 (Public Law 105-17) is beyond the scope of this book, the regulations and procedures that are most influential to children who are culturally and linguistically diverse are provided in the following sections. Questions frequently asked by practitioners are presented and addressed by direct excerpts from public law. Issues related to parental consent, native language, parental notice, evaluation procedures, eligibility determination, exclusionary factors, IEP process considerations, and non-discriminatory assessment procedures are discussed.

## WHAT DOES "INFORMED PARENTAL CONSENT" MEAN?

[§300.500(b)(1)]

**Definition of "Consent"**

Included in the meaning of "consent" is the requirement that the parent be fully informed, in his or her native language or other mode of communication, of all information relevant to the activity for which consent is sought.

Bersoff and Hofer (1990) state that three key characteristics must be present in order to establish informed consent. The person providing consent must be:

1. *Knowledgeable*. The parent or guardian must have a clear understanding of the situation for which his or her consent is requested.
2. *Legally competent*. The parent or guardian must be competent to give consent. From a legal perspective, the parent is deemed to be competent unless found to be incompetent through a formal hearing.
3. *Voluntary*. Parental consent cannot be coerced or forced. It must be given freely and voluntarily after weighing the information presented.

Federal law requires that parents be fully informed of all aspects of any activity for which consent is sought. Informed consent is not merely the act of receiving a parent's signature on a permission-to-test form, IEP form, or other official document. The signature of a parent verifying his or her understanding and consent to an activity is the culmination of a deliberate process. School-based practitioners, in the rush of the evaluation process, may approach parental consent as an initial hurdle that must be overcome as quickly and effortlessly as possible in order to move on to the true task at hand (i.e., assessment). In taking this approach, there is not only the danger of violating parental rights, but also the loss of a tremendous opportunity to encourage parents to become a knowledgeable and powerful advocate for their child. Informed consent procedures should help parents better understand the rights and responsibilities that they and their child have, the purpose of the assessment process, the sequential steps in the process, the time line of activities, and possible outcomes. The outcome of consent procedures should be a parent who is fully prepared to make an informed decision regarding his or her child's participation in the assessment process. The provision of this information in the parent's native language or other mode of communication is a critical requirement to maintain the validity of informed consent procedures (see the definition of "native language," below).

# WHAT DOES "NATIVE LANGUAGE" MEAN?

(§300.19)

### Definition of "Native Language"

The term "native language," if used with reference to an LEP individual, means:

- The language normally used by that individual, or, in the case of a child, the language normally used by the parents of the child (except as provided below).
- In all direct contact with a child (including his or her evaluation), the language normally used by the child in the home or learning environment.
- For an individual with deafness and blindness or no written language, the mode of communication is that normally used by the individual (e.g., sign language, Braille, or oral communication).

Under the 1997 revisions of the IDEA, the definition of "native language" was expanded to clarify that:

- In all direct contact with a child (including his or her evaluation), communication would be in the language normally used by the child and not that of the parents, if there is a difference between the two.
- For individuals with deafness or blindness or no written language, the mode of communication would be that normally used by the individual (e.g., sign language, Braille, or oral communication).

# ARE THERE OTHER PARENTAL NOTICE REQUIREMENTS?

[§300.561(a)(1)]

### Other Notice to Parents

The State Education Agency shall give notice that is adequate to fully inform parents that the state is required to have on file, in detail, the policies and procedures that the state has undertaken to ensure protection of the confidentiality of any personally identifiable information collected, used, or maintained for their child, including a description of the extent that the notice is given in the native languages of the various population groups in the state.

# WHAT NONDISCRIMINATORY PROCEDURES SHOULD BE FOLLOWED DURING THE EVALUATION PROCESS?

[§300.532(a)]

### Evaluation Procedures

Each public agency must ensure that tests and other evaluation materials used to assess a child under Part B of the IDEA:

- Are selected and administered so as not to discriminate on a racial or cultural basis.
- Are provided and administered in the child's native language or other mode of communication, unless it is clearly not feasible to do so.
- Are selected and administered to ensure that they measure the extent to which an LEP child has a disability and needs special education rather than measuring the child's English-language skills.

    Under Title VI of the Civil Rights Act of 1964, in order to properly evaluate a child who may be limited in English proficiency, a public agency should assess the child's proficiency in English as well as in his or her native language to distinguish language proficiency from disability needs; and an accurate assessment of the child's language proficiency should include objective assessment of reading, writing, speaking, and understanding.

Even in situations where it is clearly not feasible to provide and administer tests in the child's native language or mode of communication for a child with limited English proficiency, the public agency must still obtain and consider accurate and reliable information that will enable the agency to make an informed decision regarding:

- Whether the child has a disability.
- The effects of the disability on the child's educational needs.

In some situations, there may be no one on the staff of the public agency who is able to administer a test or other evaluation in the child's native language, but an appropriate individual is available in the surrounding area. In that case, a public agency should identify an individual in the surrounding area who is able to administer a test or other evaluation in the child's native language; locating such an individual may require contacting neighboring school districts, local universities, or professional organizations.

With the 1997 revision of the IDEA, the PEP regulations were revised and renamed for the first time since 1977. The newly established Procedures for Evaluation and Determination of Eligibility (PEDE, Section 300.532) addressed several important considerations that may arise when working with students or parents who are culturally and linguistically diverse. The complete PEDE regulations are provided in Table 3.1.

## WHAT FACTORS SHOULD BE CONSIDERED BEFORE MAKING A DETERMINATION OF ELIGIBILITY?

[§300.534(b)(1)]

### Determining Eligibility

Upon completing the administration of tests and other evaluation materials, a group of qualified professionals and the parents of the child must determine if the child is a "child with a disability." A child may not be determined to be eligible under Part B if the determining factor is the child's lack of instruction in reading or math or the child's limited English proficiency, and the child does not otherwise meet the eligibility criteria for a "child with a disability."

A public agency must ensure that a child who has a disability, as defined in 300.7, is not excluded from eligibility because the child also has limited English proficiency or has had a lack of instruction in reading or math.

## WHAT ARE EXCLUSIONARY FACTORS?

Section 4 of the exclusionary clause for Public Law 94-142 states that a child should not be identified as learning disabled if the "discrepancy between ability and achievement is primarily the result of environmental, cultural, or economic disadvantage" (U.S. Department of Education,

**TABLE 3.1. Procedures for Evaluation and Determination of Eligibility under the Individuals with Disabilities Act Amendments of 1997**

Each public agency shall ensure, at a minimum, that the following requirements are met:

(a)
  (1) Tests and other evaluation materials used to assess a child under Part B of the Act?:
      (i)  Are selected and administered so as not to be discriminatory on a racial or cultural basis; and
      (ii) Are provided and administered in the child's native language or other mode of communication, unless it is clearly not feasible to do so; and
  (2) Materials and procedures used to assess a child with limited English proficiency are selected and administered to ensure that they measure the extent to which the child has a disability and needs special education, rather than measuring the child's English language skills.

(b) A variety of assessment tools and strategies are used to gather relevant functional and developmental information about the child, including information provided by the parent, and information related to enabling the child to be involved in and progress in the general curriculum (or for a preschool child, to participate in appropriate activities), that may assist in determining:
  (1) Whether the child is a child with a disability under §300.7; and
  (2) The content of the child's IEP.

(c)
  (1) Any standardized tests that are given to a child?:
      (i)  Have been validated for the specific purpose for which they are used; and
      (ii) Are administered by trained and knowledgeable personnel in accordance with any instructions provided by the producer of the tests.
  (2) If an assessment is not conducted under standard conditions, a description of the extent to which it varied from standard conditions (e.g., the qualifications of the person administering the test, or the method of test administration) must be included in the evaluation report.

(d) Tests and other evaluation materials include those tailored to assess specific areas of educational need and not merely those that are designed to provide a single general intelligence quotient.

(e) Tests are selected and administered so as best to ensure that if a test is administered to a child with impaired sensory, manual, or speaking skills, the test results accurately reflect the child's aptitude or achievement level or whatever other factors the test purports to measure, rather than reflecting the child's impaired sensory, manual, or speaking skills (unless those skills are the factors that the test purports to measure).

(f) No single procedure is used as the sole criterion for determining whether a child is a child with a disability and for determining an appropriate educational program for the child.

(g) The child is assessed in all areas related to the suspected disability, including, if appropriate, health, vision, hearing, social and emotional status, general intelligence, academic performance, communicative status, and motor abilities.

(h) In evaluating each child with a disability under §300.531–300.536, the evaluation is sufficiently comprehensive to identify all of the child's special education and related services needs, whether or not commonly linked to the disability category in which the child has been classified.
  (i)  The public agency uses technically sound instruments that may assess the relative contribution of cognitive and behavioral factors, in addition to physical or developmental factors.
  (ii) The public agency uses assessment tools and strategies that provide relevant information that directly assists persons in determining the educational needs of the child.

*Note.* From Individuals with Disabilities Education Act, Revisions of 1997 (Public Law 105-17, Section 300.532).

1977, p. 65083). Although students who have unique environmental, cultural, or economic circumstances may be identified as having a learning disability, the extent to which these external factors affect their academic performance must be established and may not be the primary cause of the performance deficit in question. A thorough assessment of the impact of environmental, cultural, and economic factors on a student's performance is a difficult task and requires the consideration of multiple factors. Unfortunately, the majority of school psychologists have, historically, given limited attention to the assessment of these variables (see Harris, Gray, Davis, Zaremba, & Argulewicz, 1988; Ochoa, Rivera, & Powell, 1997). Chapter 7 of this text provides a practical guide for school-based practitioners to use when asking questions related to this area.

## WHAT SHOULD BE DONE TO ENHANCE PARENT PARTICIPATION DURING MEETINGS?

[§300.501(c)(5)]

### Parent Participation in Meetings

Each public agency shall ensure that the parents of each child with a disability are members of any group that makes decisions on the educational placement of their child.

The public agency shall make reasonable efforts to ensure that the parents understand, and are able to participate in, any group decisions relating to the educational placement of their child, including arranging for an interpreter for parents with deafness or whose native language is other than English.

(§300.345)

### Parent Participation in the IEP Meeting

The public agency shall take whatever action is necessary to ensure that the parent understands the proceedings of the IEP meeting, including arranging for an interpreter for parents with deafness or whose native language is other than English.

## WHAT SPECIAL FACTORS SHOULD BE CONSIDERED DURING THE IEP PROCESS?

[§300.346(a)(2)(ii) and §300.346(b) and (c)]

### Consideration of "Special Factors" When Developing, Reviewing, and Revising the IEP

With respect to an LEP child, the IEP team shall consider the language needs of the child, as those needs relate to the child's IEP, when:

- The team develops the child's IEP, and the team conducts a meeting to review and, if appropriate, revise the child's IEP.
- In considering the child's language needs (as they relate to the child's IEP), if the IEP team determines that the child needs a particular device or service (including an intervention, accommodation, or other program modification) in order for the child to receive FAPE, the IEP team must include a statement to that effect in the child's IEP.

In developing an IEP for a child with a disability, it is particularly important that the IEP team consider how the child's level of English proficiency affects the special education and related services that the child needs in order to receive FAPE. Under Title VI of the Civil Rights Act of 1964, school districts are required to provide children with alternative language services to:

- Enable them to acquire proficiency in English.
- Provide them with meaningful access to the content of the educational curriculum available to all students, including special education and related services.

A child with a disability may require special education and related services for those aspects of the educational program that address the development of English language skills and other aspects of the child's educational program. The IEP must address whether the special education and related services that the child needs will be provided in a language other than English.

## ETHICAL CODES AND GUIDELINES

Unlike legal requirements, ethical guidelines are typically aspirational in nature. They represent ideal standards set by professionals, rather than the minimum standard required by society. Jacob-Timm and Hartshorne (1998) differentiate two general types of ethics: mandatory and aspirational. Mandatory ethics guide practitioners by delineating the behaviors and actions expected of anyone practicing within a certain field. Aspirational ethics go a step further and consider the ultimate impact on the individual receiving services and assistance. Jacob-Timm and Hartshorne note that most professional ethical codes include both mandatory "standards" and aspirational "principles." Because of the variability in circumstances, environments, and services, each profession typically has its own set of ethical guidelines. Three common guidelines for ethical practice are available for school-based practitioners involved in the assessment of students who are culturally and linguistically diverse: the National Association of School Psychologists' (2000) *Professional Conduct Manual*, the American Psychological Association's (2002) *Ethical Principles of Psychologists and Code of Conduct*, and the Council for Exceptional Children's (1997) *Code of Ethics for Educators of Persons with Exceptionalities*. Figure 3.1 provides a hierarchy of legal and ethical authorities in relation to the assessment of individual students.

School-based practitioners should have an extensive knowledge of federal law, federal regulations, and state regulations before assessing any student for eligibility determination. In the vast majority of situations, legal requirements take precedence in determining the steps that practitioners are required to follow. That being said, it is important to remember that legal requirements alone may not be sufficient to address the multiplicity of needs presented by students. In order to capture the spirit of the law, as previously discussed, it is necessary to practice in an ethically responsible and professionally sound manner. Tables 3.2–3.5 provide specific ethical guidelines and professional standards for working with students who are culturally and linguistically diverse.

The IDEA is routinely updated. It is important that school-based practitioners maintain a current copy of IDEA and associated final regulations of the statute. A copy of both may be obtained by contacting Superintendent of Documents, U.S. Government Printing Office, Attn: New Orders, P.O. Box 371954, Pittsburgh, PA 15250-7954. The most recent version of IDEA and final federal regulations may also be accessed online through the Office of Special Education Programs (OSEP) at the U.S. Department of Education's website: *www.ed.gov/offices/OSERS/Policy/IDEA/*.

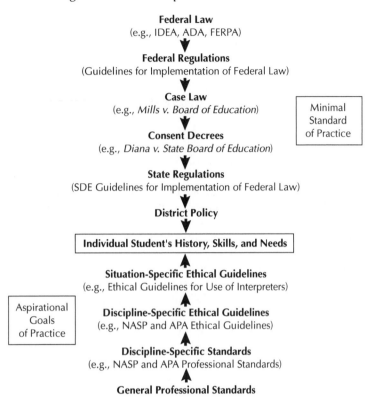

**FIGURE 3.1.** Hierarchy of legal and ethical authorities in the assessment of individual students.

## SUMMARY

The purpose of this chapter was to provide school-based practitioners with an overview of consent decrees, case law, and federal law related to the assessment of students who are culturally and linguistically diverse. Associated ethical considerations and guidelines were also discussed. The practice of individuals working with students who are culturally and linguistically diverse should be based upon an understanding of the historical context of legal and ethical requirements and current federal law, ethical guidelines, and professional standards.

**TABLE 3.2.** Excerpts from the National Association of School Psychologists' (2000) *Professional Conduct Manual*

The following excerpts from the National Association of School Psychologists' *Professional Conduct Manual* represent ethical principles and standards of practice related to issues of cultural and linguistic diversity.

## PRINCIPLES FOR PROFESSIONAL ETHICS

### Professional Relationships

(A.2.) School psychologists respect all persons and are sensitive to physical, mental, emotional, political, economic, social, cultural, ethnic and racial characteristics, gender, sexual orientation, and religion.

(A.3.) School psychologists in all settings maintain professional relationships with children, parents, and the school community. Consequently, parents and children are to be fully informed about all relevant aspects of school psychological services in advance. The explanation should take into account language and cultural differences, cognitive capabilities, developmental level, and age so that it may be understood by the child, parent, or guardian.

(C.3.) School psychologists encourage and promote parental participation in designing services provided to their children. When appropriate, this includes linking interventions between the school and the home, tailoring parental involvement to the skills of the family, and helping parents gain the skills needed to help their children.

(C.5.) School psychologists discuss with parents the recommendations and plans for assisting their children. The discussion includes alternatives associated with each set of plans, which show respect for the ethnic/cultural values of the family. The parents are informed of sources of help available at school and in the community.

### Professional Practices

(C.1.b.) School psychologists respect differences in age, gender, sexual orientation, and socioeconomic, cultural, and ethnic backgrounds. They select and use appropriate assessment or treatment procedures, techniques, and strategies. Decision-making related to assessment and subsequent interventions is primarily data-based.

## GUIDELINES FOR THE PROVISION OF SCHOOL PSYCHOLOGICAL SERVICES

**Practice Guideline 5:** School psychologists have the sensitivity, knowledge, and skills to work with individuals and groups with a diverse range of strengths and needs from a variety of racial, cultural, ethnic, experiential, and linguistic backgrounds.

(5.2) School psychologists recognize (in themselves and others and in the techniques and instruments that they use for assessment and intervention) the subtle racial, class, gender, and cultural biases they may bring to their work and the way these biases influence decision-making, instruction, behavior, and long-term outcomes for students. School psychologists work to reduce and eliminate these biases where they occur.

(5.4) School psychologists incorporate their understanding of the influence of culture, background, and individual learning characteristics when designing and implementing interventions to achieve learning and behavioral outcomes.

**TABLE 3.3. Excerpts from the American Psychological Association's (2002) *Ethical Principles of Psychologists and Code of Conduct***

The following excerpts from the American Psychological Association's *Ethical Principles of Psychologists and Code of Conduct* address ethical principles related to issues of cultural and linguistic diversity.

### Boundaries of Competence (2.01)

Psychologists provide services, teach, and conduct research with populations and in areas only within the boundaries of their competence, based on their education, training, supervised experience, consultation, study, or professional experience.

Where scientific or professional knowledge in the discipline of psychology establishes that an understanding of factors associated with age, gender, gender identity, race, ethnicity, culture, national origin, religion, sexual orientation, disability, language, or socioeconomic status is essential for effective implementation of their services or research, psychologists have to obtain the training, experience, consultation, or supervision necessary to ensure the competence of their services, or they make appropriate referrals, except as provided elsewhere in the Standards regarding Providing Services in Emergencies.

### Informed Consent (3.10)

When psychologists conduct research or provide assessment, therapy, counseling, or consulting services in person or via electronic transmission or other forms of communication, they obtain the informed consent of the individual or individuals using language that is reasonably understandable to that person or persons except when conducting such activities without consent is mandated by law or governmental regulation or as otherwise provided in this ethics code.

### Informed Consent in Assessments (9.03)

Psychologists obtain informed consent for assessments, evaluations, or diagnostic services, as described in Standard 3.10, Informed Consent, except when (1) testing is mandated by law or governmental regulations; (2) informed consent is implied because testing is conducted as a routine educational, institutional, or organizational activity (e.g., when participants voluntarily agree to assessment when applying for a job); or (3) one purpose of the testing is to evaluate decisional capacity. Informed consent includes an explanation of the nature and purpose of the assessment, fees, involvement of third parties, and limits of confidentiality and sufficient opportunity for the client/patient to ask questions and receive answers.

Psychologists inform persons with questionable capacity to consent or for whom testing is mandated by law or governmental regulations about the nature and purpose of the proposed assessment services, using language that is reasonably understandable to the person being assessed.

Psychologists using the services of an interpreter obtain informed consent from the client/patient to use that interpreter, ensure that confidentiality of test results and test security are maintained, and include in their recommendations, reports, and diagnostic or evaluative statements, including forensic testimony, discussion of any limitations on the data obtained.

### Use of Assessments (9.02)

Psychologists administer, adapt, score, interpret, or use assessment techniques, interviews, tests, or instruments in a manner and for purposes that are appropriate in light of the research on or evidence of the usefulness and proper application of the techniques.

Psychologists use assessment instruments whose validity and reliability have been established for use with members of the population tested. When such validity or reliability has not been established, psychologists describe the strengths and limitations of test results and interpretation.

Psychologists use assessment methods that are appropriate to an individual's language preference and competence, unless the use of an alternative language is relevant to the assessment issues.

### Interpeting Assessment Results (9.06)

When interpreting assessment results, including automated interpretations, psychologists take into account the purpose of the assessment as well as the various test factors, test-taking abilities, and other characteristics of the person being assessed, such as situational, personal, linguistic, and cultural differences, that might affect psychologists' judgments or reduce the accuracy of their interpretations. They indicate any significant limitations of their interpretations.

**TABLE 3.4. Excerpts from the Council for Exceptional Children's (1997) *Code of Ethics for Educators of Persons with Exceptionalities***

The following excerpts from the Council for Exceptional Children's *Code of Ethics for Educators of Persons with Exceptionalities* address ethical principles related to issues of cultural and linguistic diversity.

**Instructional Responsibilities**

Special education personnel are committed to the application of professional expertise to ensure the provision of quality education for all individuals with exceptionalities. Professionals strive to:

5. Use assessment instruments and procedures that do not discriminate against persons with exceptionalities on the basis of race, color, creed, sex, national origin, age, political practices, family or social background, sexual orientation, or exceptionality.

**Parent Relationships**

Professionals seek to develop relationships with parents based on mutual respect for their roles in achieving benefits for the exceptional person. Special education professionals:

1. Develop effective communication with parents, avoiding technical terminology, using the primary language of the home, and other modes of communication when appropriate, and
6. Recognize and respect cultural diversities which exist in some families with persons with exceptionalities.

**TABLE 3.5. Excerpts from the American Educational Research Association, American Psychological Association, and National Council on Measurement in Education's (1999) *Standards for Educational and Psychological Testing***

9.1 Testing practice should be designed to reduce threats to reliability and validity of test score inferences that may arise from language difference.

9.2 When credible research evidence reports that test scores differ in meaning across subgroups of linguistically diverse test takers, then to the extent feasible, test developers should collect for each linguistic subgroup studied the same form of validity evidence collected for the examinee population as a whole.

9.3 When testing an examinee proficient in two or more languages for which the test is available, the examinee's relative language proficiencies should be determined. The test generally should be administered in the test taker's most proficient language, unless proficiency in the less proficient language is part of the assessment.

9.4 Linguistic modifications recommended by test publishers, as well as the rationale for the modifications, should be described in detail in the test manual.

9.5 When there is credible evidence of score comparability across regular and modified tests or administrators, no flag should be attached to a score. When such evidence is lacking, specific information about the nature of the modification should be provided, if permitted by law, to assist test users properly to interpret and act on test scores.

9.6 When a test is recommended for use with linguistically diverse test takers, test developers and publishers should provide the information necessary for appropriate test use and interpretation.

9.7 When a test is translated from one language to another, the methods used in establishing the adequacy of the translation should be described, and empirical and logical evidence should be provided for score reliability and the validity of the translated test's score inferences for the use intended in the linguistic groups to be tested.

9.8 In employment and credentialing testing, the proficiency level required in the language of the test should not exceed that appropriate to the relevant occupation or profession.

9.9 When multiple language versions of a test are intended to be comparable, test developers should report evidence of test comparability.

9.10 Inferences about test takers' general language proficiency should be based on tests that measure a range of language features, and not a single linguistic skill.

9.11 When an interpreter is used in testing, the interpreter should be fluent in both the language of the test and the examinee's native language, should have expertise in translating, and should have a basic understanding of the assessment process.

# 4

## Bilingual Education and Second-Language Acquisition

### *Implications for Assessment and School-Based Practice*

School-based practitioners who assess second-language learners need to have a theoretical background in regard to critical factors related to dual-language instructional programming and second-language acquisition. In order to provide this theoretical context, this chapter addresses the following seven factors: (1) reasons why having this theoretical context is important; (2) current educational attainment status of second-language learners in the United States; (3) states that offer bilingual programs and require teacher certification in this area; (4) an explanation of the different types of bilingual education programs available in the United States; (5) research on the effectiveness of bilingual education; (6) second-language acquisition; and (7) common linguistic characteristics frequently observed in second-language learners. Knowledge about each of these seven factors enables school psychologists and other school personnel to incorporate language-sensitive procedures into their assessment practices and the eligibility decision-making process.

## WHY SHOULD SCHOOL-BASED PRACTITIONERS HAVE A THEORETICAL BACKGROUND IN SECOND-LANGUAGE ACQUISITION AND BILINGUAL EDUCATION?

There are several reasons why school-based practitioners need to have a theoretical background in second-language acquisition and bilingual education. Four main reasons are provided here, along with the implications of these reasons for school psychologists and other school personnel who assess second-language learners.

First, many myths are held by many educators and psychologists about bilingual education and how children can best acquire a second language. Cummins (1983) states that "many (but by

This chapter is by Salvador Hector Ochoa.

no means all) of the difficulties minority students experience in school are the result of both inappropriate pedagogy and misconceptions about the nature of bilingualism among educational professionals" (p. 384). Bilingual education is a controversial educational topic in the United States. One misconception held by many individuals is that bilingual education delays, if not prevents, LEP students from learning English. Many believe that it is best for an LEP child to be completely immersed in English because the best way to learn English is to spend significant amounts of time using it. This myth is held by many people in the general public, non- or limited-English-speaking parents, school officials, and school psychologists. As a result, some parents of LEP students will reject bilingual education services because they fear that their child will only learn to use their native language and fear that their child will be limited English proficient like some of them. Some parents have commented to this author that they never want their child to encounter the discrimination they themselves experienced as a result of not being able to speak English well. In these situations, school personnel (including school psychologists) often fail to provide these parents with accurate information about how best to proceed with regard to their child's mastery of the English language. It is also not uncommon for school officials who espouse the immersion myth to recommend to non- or limited-English-speaking parents that they *not* place their child in a bilingual education program.

The decision to reject bilingual education, whether parent initiated or school induced, can have significant implications concerning second-language acquisition (i.e., English) and the academic trajectory of a given LEP student. These implications are discussed in more detail later in this chapter. It is crucial that school personnel and psychologists make decisions about LEP students that are based on theory and empirical research rather than personal opinions, biases, or myths.

Second, research (Ochoa, Robles-Piña, Garcia, & Breunig, 1999; Ortiz & Polyzoi, 1986; Rueda, Cardoza, Mercer, & Carpenter, 1985) indicates that LEP children are frequently referred for special education because of oral-language-related factors. In these situations, it is important for school psychologists to ascertain whether the apparent language-related difficulty commonly exists among second-language learners. Additionally, school psychologists need to examine whether the behavioral difficulties that the LEP student is displaying stem from his or her limited English skills. Some behavioral similarities exist between the LEP student population and the LD student population (Hoover & Collier, 1985; Ortiz & Maldonado-Colon, 1986). Many school psychologists, however, do not have the training to make these types of differentiations. Ochoa, Rivera, and Ford (1997) found that less than 25% of school psychologists employed in states that have large numbers of second-language learners self-reported that they were adequately trained by their university program "to understand second language acquisition factors and their relationship to assessment of culturally and linguistically diverse pupils" (p. 338). Moreover, more than 88% of the school psychologists who reported assessing second-language learners also self-reported that they were less than adequately trained on this same factor.

Third, as discussed in Chapters 2 and 3, legal provisions outlined in IDEA 1997 require that a lack of educational opportunity and limited English proficiency be ruled out as determining factors of the child's academic failure prior to qualifying him or her as having a disability. Kovaleski and Prasse (1999) define lack of educational opportunity to include academic problems that are "a direct result of ineffective instruction or the lack of opportunity to receive effective instruction" (p. 24). How can school-based practitioners truly meet the egalitarian intent of these legal provisions if they do not have knowledge about the second-language acquisition process and what types of bilingual education programming result in positive achievement outcomes?

Fourth, IDEA 1997 also stipulates that children be assessed in their native language unless it is clearly unfeasible to do so. School psychologists need to know when it is appropriate to test LEP/bilingual students in both languages, in their native language only, or in English only. It is not uncommon for school psychologists to assess an LEP student in English only because he or she is able to converse with them in English or because the child has exited the bilingual education program. In the former situation, school psychologists overestimate the child's English-language skills. Although the LEP/bilingual child can carry a conversation in English in informal social interactions with the school psychologist, teachers, and peers, this facility does not necessarily guarantee that his or her skills in this language are sufficiently adequate to be given an intelligence measure in English. In the latter situation, school psychologists should not assume that just because the child is no longer in bilingual education that he or she possesses adequate English skills. The LEP child could have been removed from bilingual education instruction because the school that he or she attends only offers the program up to a certain grade level. Moreover, the LEP child may have been illegally exited from a bilingual education program because he or she failed to meet established exit criteria. States have guidelines specifying the criteria an LEP child must meet in order to exit the bilingual program. School psychologists need to become familiar with their respective state's criteria to ensure that second-language learners have, in fact, met this criteria. Often, school administrators are not aware of these criteria; nevertheless, they are a part of the team that makes the decision to have the LEP child removed from a bilingual program. If an LEP student has not met the state's established exit criteria, how can we conclude that the limited English proficiency or lack of educational opportunity might not be a determining factor in this student's academic difficulties?

## CURRENT EDUCATIONAL ATTAINMENT STATUS OF SECOND-LANGUAGE LEARNERS IN THE UNITED STATES

There are ample data to suggest that the collective academic performance of LEP students is significantly below that of their monolingual English-speaking peers. Data are consistent across different measures of academic performance, including performance on reading comprehension tests in native-language and English reading tests, retention, and the number of dropouts. Kindler's (2002) study on data obtained from 35 state education agencies and 3 U.S. territories (Guam, Palau, and Virgin Islands) found that only "16% of LEP students assessed scored above the state-established norm" on English reading comprehension measures (p. 8). Moreover, Kindler reported that data from 8 state educational agencies (Alaska, Iowa, Nebraska, New Jersey, New Mexico, Oklahoma, Rhode Island, and Texas) and the Virgin Islands indicated that "30% of LEP students assessed scored above the state-established norm" on Spanish reading comprehension measures (p. 9). This student population also evidences high retention rates (e.g., repeating a grade level). With regard to retention rates, Kindler's study on data obtained from 39 states, Guam, Northern Mariana Islands, and the Virgin Islands reported that 8.7% of LEP students in grades 7 to 12 had been retained.

The National Center for Educational Statistics (NCES, 1997b) reported major differences in the dropout rates between LEP students versus monolingual English-speaking students and students with learning disabilities (all study individuals were between the ages of 16 and 24 years in

1995). The NCES (1997) found that 24.2% students who came from homes in which English was not spoken (i.e., LEP students) dropped out of school. The dropout rate for students of the same ages who came from homes in which English was spoken was considerably lower: 9.6%. Notably, the dropout rate for students with learning disabilities was 17.6%. Thus, the dropout rate for LEP students was higher than it was for students with disabilities. As evidenced by their passing rates at or above their respective state norm on native-language and English reading comprehension tests, these data clearly indicate that a significant number of LEP students is experiencing academic difficulties. Moreover, approximately one-fourth of LEP students drop out of school. Given these data, it is not surprising that LEP students are referred for special education. The critical question to ask, however, is: "To what degree is the second-language learner's academic difficulty or failure due to an inherent disability versus pedagogically induced factors?" These data appear to reveal more about the instruction these students receive than their individual or collective academic potential. Thus, a review of the instructional pedagogy these students received is warranted.

## AVAILABILITY OF BILINGUAL EDUCATION, ENGLISH AS A SECOND LANGUAGE, AND CERTIFIED TEACHERS

There is considerable variability across states with regard to the availability of bilingual education and ESL programs as well as certified teachers to staff them. Table 4.1 displays the results of McKnight and Antunez's (1999) study of state education agencies, in which they examined teacher certification for working with LEP students. As can be seen in Table 4.1, only 19 states provide certification or endorsement for teachers in the field of bilingual education, and only 17 states legally mandate that this training be provided. Nearly twice as many more states ($n = 37$) provide endorsement or certification in ESL, but it is only legally mandated in 23 states.

There is a shortage of trained bilingual education and ESL teachers in the United States. Kindler (2002) reports that "there is an average of one teacher certified in ESL for approximately every 30 students . . . and an average of one teacher certified in bilingual education for every 76 LEP students" (p. 10). Ratios of certified bilingual and ESL teachers to LEP students vary considerably by state. According to Kindler, the following states had a certified bilingual education teacher-to-LEP student ratio that was larger than 1:1,000: Kansas, Maryland, Nebraska, Oregon, and South Dakota (Kindler, 2002). The following states had a ratio between 1:375 and 1:600: Minnesota, New Hampshire, North Dakota, Oklahoma, Tennessee, Utah, and Wyoming. Fourteen states had a ratio between 1:100 and 1:300, and 11 states had a ratio between 1:25 and 1:99. The two states with the lowest ratio were Massachusetts and Vermont (1:12). Kindler was unable to obtain ratios for 11 states and the District of Columbia.

The shortage of bilingual education teachers also exists in urban areas (Urban Teacher Collaborative, 2000). The Urban Teacher Collaborative's (2000) survey of 40 large urban school districts across the country revealed that there was an immediate demand for elementary level bilingual teachers in 67.5% of the districts and for both middle school level and high school level bilingual teachers in 57.5% of the districts.

Regarding the ratio of certified ESL teachers to LEP students, Kindler (2002) reported that eight states had a ratio that was larger than 1:2,000 (Alabama, Alaska, Michigan, Montana, North Dakota, New York, North Dakota, and Oklahoma). Five states (Hawaii, Mississippi, New Mexico,

TABLE 4.1. State Legislative Requirements

| State | Does the state have legislative provisions for: | | Does the state offer teacher certification/endorsement for: | |
| --- | --- | --- | --- | --- |
| | LEP student instructional programs? | Instructional program funding for LEP students? | English as a second language? | Bilingual/dual language? |
| Alabama | No | No | Yes | Yes |
| Alaska | Yes | Yes | No | No |
| Arizona | Yes | Yes | Yes | Yes |
| Arkansas | Yes | Yes | Yes | No |
| California | Yes | Yes | Yes[a] | Yes[a] |
| Colorado | Yes | Yes | Yes[a] | Yes[a] |
| Connecticut | Yes | Yes | Yes[a] | Yes[a] |
| Delaware | Yes | Yes | Yes | Yes |
| District of Columbia | Yes | No | Yes | Yes |
| Florida | Yes | Yes | Yes | No |
| Georgia | Yes | Yes | Yes | No |
| Hawaii | No | No | Yes | No |
| Idaho | Yes | Yes | No | No |
| Illinois | Yes | Yes | Yes[a] | Yes[a] |
| Indiana | Yes | Yes | Yes[a] | Yes[a] |
| Iowa | Yes | Yes | Yes | No |
| Kansas | Yes | Yes | Yes[a] | Yes[a] |
| Kentucky | Yes | No | Yes[a] | No |
| Louisiana | No | No | No | No |
| Maine | Yes | Yes | Yes | Yes |
| Maryland | Yes | Yes | Yes[a] | No |
| Massachusetts | Yes | Yes | Yes[a] | Yes[a] |
| Michigan | Yes | Yes | No | Yes[a] |
| Minnesota | Yes | Yes | Yes[a] | Yes[a] |
| Mississippi | No | No | No | No |
| Missouri | Yes | Yes | Yes[a] | No |
| Montana | Yes | No | Yes[a] | No |
| Nebraska | Yes | Yes | Yes[a] | No |
| Nevada | Yes | Yes | Yes[a] | Yes[a] |
| New Hampshire | Yes | Yes | Yes | No |
| New Jersey | Yes | Yes | Yes[a] | Yes[a] |
| New Mexico | Yes | Yes | Yes | Yes |
| New York | Yes | Yes | Yes[a] | Yes[a] |
| North Carolina | Yes | Yes | Yes[a] | No |
| North Dakota | Yes | Yes | No | Yes |
| Ohio | Yes | No | Yes[a] | Yes[a] |
| Oklahoma | Yes | Yes | No | No |
| Oregon | Yes | Yes | Yes | No |
| Pennsylvania | Yes | No | No | No |
| Rhode Island | Yes | Yes | No | No |
| South Carolina | No | No | No | No |
| South Dakota | Yes | No | No | No |
| Tennessee | No | No | Yes | No |
| Texas | Yes | Yes | Yes[a] | Yes[a] |
| Utah | Yes | Yes | Yes[a] | Yes[a] |
| Vermont | Yes | Yes | No | No |
| Virginia | Yes | Yes | Yes[a] | No |
| Washington | Yes | Yes | Yes[a] | Yes[a] |
| West Virginia | No | No | No | |
| Wisconsin | Yes | Yes | Yes[a] | Yes[a] |
| Wyoming | Yes | No | No | Yes |

*Note.* From McKnight and Antunez (1999). Reprinted by permission from the National Clearinghouse for Language Acquisition and Language Instruction Educational Programs.
[a]State has a legal *mandate* to provide certification or endorsement.

Oregon and Wyoming) had ratios between 1:100 and 1:199; 27 states had ratios between 1:25 and 1:99; only four states had a ratio below 1:25 (Rhode Island at 1:20, Texas at 1:16, Louisiana at 1:11, and Virginia at 1:9). Kindler's study was unable to obtain ratios for six states and the District of Columbia.

These data clearly indicate that a significant number of LEP students in the United States is not being taught by teachers who have certification in ESL and bilingual education. For example, in Texas, many of the teachers who were hired in 2000–2001 (48%) and 2001–2002 (40%) in the elementary bilingual/ESL field were "less than fully certified" (Texas A&M University System, 2002). Moreover, the teachers who were hired in the secondary bilingual/ESL field in 2000–2001 (41%) and 2001–2002 (35%) were "less than fully certified" (Texas A&M University System, 2002). The impact of not being taught by a certified teacher should not be ignored by school-based practitioners when second-language learners are referred for special education testing due to low academic performance.

## INSTRUCTIONAL PROGRAMS PROVIDED TO LEP STUDENTS

Instructional programs for LEP students in the United States have existed for well over 200 years (Weaver & Padron, 1999). Bilingual education has a long history in our country, which was a country of immigrants when it was founded. However, despite this long history bilingual education has not gone without controversy. Indeed, bilingual education was not permitted in U.S. schools in the earlier part of the 20th century (Crawford, 1995). In 1968 President Johnson signed the Bilingual Education Act that appropriated funds for the development of dual-language programs. In 1974, the Supreme Court ruled on the case of *Lau v. Nichols* that pertained to education of LEP students. In this case Chinese pupils in the San Francisco School District contended that they did not have equal educational opportunity as a result of not being educated in their native language. The Supreme Court ruled that equal educational opportunity did not exist if students were not educated in a language which they understood. "While the Supreme Court ruling did not specifically mandate the implementation of bilingual programs, it did offer bilingual education as one means by which a school could provide an educational opportunity for its non-English speaking population students" (Weaver & Padron, 1999, p. 80). In the 1980s, the English Only movement attempted to make English the official language in the country. In the mid to late 1990s, the Unz movement started in California, the goal of which was to get voter approval for Proposition 227 that would abolish most types of bilingual education in California. Residents of California approved Proposition 227.

Currently, there are five types of instructional programs provided to LEP students. These five programs can be classified into one of two categories: bilingual education or ESL. Bilingual education differs from ESL in that instruction is provided in both native and English languages; ESL programs provide instruction in English only. There are three types of bilingual education programs and two types of ESL programs in the United States. Many of the different types of instructional programs provided to LEP students have multiple names. As each of the five types of programs is described below, the various names given for it are provided to minimize confusion. It is also important to note that each type of program can vary with regard to how it is implemented.

## Transitional/Early-Exit Bilingual Education Program

The first type of bilingual education program offered to LEP students is an early-exit or transitional program. Transitional bilingual education classrooms are primarily, if not exclusively, comprised of LEP students who are from the same language group. This program varies in length but generally is provided for 2–4 years. The philosophy of a transitional program is to initially use the child's native language as a foundation from which to transition him or her to an English-speaking learning environment. Both English and the child's native language are used for instructional purposes at the beginning of this program. Spanish language arts instruction is provided for a short period of time and eventually terminated and replaced with language arts instruction in English. The use of the child's native language during instruction in other content areas is severely limited or terminated within a short period of time. The goal of this program is to teach the child a second language, English, at the expense of his or her native language. Thus, this program is considered to be a *subtractive* bilingual education program.

Many individuals philosophically support transitional programs because they recognize that LEP students need some period of time in which to adjust to the culture of a U.S. school, which can be significantly different from their home culture and language. However, they believe that this transition period should be brief because the child needs to be exposed to English as quickly and as often as possible in order to master it. The validity of this view is examined later in this chapter.

## Maintenance/Late-Exit/Developmental Bilingual Education Program

Maintenance programs are similar to, yet different from, transitional programs in several important ways. A maintenance program is similar to a transitional bilingual program in that classrooms implementing this approach are primarily, if not exclusively, comprised of LEP students who are from the same language group. However, maintenance education programs are offered to LEP students for a greater length of time than transitional programs: generally 4–6 years. Maintenance programs also use the child's native language for instructional purposes to a greater extent and for a longer period of time than transitional programs. Maintenance programs vary in the amount of time they provide instruction in the child's native language and English. Various models exist. Two of the more common models use language ratios of 90:10 and 50:50. The 90:10 model initially offers 90% of the instructional time in the child's native language and 10% in English. With time (across grade levels), the amount of instructional time in the child's native language is reduced as the amount of time in English is increased. The 50:50 model provides approximately equal amounts of instruction in English and the native language. It should be noted that language arts instruction occurs in both languages throughout a maintenance program. The goal of this program is to help the child maintain his or her first language as he or she acquires a second language, English. Thus, this program is considered *additive* in nature, because the child adds a second language to his or her linguistic repertoire.

Educators and the general public view this type of program both positively and negatively. Those in favor contend that this type of program allows the child to recognize the strengths of his or her culture and language. Moreover, proponents also recognize the economic value of being bilingual. Those who view this program unfavorably state that not enough time is devoted to instruction in English, which will result in lower academic achievement in English. The validity of these views is discussed in the section that discusses the effectiveness of bilingual education.

## Two-Way/Dual-Language Bilingual Education Program

Two-way programs differ from the preceding two types of programs in that these children are either English speakers or LEP students. The goal of this program is for the English-speaking student to become bilingual by developing English and the language spoken by his or her LEP classmates. The goal for the LEP student is to become bilingual by developing his or her native language and English. Thus, this program is an *additive* bilingual program. Both of these groups are approximately equally represented in a two-way/dual language bilingual education classroom. The makeup of each language group, however, can vary from one-third to two-thirds of the entire classroom (Center for Applied Linguistics, 2001). LEP students take part in this program because of their limited English skills. Parents of English-speaking children are recruited for the program on a volunteer basis or go through a lottery system. This program is provided for at least 4–6 years. Students who participate usually enter at the kindergarten level and are encouraged to remain in the program until it is no longer offered. As in the maintenance program, two popular models, among others, are the 90:10 and 50:50 model. Language arts is provided in both English and the native language of the LEP student group in the class. Some two-way bilingual programs alternate the language in which an academic subject is taught. For example, math is taught in Spanish in kindergarten, second, and fourth grades and in English in first, third, and fifth grades.

Dual-language programs are generally viewed positively. Many English-speaking parents want their children to learn a second language as long as it does not have a detrimental effect on their English skills. Moreover, these parents recognize the benefits of their children obtaining information about different cultures and developing multicultural sensitivity and understanding. Many non-English-speaking parents appreciate the fact that their child will not be segregated along with other LEP students but, rather, interact with children who are from the dominant culture and who are good English-language models for their children.

## Content-Based ESL/Sheltered English

This program model differs from the aforementioned bilingual models in that students receive instruction in English only. ESL classrooms can consist entirely of students from the same language subgroup or can be comprised of pupils from many different language groups. This type of program focuses on teaching academic material in English by using the total physical response (TPR). TPR consists of physical gestures and visual cues that are used to facilitate the second-language learner's understanding of the curriculum context. In sheltered English, "students receive subject matter instruction in English, modified so that is understandable to them at their level of English proficiency" (August & Hakuta, 1998, p. 6). The amount of time the child spends in a content-based ESL classroom can vary from approximately 50 to 100% of the day (Thomas & Collier, 1997). The intent of this program is for the LEP student to acquire English and not to maintain his or her native language.

## Pullout ESL

This program is very similar to the content-based ESL model but differs in three important dimensions. First, the focus of instruction in this ESL model is not on teaching academic material but rather on developing the student's English-language skills. Second, LEP students leave their classroom and receive instruction from a teacher who is (hopefully) certified in the ESL field. Third, the length of time the student is educated in this setting varies but is generally less than half a day (Thomas & Collier, 1997).

## Prevalence of Each Type of Program

Pullout and content-based ESL programs are common. Of the three types of bilingual education programs, transitional programs are the most frequently offered to LEP students, and maintenance programs are not common (August & Hakuta, 1998). Two-way bilingual programs are also not very common. According to data maintained by the Center of Applied Linguistics (2001), there are 260 schools that have dual-language bilingual programs located in 23 states and the District of Columbia. This number is considered to be an underestimate, because many programs are not registered with CAL. The overwhelming majority of these programs is Spanish/English (Center for Applied Linguistics, 2001). Two-way bilingual programs are also offered in French/English, Chinese/English, Korean/English, and Navajo/English.

## RESEARCH ON THE EFFECTIVENESS OF BILINGUAL EDUCATION

There has been much controversy surrounding the effectiveness of bilingual education. Research in this area has been conducted on both small- and national-scale bases (August & Hakuta, 1998). The results of studies conducted on a small-scale basis have shown conflicting results (Baker & de Kanter, 1981, 1983; Greene, 1998; Rossell & Baker, 1996; Willig, 1985; Zappert & Cruz, 1977). Each of these small-scale studies has aggregated studies examining the effects of bilingual education. This aggregation was achieved via the use of the vote-counting method (Baker & de Kanter, 1981, 1983; Rossell & Baker, 1996; Zappert & Cruz, 1977) and meta-analysis (Greene, 1998). With regard to the vote-counting studies, Baker and de Kanter (1981, 1983) reported unfavorable results for bilingual education, whereas Rossell and Baker (1996) found no significant achievement differences for LEP students who were in transitional bilingual programs versus those who were not. Zappert and Cruz (1977), however, found that in 58% of the cases examined, pupils in bilingual education had higher educational achievement than those who were not enrolled in a bilingual education program. Thomas and Collier (1997) have criticized these three studies because they used the "vote counting method . . . that divide[d] studies into 'significant positive', 'significant negative', and 'non-significant' outcomes and then count[ed] the numbers in each category to arrive at an overall summary" (p. 24).

Meta-analytic studies contradict the results provided by the majority of the vote-counting studies (Baker & de Kanter, 1981, 1983; Rossell & Baker, 1996). This research procedure is superior to the vote-counting method. Willig's (1985) meta-analysis included some of the studies that were included in Baker and de Kanter's (1981) study. Willig (1985) found "positive effects for bilingual education" (p. 297) and noted "that the average student in bilingual programs scored higher than 74% of the students in the traditional program when all test scores were aggregated" (p. 291). Positive effects were noted in total English achievement and in reading and math. Greene's (1998) meta-analysis also found positive support for bilingual education and the findings were consistent with those obtained by Willig (1985).

## Danoff (1978)

Several large-scale studies have examined the effectiveness of bilingual education (Danoff, 1978; Ramirez, Yuen, & Ramey, 1991; Thomas & Collier, 1997, 2002), and only one of these studies (Danoff, 1978) did not find positive results. This study (Danoff, 1978), however, has significant methodological limitations (August & Hakuta, 1998; O'Malley, 1978; Weaver & Padron, 1999; Willig, 1985). In particular, it "did not compare bilingual education with no bilingual education because two-thirds of the children in the control group has previously been in bilingual programs" (August & Hakuta, 1998, p. 56).

## Ramirez, Yuen, and Ramey (1991)

A second large-scale study was conducted by Ramirez et al. (1991). This study examined how second-language learners' academic performance varied in different educational settings. The settings included English immersion as well as transitional and maintenance bilingual education programs. The researchers reported that the academic performance of third-grade LEP students taught in English-immersion settings attained similar achievement outcomes to those instructed in transitional bilingual education programs. However, the researchers noted positive educational attainment for LEP students enrolled in maintenance programs.

## Thomas and Collier (1997)

This study is significant in that it was one of the first to examine second-language learners' long-term performance perspective by type of bilingual program being offered. Using a cross-sectional and longitudinal design, Thomas and Collier examined the academic achievement of 42,317 second-language learners in five large school districts from 1982 to 1996. Specifically, they examined the "long-term achievement" (kindergarten through 12th grade) of LEP students in the following six types of bilingual programs: dual language, maintenance, transitional bilingual along with content-based ESL, transitional bilingual along with pullout ESL, content-based ESL only, and pullout ESL only (p. 53). Figure 4.1 displays the results of the their study. Thomas and Collier found that second-language learners across all types of bilingual programs made positive gains in English reading skills from the start of their educational career to around third to fourth grade. Thus, all programs produced initial, positive, short-term gains. These gains, however, did not continue across all programs on a long-term basis. The researchers reported the following English-reading normal curve equivalent (NCE) scores obtained from standardized tests for LEP students in 12th grade for each of the six bilingual programs: dual language = NCE of 61; maintenance = NCE of 52; transitional bilingual along with content-based ESL = NCE of 40; transitional bilingual along with pullout ESL = NCE of 35; content-based ESL only = NCE of 34; and pullout ESL only = NCE of 24. This pattern of performance was consistent across academic settings in

Results aggregated from a series of 4- to 8-year longitudinal studies from well-implemented, mature programs in five school districts. Program 1: two-way developmental bilingual education (BE); Program 2: one-way developmental BE, including ESL taught through academic content; Program 3: transitional BE, including ESL taught through academic content; Program 4: transitional BE, including ESL, both taught traditionally; Program 5: ESL taught through academic content using current approaches; Program 6: ESL pullout taught traditionally.

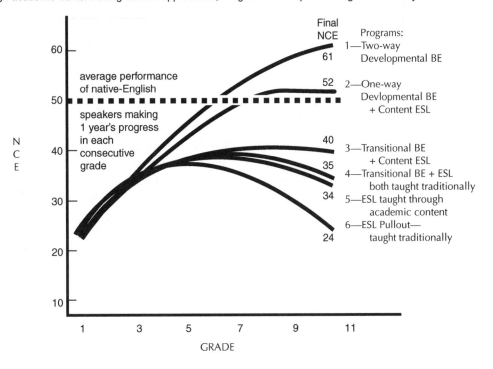

**FIGURE 4.1.** Patterns of K–12 English learners' long-term achievement in NCEs on standardized tests in English reading compared across six program models. From Thomas and Collier (1997, p. 53). Copyright 1997 by Wayne P. Thomas and Virginia P. Collier. Reprinted by permission from Wayne P. Thomas and Virginia P. Collier.

the five districts that were included in the study. Moreover, this pattern of academic performance was noted in science and social studies. Thomas and Collier (1997) also noted that:

> mathematics and English language arts achievement of language minority students is slightly higher than their performance on the English reading, science and social studies tests, but the same general pattern of performance, as well as the same ranking of long-term achievement influenced by program participation is present in the mathematics and language arts data. (p. 52)

Thomas and Collier (1997) also noted that LEP students in ESL programs were the "most likely" to drop out, whereas those enrolled in a maintenance or dual-language program were the "least likely" to drop out of school (p. 68).

## Thomas and Collier (2002)

This study, conducted between 1996 and 2001 in five school sites located in Maine ($n = 2$), Oregon, Texas, and Florida, examined the English and Spanish academic performance of second-language learners in a variety of different types of bilingual education programs. Given that the study was conducted in five sites, different measures were used to assess English and Spanish academic performance. The English measures included the Iowa Test of Basic Skills, Stanford 9, Terra Nova, and the California Test of Basic Skills. The Spanish measures used were the Aprenda 2 and the SABE. This study differed from the previous Thomas and Collier (1997) study in that it examined second-language learners' performance in immersion settings and in transitional, maintenance, and dual-language programs that varied in the amount of English and Spanish instruction being provided.

LEP students in immersion settings—which meant that their parents did not want their child to receive bilingual education services and elected an English-only instructional setting— obtained a NCE score of 25 in English reading in 11th grade. LEP students enrolled in content-based ESL programs obtained a median NCE score of 34 in total English reading in 12th grade. These exact findings were obtained in their 1997 study. The study also found positive results for LEP students enrolled in maintenance and dual-language programs in English-reading skills. Second-language learners in maintenance and dual-language programs also obtained positive results in Spanish-reading skills. Interestingly, Thomas and Collier reported that monolingual English-speaking students enrolled in a dual-language program performed above the national average on standardized English achievement measures and had acquired a second language.

## Implications of Effectiveness Research on Assessment

Very few individuals, if any, would disagree that in order to be academically successful in U.S. schools, all students need to be proficient in English. The question that causes much disagreement is: From an educational programming perspective, how can second-language learners best learn English? As mentioned previously, many individuals believe that the best way to achieve this goal is to immerse students in an English-only academic setting that results in the LEP child being exposed to and forced to use English. Thus, they advocate that LEP students be placed in a regular English-speaking classroom (e.g., immersion) or an ESL pullout or content-based ESL setting. Many individuals who espouse this view state that LEP students in these academic settings acquire English very quickly and that their performance on English academic measures reveals early significant gains. Thomas and Collier's (1997) study found that LEP students make early significant academic strides in all types of bilingual education programs. So, although these individuals are correct when they make these claims about the early promising results of second-language learners' performance, Thomas and Collier (1997) ask school personnel to question if these early gains will continue throughout the child's educational trajectory into high school. Thomas and Collier's (1997, 2002) studies clearly reveal that the gains do not hold. At best, LEP students in these academic settings achieve at approximately the 25th NCE in immersion and ESL pullout classrooms and at around the 34th NCE in content-based ESL programs toward the end of high school. Moreover, Thomas and Collier found that LEP students who were in ESL or immersion settings in their elementary years were "more likely" to drop out of school.

It should be noted that LEP students in the United States are frequently educated in English-only immersion settings or ESL settings. These programs, however, do not produce positive academic outcomes when examined from a long-term perspective. Data from the NCES (1997) and Kindler (2002) studies also provide support for the fact that second-language learners' performance is not commensurate with their English-speaking peers. The implications these studies (in particular, the Thomas and Collier studies) have on determining whether the academic difficulties of elementary LEP students are a within-child phenomenon versus a within-system (i.e., pedagogically induced) one cannot be overlooked. In other words, from a practical perspective, are LEP students in ESL and English-only immersion settings more likely to be referred to special education? With NCE scores in the bottom third or lower for English-reading skills on standardized measures, it would not be unusual for these students to be referred to special education. In fact, monolingual English-speaking students with similar levels of performance would be likely to be referred. Moreover, from a legal perspective, how do school-based practitioners comply with the new provisions added to the IDEA 1997 pertaining to lack of educational opportunity? This is not to say that an LEP student who has been instructed in immersion or ESL settings should not be referred to special education and subsequently identified as having a disability. For LEP students who have been educated in immersion or ESL settings during their elementary years, however, it is critical for school psychologists and other educators involved in the referral and assessment process to critically examine whether, or the extent to which, these instructional arrangements have contributed to the students' academic difficulties.

Research on the academic trajectory of LEP students enrolled in various forms of transitional programs reveal that they fail to achieve the national norm. Thomas and Collier (1997) found that LEP students enrolled in transitional programs scored in the 35th- to 40th-NCE range at the end of high school. In their 2002 study, LEP students in a 50:50 transitional program were at the 47th NCE in English reading. Although these students fare better than those enrolled in ESL or immersion settings, their level of academic performance puts them at risk for referral to special education. Such a referral is more likely to occur once these students are no longer receiving first-language instructional support and simultaneously are exposed to more cognitively complex academic content.

Overall results of Thomas and Collier's studies (1997, 2002) indicate positive academic performance on English standardized measures of LEP students who are instructed in maintenance and dual-language programs. These students have maintained their first language and achieve at, or above, the national norm on standardized tests in the areas of English reading, language arts, math, and science. Unfortunately, relatively few LEP students are educated in either type of program, in comparison to those taught in ESL, transitional, and immersion settings. Given the collective academic performance of second-language learners in these two types of programs, one would not expect as many LEP students in these programs to be referred for special education.

It is important that school-based practitioners ascertain which type of bilingual program the LEP student has received. Research clearly indicates that participation in a particular type of bilingual program can have a significant impact on long-tern academic performance. In other words, not all types of bilingual programs are alike and equal.

## SECOND-LANGUAGE ACQUISITION PROCESS AND RELATED CRITICAL CONSTRUCTS

Prior to reviewing the process of second-language acquisition, a very brief review about first-language acquisition process is provided. McLaughlin (1984, as cited in Collier, 1989) states that it takes at least 12 years for students to acquire their first language:

From birth through age 5, children acquire enormous amounts of L1 [first language] phonology, vocabulary, grammar, semantics, and pragmatics, but the process is not at all complete by the time children reach school age. From ages 6 to 12, children still have to develop in their first language the complex skills of reading and writing, in addition to the complex rules of morphology and syntax, elaboration of speech acts, expansion of vocabulary (which continues throughout a person's lifetime), semantic development, and even some aspects of phonological development. (Collier, 1989, p. 510)

## Second-Language Acquisition Process

There are four stages through which LEP pupils proceed during the lengthy process of second-language acquisition: preproduction, early production, speech emergence, and intermediate fluency (Hearne, 2000; Roseberry-McKibbin, 2002; Ortiz & Kushner, 1997). An explanation of these four stages and common characteristics displayed by second-language learners are described in Table 4.2. Moreover, this table provides appropriate intervention considerations for each of the four stages of second-language acquisition.

## Basic Interpersonal Communication Skills and Cognitive Academic Language Proficiency

The research on the effectiveness of bilingual education provides empirical support for the theories many linguistics have proposed regarding the process of second-language acquisition. Cummins (1984) proposed that there are two types of language proficiencies: basic interpersonal communication skills (BICS) and cognitive academic language proficiency (CALP). Cummins describe BICS as the type of language proficiency typically utilized in social and informal settings to carry a conversation with another person. In school situations, it would be characteristic of a conversation between classmates on the playground or informal greetings and conversations between the LEP student and his or her teacher. Cummins proposed that it usually takes a second-language learner around 2 or 3 years to acquire BICS. The second type of language skills, CALP, consists of the language skills needed to do schoolwork. Attaining this type of proficiency is critical in order for the LEP child to make academic progress. CALP can be attained by second-language learners within 5 to 7 years (Cummins, 1984).

In order for language-minority youth to be successful in U.S. schools, their attainment of CALP in English (their second language) is paramount. The critical question then becomes: How do second-language learners develop CALP in English? Cummins (1984) noted that this can be best accomplished when LEP students first attain CALP in their native language. LEP students need to attain a minimum threshold level in their first language before they can develop CALP in a second language (Cummins, 1984). In other words, the greater the development of the second-language learner's first language, the greater the probability that the child will develop a second language. If LEP students are not given a sufficient opportunity to develop their first language, the omission will have negative consequences on their second-language development and on their school performance (Collier, 1989). "One important finding is that the lack of continuing L1 [first language] cognitive development during second language acquisition may lead to lowered proficiency levels in the second language and in cognitive academic growth" (Collier, 1989, p. 511).

**TABLE 4.2. Matching Intervention to Second-Language (L2) Acquisition Stages**

| Stage I: Preproduction (first 3 months of L2 exposure) | Stage II: Early production (3–6 months) | Stage III: Speech emergence (6 months– 2 years) | Stage IV: Intermediate fluency (2–3 years) |
| --- | --- | --- | --- |
| Student characteristics | | | |
| • Silent period<br>• Focusing on comprehension | • Focusing on comprehension<br>• Using 1- to 3-word phrases<br>• May be using routines/formulas (e.g., "gimme five") | • Increased comprehension<br>• Using simple sentences<br>• Expanded vocabulary<br>• Continued grammatical errors | • Improved comprehension<br>• Adequate face-to-face conversational proficiency<br>• More extensive vocabulary<br>• Few grammatical errors |
| Goals: Oral responses | | | |
| • Yes–No responses in English<br>• One-word answers | • 1- to 3-word responses<br>• Naming/labeling items<br>• Choral responses<br>• Answering questions: either/or, who/what/ where, sentence completion | • Recalling<br>• Telling/retelling<br>• Describing/explaining<br>• Comparing<br>• Sequencing<br>• Carrying on dialogues | • Predicting<br>• Narrating<br>• Describing/explaining<br>• Summarizing<br>• Giving opinions<br>• Debating/defending |
| Goals: Visual/written responses | | | |
| • Drawing/painting<br>• Graphic designs<br>• Copying | • Drawing/painting, graphic designs<br>• Copying<br>• Grouping and labeling<br>• Simple rebus responses | • Written responses<br>• Drawing, painting, graphics | • Creative writing (e.g., stories)<br>• Essays, summaries<br>• Drawing, painting, graphics<br>• Comprehensible written tests |
| Goals: Physical responses | | | |
| • Pointing<br>• Circling, underlining<br>• Choosing among items<br>• Matching objects/ pictures | • Pointing<br>• Selecting<br>• Matching<br>• Constructing<br>• Miming/acting-out responses | • Demonstrating<br>• Creating/constructing<br>• Role playing/acting<br>• Cooperative group tasks | • Demonstrating<br>• Creating/constructing<br>• Role playing<br>• Cooperative group work<br>• Videotaped presentations |

*Note.* Adapted from Hearne (2000, Table 10.4), further adapted by Roseberry-McKibbin (2002, Table 15.1). Copyright 2000 and 2002 by Academic Communication Associates. Adapted by permission.

There is research to support the existence of Cummins's BICS/CALP language constructs (Collier, 1987, 1989). Thomas and Collier's (1997, 2002) studies also lend support to the construct of CALP and the amount of time it takes to develop it. They found that "the deeper a student's level of L1 [first language] cognitive and academic development (which includes L1 proficiency), the faster students will progress in L2 [second language]" (p. 38). Thomas and Collier (1997) examined the amount of time it takes second-language learners to attain the 50th NCE score on standardized English-reading measures. They reported that

> it takes typically bilingually schooled students, who are achieving on grade level in L1 [first language], from 4–7 years to make it to the 50th NCE in L2 [second language]. It takes typical "advantaged" immigrants with 2–5 years of on grade-level home country schooling in L1 from 5–7 years to reach the 50th NCE in L2, when schooled all in L2 in the U.S. It takes the typical young immigrant schooled all in L2 in the U.S. 7–10 years or more to reach the 50th NCE, and the majority of these students do not ever make it to the 50th NCE, unless they receive support for L1 academic and cognitive development at home. (p. 36)

Interestingly, Thomas and Collier (1997) also found that it takes monolingual English-speaking students who are enrolled in dual-language bilingual programs approximately 4 to 7 years to attain the 50th NCE mark on academic measures in the second language.

Thomas and Collier (1997, 2002) noted some important factors influencing the academic performance of students with LEP. They found that "the strongest predictor of L2 achievement is amount of L1 schooling. The more L1 grade level schooling, the higher L2 achievement" (Thomas & Collier, 2002, p. 334). Moreover, in regard to academic achievement Thomas and Collier (2002) found that "number of years of primary language schooling . . . had more influence than socioeconomic status when the number of years of schooling was 4 or more years" (p. 332).

## Implications of Second-Language Acquisition Process and Related Critical Concepts on Assessment

It is critical that school psychologists and other school personnel have a theoretical understanding of the second-language acquisition process in order to avoid reaching inappropriate conclusions about the English-language learner's linguistic abilities or his or her lack of adequate academic progress. Cummins (1984) stressed the importance of differentiating between the BICS and CALP constructs. His research found that many school psychologists do not differentiate while conducting assessment. The important factor to consider is that even if an LEP student is able to carry on a social conversation with peers, teachers, and a psychologist in English, it does not necessarily mean that he or she has sufficient English-language skills to perform academic tasks or to be assessed accurately if given an intellectual measure in English. School-based practitioners need to ascertain, to the extent possible, whether the LEP child has attained CALP in both his or her native language and English. (This topic is discussed in Chapter 9.)

Given the research (Thomas & Collier, 1997) stating that it takes, on average, 4 to 7 years for LEP students who have received instruction in their native language to reach national norms on English achievement measures, it is important that school psychologists and other school personnel consider this time element when attempting to explain second-language learners' low academic performance. Moreover, Cummins (1984) noted:

Minority language students are frequently transferred from bilingual to English-only classrooms when they have developed superficially fluent English communicative skills. Despite being classified as "English proficient" many such students fall progressively further behind grade norms in the development of English academic skills. (p. 131)

This is not to say that school psychologists and other personnel need to necessarily wait this length of time to refer a child. Instead, the school psychologist should compare the educational trajectory of an LEP student in question with those of his or her same grade-level LEP peers. If the educational trajectories are similar and are below the 50th NCE because they are within the time period noted above, it might be a possible reason to consider length of native language instructional programming as a critical factor in the student's performance. However, if the educational trajectory of an LEP student across several years is notably different from his or her LEP classmates who have been educated in a similar bilingual program for approximately the same number of years, this might be a cause of concern.

The following are critical questions that school-based practitioners need to ask concerning second-language acquisition and its relationship to dual-language instructions:

- Can the student's difficulty in acquiring English proficiency be attributed to his or her insufficient development in his or her first language?
- Can the student's academic difficulties or failure in an English-only academic setting be attributed to his or her not having attained CALP in English?
- Was the student given ample instructional time in his or her first language to (1) develop CALP in this language and (2) demonstrate ability somewhat within the average range of academic performance?

## LANGUAGE CHARACTERISTICS FREQUENTLY OBSERVED IN SECOND-LANGUAGE LEARNERS

Roseberry-McKibbin (2002) states that there are "normal processes of second language acquisition [that] . . . need to be recognized as normal behaviors for students who are not yet proficient in English" (p. 193). Some of these processes include interference, interlanguage, silent period, code switching, and language loss (Roseberry-McKibbin, 2002). Understanding these learning processes will help psychologists, speech–language pathologists, and other school personnel not to automatically assume that the second-language learner is exhibiting deficiencies.

### Interference

Interference . . . refers to a process in which a communicative behavior for the first language is carried over into the second language. . . . A student is more likely to demonstrate interference when using English in a formal setting, such as a testing situation, than on the playground. . . . Thus, when second language learners produce errors in English, it is important to consider the possibility that these errors result from language interference or from the student's limited experience in English. (Roseberry-McKibbin, 2002, p. 193)

An example of interference might be when an LEP student tells a peer that she wants him to "have a seat" next to her. In Spanish, this request would be worded *"tome una silla."* When this phrase is literally translated, it means "take a seat." If the LEP child said "take a seat" in this situation, interference would be the reason.

## Interlanguage

Hamayan and Damico (1991b) and Roseberry-McKibbin (2002) contend that "interlanguage" is a common language characteristic noted in second-language learners. While a second-language learner is attempting to learn English, he or she develops a new language system that incorporates part of his or her native language and part of the newly learned English. "The [second] language learner tests hypotheses about how language works and forms a personal set of rules for using language" (Roseberry-McKibbin, 2002, p. 194). This language system will change (Roseberry-McKibbin, 2002) and more closely resemble the second language (English) as the LEP student develops a better mastery of English (Hamayan & Damico, 1991b).

## Silent Period

As noted in Table 4.2, we can expect second-language learners to experience a silent period when they are initially exposed to a second language. The length of this time varies from 3 to 6 months, depending on the age of the student (Roseberry-McKibbin, 2002). During this time, the second-language learners' oral communication is very limited.

## Code Switching

Experts (Hamayan & Damico, 1991b; Ortiz & Maldonado-Colon, 1986; Roseberry-McKibbin, 2002) have noted that code switching is a common language pattern observed in second-language learners. Code switching occurs when an LEP child switches from one language to another language when conversing, usually between sentences. An example of an LEP student using code switching is illustrated in the following statement: *"Fuimos al cine* (we went to the movies). The Spider Man movie was great!"

## Language Loss

Several experts have noted that language loss can occur in second-language learners (Mattes & Omark, 1991; Roseberry-McKibbon, 2002; Schiff-Myers, 1992; Schiff-Myers, Djukic, McGovern-Lawler, & Perez, 1993). Language loss is "the weakening of an individual's first language because of a concentrated focus on the development of L2 (English)" (Schiff-Myers, 1992, p. 28). Thus, second-language learners who do not receive native-language instruction in school can possibly experience language loss.

## Language Differences

Roseberry-McKibbon (2002) states: "It is important for professionals who work with Spanish speaking students to understand the language differences commonly observed when these stu-

**TABLE 4.3. Language Differences Commonly Observed among Spanish Speakers**

| Language characteristics | Sample English utterances |
| --- | --- |
| 1. Adjective comes after noun. | The house green. |
| 2. 's is often omitted in plurals and possessives. | The girl book is . . . Juan hat is red. |
| 3. Past tense -*ed* is often omitted. | We walk yesterday. |
| 4. Double negatives are required. | I don't have no more. |
| 5. Superiority is demonstrated by using *mas*. | This cake is more big. |
| 6. The adverb often follows the verb. | He drives very fast his motorcycle. |

*Note.* From Roseberry-McKibbin (2002, Table 5.1). Copyright 2002 by Academic Communication Associates. Reprinted by permission.

dents learn English" (p. 84). Table 4.3 displays some of the language differences noted in Spanish-speaking students who are learning English as a second language.

## SUMMARY

This chapter has reviewed many critical factors concerning bilingual education and second-language acquisition that psychologists, educators, and other related school personnel need to consider during the assessment, interpretation, and eligibility process involving second-language learners. Keys issues include (1) knowing the different types of bilingual education and their respective long-term educational outcomes; (2) understanding the process of second-language acquisition; (3) differentiating between BICS and CALP; and (4) recognizing common language characteristics observed in second-language learners. School-based practitioners who assess culturally and linguistically diverse students, without considering these key issues, may reach inaccurate conclusions regarding the language abilities and academic difficulties of LEP students.

# 5

# Prereferral Considerations for Culturally and Linguistically Diverse Students

There is considerable variability in how prereferral teams are constituted, perceived, and allowed to function across schools. These three factors can have an impact on the number of children who eventually get referred to special education. With respect to the composition of prereferral teams, membership can play an important role. Some teams are exclusively comprised of teachers who work collaboratively within a problem-solving framework to assist one of their peers who is seeking assistance with a given child. Other teams may have additional members that include an administrator, special education personnel, or related service personnel. When the child in question is a second-language learner, at least one member, if not more, should have a knowledge base about cultural, linguistic, and instructional factors that can have a significant impact on the pupil's performance or behavior. Prereferral teams that have a member with this expertise increase the probability that the factors that impact student performance and behavior will be given due consideration prior to referring the second-language learner for special education. Moreover, this expertise will help to ensure that limited English proficiency, as the determining factor of the student's academic failure, is addressed from the beginning of the process. Thus, one critical variable that needs to be considered regarding team composition is whether anyone currently serving on the prereferral teams has this expertise. Ochoa, Robles-Piña, Garcia, and Breunig (1999) found that a professional with this expertise (e.g., personnel from bilingual education) was reported to be a member in only half of the prereferral teams across eight states with large LEP student populations. In Colorado and New York, for example, a bilingual education representative was reported to be a member in approximately one-third of the prereferral teams. When teams do not have a member who has expertise in second-language acquisition, cultural differences, bilingual education, and ESL programming, it is imperative that they consider the information included in this

This chapter is by Salvador Hector Ochoa.

book when designing interventions and making decisions about whether to proceed in referring a child.

A second critical factor that influences the number of children who are referred is how school personnel perceive prereferral teams. In some schools, prereferral teams are viewed as a valued resource by teachers and other school personnel. These teams are comprised of teachers who possess additional skills, knowledge, understanding, and teaching strategies/interventions that pertain to children who are at risk for academic failure. In other schools, prereferral teams are perceived to be an obstacle in either getting the child needed help or removing the child from the general education classroom. In these situations, school personnel may want to proceed quickly for a variety of reasons. These reasons, among others, can include the following: (1) wanting to exclude the child in question from taking the state accountability academic test, because his or her score could lower the school's rating; (2) "saving" the child from "drowning" in the general education environment and believing that it won't hurt him or her to be in special education; (3) recognizing that the school does not provide the instructional services needed to address the child's linguistic needs. Uninformed team members may conclude that a special education instructional environment that has a teacher with his or her "special bag of instructional strategies or tricks" along with a smaller teacher ratio is a preferable option than the general education classroom.

None of these reasons is an acceptable reason for referring any child to special education. With regard to the first reason of avoiding state tests, this author (S.H.O.) has heard stories from assessment personnel who reported that their school administrator told them that they needed "just a few more kids" to pass the state accountability test to obtain a higher rating for their schools. (Sometimes the converse is reported: that their campus would have obtained a higher rating if more "minority" children would have passed the test.) To preclude this situation, more children were referred to special education. (See the section in Chapter 2 on school accountability for more detail.)

Referring a child to special education should never be based on the notion of "saving" the child from regular education or trying to compensate for inadequate instruction. It is important for educators (both general and special education), administrators, psychologists, and all members who serve on prereferral teams to understand that special education was never meant to solve all of the problems that occur in general education. Instead, special education should be perceived as a service that is provided to students with genuine, inherent disabilities. Special education should not be perceived as an acceptable alternative for the slow learner, the at-risk child, or the culturally and linguistically diverse learner, simply because general education personnel do not know how to effectively educate these children. Instead, prereferral teams need to examine how they can help teachers acquire whatever skills and materials are needed to provide the necessary, and if applicable, improved quality of educational services the child needs.

To improve the quality of educational services first requires a review of classroom practices. This review can produce findings that are difficult to address because of the human factor. For example, the qualitative research of Harry, Klinger, Sturges, and Moore (2002) found that pupils were sometimes referred because of "the teacher's lack of skills" (p. 82). Harry et al. also noted: "It appears from the informal conversations with teachers that it is well known among them who are perceived to be strong and weak teachers, but colleagues are reluctant to jeopardize their relationships with one another" (p. 82). It may be up to the school psychologist to break this code of silence and directly help those weaker teachers.

Referring a child to special education should not be contingent upon the unavailability of necessary general education services. Special education should not be perceived as acceptable educational alternative when the school does not provide bilingual educational programs. Bilingual education is a part of general education and not a remedial program. Ortiz (1997) states:

> If student failure can be attributed to the teacher's lack of understanding of diversity, the use of inappropriate curriculum or materials, or ineffective instructional practices, then referrals to special education are unwarranted. Efforts, instead, should focus on modifying the school context and instructional programs. (p. 324)

Special education should not be considered as a no-risk or even low-risk placement for the LEP student. Some educators may believe "it will not hurt," but research suggests otherwise. "An issue more basic than whether students profit from special education is whether they are eligible for such services in the first place" (Ortiz, 1992, p. 2). Moreover, Wilkinson and Ortiz (1986) reported that Hispanics who were placed in special education did not make academic strides. Perhaps the bottom line is for school-based practitioners and educators to apply this argument to their own child and honestly consider how they would feel if their child were referred to special education because (1) it will not hurt him or her; (2) their child could get "extra" help; (3) general education does not provide the actual program that could result in their child improving their educational performance; or (4) the teacher does not have the skills to work with their child. Given their professional training and experience, this author (S.H.O.) sincerely believes that most psychologists and educators would not agree to have their child referred on the basis of any of these arguments. Unfortunately, many families, especially those from culturally and linguistically diverse backgrounds, do not have the expertise to address these factors. Thus, school-based practitioners who are involved in the prereferral or assessment process need to undertake an advocacy-oriented role (see also Cummins, 1986; Damico & Hamayan, 1991).

A third critical factor in the number of children who get referred is how the prereferral teams function. In some schools, prereferral teams are nothing more than a rubber stamp, a formality that a teacher must go through to get the child tested. In other schools, the prereferral team provides consultative services to the teacher, who, in turn, provides needed intervention. Research indicates that there is variability in how prereferral teams function and in the number of students who are typically referred. Drane (2002) found that teachers were more inclined to refer students to special education when there was no "clearly defined prereferral model" on their campus than when there was a well-defined model (p. 49).

There also is empirical data to suggest that the teacher's decision to refer the child to the prereferral team is very important, given the percentage of children who are eventually placed in special education. Algozzinne, Christenson, and Ysseldyke (1982) found that 92% of cases brought before the referral team were eventually referred for an evaluation. In a follow-up study, Ysseldyke, Vanderwood, and Shriner (1997) found that 90–92% of cases brought before the referral teams were eventually referred for an evaluation across a 3-year period. These two studies, along with others, have examined the percentage of children who were eventually placed in special education. Algozzine et al. (1982) and Ysseldyke et al. (1997) found that 73% and 70–74%, respectively, of students referred were deemed eligible for special education services. The ratio of referral to special education placement varied across studies: Foster, Ysseldyke, Casey, and Thurlow (1984) reported 72%; Furlong (1988) reported 60.5%; and Fugate, Clarizio, and Phillips (1993) reported 54%. Rueda et al. (1985) found that 86% of referred Hispanics pupils were deemed eligible for special education.

These data clearly indicate that if teachers decide to bring children's cases before their prereferral committees, the children will most likely be referred. Thus, the effectiveness of these teams can be questioned. All the aforementioned studies revealed that once the child is referred, there is a greater than 50% probability that the child will be placed. Some individuals would interpret these data as indicating a need to improve prereferral interventions and practices. Data from two large-scale studies indicate that the quality of prereferral intervention is poor (Flugum & Reschly, 1994; Telzrow, McNamara, & Hollinger, 2000). Thus, school-based practitioners must consider whether the lack of quality prereferral interventions contributes to the referral of students.

Clearly, there is a need for improvement along two major fronts. The first area of improvement would place greater emphasis on prevention efforts (Ortiz, 1992, 1997). These preventive efforts should consist of ensuring that high-quality instructional programs are provided for students in general education. Such programs would reduce the probability that LEP children experience failure and subsequently become the subject of review by the prereferral team. Psychologists as well as members of the prereferral team need to be aware of the indicators of effective instructional practices for second-language learners. Obtaining a knowledge base in this area also enables members of prereferral teams to conduct an ecological assessment of classroom practices.

The second area of improvement, as it relates to second-language learners, involves improving prereferral interventions and determining which factors need to be considered by the prereferral team before making a decision to recommend testing. Ortiz (1992, 1997) cites prereferral intervention as a second component of the prereferrral process. The following sections discuss three important factors that need to be considered by prereferral teams: the school and classroom environment, language acquisition, and cultural variables pertaining to the child and their families.

## PREVENTION EFFORTS: COMPONENTS OF EFFECTIVE LEARNING ENVIRONMENTS FOR SECOND-LANGUAGE LEARNERS

As noted in Chapter 4, research indicates that the different types of bilingual programs yield substantially different achievement outcomes when examined from a long-term perspective. In addition, differences or variability may occur within certain types of bilingual education programs. Several critical components have been identified in effective learning environments for second-language learners: (1) instruction in children's native languages is provided; (2) content-based instruction in English is provided; (3) students are treated as active learners; (4) students' languages and cultures are valued; (5) interaction with monolingual English-speaking peers occurs; and (6) the bilingual education program is an integral rather than tangential part of the school. It should be noted that these are some, but by no means all, of the critical components that need to be considered. It is important for school psychologists and other school personnel to ascertain whether, or the degree to which, these components are evident in their instructional settings. If most or all of these components are evident in learning environments for second-language learners, then the probability that the LEP child has received quality instruction in general education substantially increases. However, if very few of these components are evident in classrooms for linguistically diverse students, then those in positions of authority need to question whether the absence of such components has an impact on children's academic performance.

## Instruction in the Child's Native Language

Thomas and Collier (1997) cite instruction in the child's native language as the most important component. They state that students need to receive challenging academic content (e.g., "on-grade-level academic" work) for "as long as possible" (pp. 49, 64) and stress the importance of this factor:

> Without L1 [first language] academic support, even when all the other four variables [points 2–5 above] are provided, this is not sufficient assistance for English language learners eventually to close the achievement gap. . . . Of all the five program variables, L1 support explains the most variance in student achievement and is the most powerful influence on language minority students' long term academic success. (p. 64)

## Content-Based Instruction in English

When English instruction is provided to second-language learners, it should not exclusively focus on teaching just English (Thomas & Collier, 1997). Instead, the focus of instruction should be on teaching academic content at the student's respective grade level in English and simultaneously making the necessary modifications to adjust for the student's English proficiency (Thomas & Collier, 1997).

## Students as Active Learners

Second-language learners should be treated as active, rather than passive, learners, which means that LEP students must be given the opportunity to interact with one another. Thomas and Collier (1997) found that "students who participate[d] in classes that [were] very interactive, with discovery learning facilitated by teachers so that students work cooperatively together in a socioculturally supportive environment, [did] better than those attending classes taught more traditionally" (p. 50). Cummins (1986) describes this process as one of reciprocal instruction; much conversation takes place among students and between students and their teacher.

## Valuing Students' Languages and Cultures

Thomas and Collier (1997) found that recognizing second-language learners' strengths, such as their cultural and linguistic backgrounds, is important in an effective instructional environment. August and Hakuta (1998) also found that these two factors were valued in effective learning environments for second-language learners, as did Cummins (1986), who stated that culture and language are important aspects that need to be included in the curriculum for second-language learners.

## Interaction with Monolingual English-Speaking Peers

Second-language learners need to be exposed to good English-language models in order to learn English, and "same-age peers are a crucial source of L2 [second-language] input" (Thomas & Collier, 1997, p. 51). August and Hakuta (1998) also found that second-language learners benefit from "opportunities to practice" with their monolingual English-speaking peers (p. 80).

## Bilingual Education Program Is Valued as an Integral Part of the School

Support for bilingual education programs from their fellow educators and administrators in effective learning environments is essential for their success (August & Hakuta, 1998; Thomas & Collier, 1997). Perez and Ochoa (1993) found that support for bilingual education programs was more likely to exist in effective schools as compared to schools that were not characterized as effective. Curriculum-planning coordination is essential between bilingual education and general education in order to prepare for the eventual transition of the second-language learners (August & Hakuta, 1998).

## REASONS WHY SECOND-LANGUAGE LEARNERS ARE REFERRED: POSSIBLE CONNECTIONS WITH CULTURE AND LANGUAGE

There has been limited research examining the reasons why LEP students are referred to special education. Two of these studies were small-scale investigations that included three school districts in Texas (Ortiz & Polyzoi, 1986) and four school districts in California (Rueda et al., 1985). A third study involved a large-scale investigation of the reasons why LEP students were referred in eight states (Arizona, California, Colorado, Florida, New Jersey, New Mexico, New York, and Texas) with high LEP student populations (Ochoa, Robles-Piña, Garcia, & Breunig, 1999). In this study 1,384 school psychologists identified up to three most common referral reasons noted in the referral packets of LEP students. The top 10 most frequent reasons given for LEP pupils being referred to special education were (1) "poor/low achievement," (2) "behavioral problems," (3) "oral-language-related (i.e., acquisition delay)," (4) "reading problems," (5) "learning difficulties," (6) "socio-emotional difficulties," (7) "diagnosis for particular disability condition," (8) "written language," (9) "low attention span," and (10) "unable to understand and/or follow directions" (Ochoa, Robles-Piña, Garcia, & Breunig, 1999, p. 7). There was consistency across these three studies: Poor academic performance, behavioral problems, low attention, and oral language factors were noted to be common reasons for referral across all three studies.

Ochoa, Robles-Piña, Garcia, and Breunig (1999) stated that 7 of the 10 most frequent reasons for referral, noted above, could "have a plausible linkage with language/and or culture" (p. 7). One of the seven reasons that can be linked to language is obviously the oral-language-related variable noted above. Approximately one-third of school psychologists in their study reported that oral language is one of the top three reasons why LEP students are referred. If a student is referred for oral-language-related types of problems, it is important to consider several factors. One factor is the child's linguistic abilities and deficits in both his or her native and second languages. Is the problem apparent in both languages? If the apparent problem is noted only in English and not in the child's first language, it is most likely due to factors associated with second-language acquisition than with a problem inherent in the child.

Second, the impact of the child's placement in relation to the development of CALP and its subsequent influence on academic-related problems must be considered. If the child is being taught in an English-only academic setting, did the child develop CALP in his or her first language? If the student did not develop a minimum threshold in his or her first language, this lack will greatly impact his or her development of English academic language skills. Moreover, "a strong foundation of oral language skills is essential to the development of literacy in general" (Ochoa, Robles-Piña, Garcia, & Breunig, 1999, p. 10). Thus, if the student is referred for reading problems (reason 4 noted above) or written language difficulties (reason 8 noted above), the extent to which CALP was, or was not, developed in the child's first language and whether the pedagogy he or she received was designed to foster CALP in the first language must be considered.

Third, the degree to which the language-related concerns are commonly found in LEP students should also be considered: Is the student displaying any of the common language patterns observed in students with LEP? These patterns include interference, interlanguage, code switching, silent period, language loss, and language differences. (See Chapter 4 for more information about these common language patterns.) Does the student display common language-usage characteristics noted in second-language learners. Common language characteristics/behaviors noted in LEP students include the following:

> Speaks infrequently, uses gestures, speaks in single words or phrases, refuses to answer questions, does not volunteer information, comments inappropriately, poor recall, poor comprehension, poor vocabulary, difficulty sequencing events, unable to tell or retell stories, confuses similar sounding words, poor pronunciation, [and] poor syntax/grammar. (Ortiz & Maldonado-Colon, 1986, p. 45)

Second-language learners' problematic behaviors can also be associated with, or linked to, learning a second language or culture. Ochoa, Robles-Piña, et al. (1999) reported that LEP students are referred as a result of behavioral problems (reason 2 noted above). Second-language learners may display "defensive," "withdrawn," and "disorganized" behaviors (Hoover & Collier, 1985). Social–emotional difficulties (reason 6 noted above) have also been noted in second-language learners. LEP students may be shy, timid, and fearful when striving to acquire a second language (Ortiz and Maldonado-Colon, 1986). Culturally and linguistically diverse pupils may display "heightened anxiety" and "low self-esteem" when they are placed in environments that are different from their home culture (Collier & Hoover, 1987). Low attention span (reason 9 noted above) is another expected occurrence in some second-language learners (Collier & Hoover, 1987; Ortiz & Maldonado-Colon, 1986), as is an inability to understand or follow directions (reason 10). Hoover and Collier (1985) note that "a child with some English proficiency may appear to understand directions or rules but in reality lacks enough conceptual knowledge to sufficiently comprehend certain ideas" (p. 508).

The behavioral difficulties that are linked to second-language acquisition can significantly impact students' performance. Teachers may be concerned when they observe these behaviors in LEP students because they most likely have seen similar characteristics in monolingual students who have previously been placed in special education. There are several key questions to consider in these situations:

1. Are these behaviors noted when instruction is provided in the child's native language?
2. Are these same behaviors observed at home and in the child's community?
3. How do the severity and frequency of the behaviors that are a cause of concern differ when compared to peers who are from culturally and linguistically diverse backgrounds?

The answers to these questions can shed light on the influence of culture and language on the LEP student's behavior.

## PREREFERRAL SALIENT FACTORS

Many factors need to be considered when a second-language learner is brought before the prereferral team. These factors include general educational background history, preschool experiences, many variables associated with schooling, student performance, and considerations pertaining to language, family, and culture. Form 5.1 at the end of the chapter includes over 100 questions that psychologists, school personnel, and prereferral team members should consider when reviewing what might be contributing to the second-language learner's academic difficulties and exploring options on how to intervene with the student.

Several important factors need to be stressed when using the questions included in the table. First, not all questions will be applicable to every case involving every second-language learner. Second, not all questions carry equal weight. A response to particular questions should not automatically preclude a second-language learner from being referred for testing. What is important to consider is the appearance of consistent patterns across questions. When reviewing the information obtained by answering these questions, it is important to ask the following series of questions:

1. Are there consistent pieces of data that suggest that limited English proficiency/second-language acquisition might be a significant contributing factor in the child's academic performance?
2. Are there consistent pieces of data that indicate that the student has, or has not, received effective instruction?
3. Are there consistent pieces of data that suggest that cultural differences or family factors might be significantly impacting student performance and behavior?
4. Are there consistent pieces of data that indicate that the student's language growth and academic performance in both the native language and English are significantly different from his or her second-language learner peers? *Note*: This question assumes that a comparison is being made with other LEP students who have been instructed in the same type of bilingual/ESL program for approximately the same length of time.

After reviewing the questions on the table, one might conclude that it would be very difficult to refer a second-language learner for testing. Although it is important to consider all options and factors before recommending testing, it is critical to acknowledge that there are second-language learners who have special needs and that these students do require special education services. The questions should not be used to automatically prevent students from being referred. Some schools may "discourage" or "prohibit referrals" of second-language learners for a certain period of time (Ortiz, 1997, p. 332). In our view, this practice is not appropriate. The goal of answering the questions on Form 5.1 is to see if consistent patterns emerge in order to help differentiate cultural and linguistic differences from genuine disabilities. If used in this manner, the answers obtained will help to provide a rationale as to why the student was, or was not, referred. This information should be shared with the psychologist conducting the bilingual psychoeducational assessment.

## SUMMARY

This chapter has explored the variability in how prereferral teams are constituted and perceived and in how they function. An individual with expertise in second-language acquisition and dual-language programming is needed on the prereferral team when a second-language learner is referred. Many of the most common reasons that LEP students are referred to these teams have a plausible link to language and culture. Therefore, the impact of these factors, along with others not in this chapter, must be thoroughly reviewed in order to determine if patterns exist across the data and information collected and reviewed. It is critical for prereferral team members to evaluate if these patterns suggest/indicate a need to consider other alternatives within the general education environment or to recommend testing.

FORM 5.1. Prereferral Team Considerations: Questions Pertaining
to Second-Language Learners

Teacher's reason(s) for concern: Why has the teacher brought this student before the prereferral team?

## GENERAL EDUCATIONAL BACKGROUND HISTORY

1. Did child start his or her formal schooling in the United States?
   If yes, proceed to next section. If no, ask the following questions:
2. How many years did the child attend school in his or her native country?
3. How is school structured in the child's native country? Ask parents to describe a typical school day in their native country.
4. Are there differences between the schools in the native country and in the United States? If yes, describe these differences and consider how these differences might impact the student's performance.
5. What do we know about the language system used in the native country? For example, does it have a written form and is it read from left to right, or vice versa?
6. Was the school that the child attended in his or her native country located in an urban or rural area?
7. Did child regularly attend school in his or her native country?
8. Did the student evidence any academic difficulties/problems while attending school in the native country?
9. Do parents have written documentation about their child's school performance in their native country? Have these been translated and reviewed?

## PRESCHOOL EXPERIENCES

10. Who was/were the child's primary caregiver(s)? What language(s) did each caregiver speak to the child? Obtain a percentage for each language spoken to the child by each caregiver.
11. Did the child receive any preschool educational services (i.e., Head Start or private center)? If no, proceed to next section.
12. For how long did the child receive these preschool educational services?
13. Were the preschool services offered in the child's native language, in English, or in both languages?
14. Did personnel in these preschool settings note any concerns about this child? If yes, please describe.

*(continued)*

## SCHOOLING FACTORS

Entrance to Bilingual Education and/or ESL Program Considerations

15. What does the child's home language survey indicate?
16. Did bilingual education/ESL program personnel give language proficiency measures to the child? If no, why not? If no, proceed to Question 20.
17. What language measure(s) was/were given?
18. What results were obtained from this/these measure(s)?
19. Was/were the person(s) who administered this/these measure(s) trained to do so?
20. Did parents deny bilingual education/ESL program? If yes, why?
21. Was child placed in bilingual education/ESL program? If no, why not?
    If no, proceed to Question 37.

Bilingual Education Program Factors

22. What type of bilingual education and/or ESL program does the school offer?
23. In what grades is bilingual education/ESL provided in this school?
24. What percent of instruction is provided in the non-English language and in English across the grade levels that have bilingual education/ESL programs?
25. How many of the teachers that instructed the child have been certified in bilingual and/or ESL program? How many have not?
26. Do/did all bilingual education teachers who have taught the child have sufficient proficiency in English and Spanish (or other language) to provide academic instruction?
27. Is there school district and campus administrative support for bilingual education and ESL program?
28. Are bilingual education and ESL program perceived to be appropriate instructional methodology that should be used with second-language learners?
29. Is curriculum offered in bilingual education/ESL program comparable to that provided to monolingual English-speaking students in other general education settings?
30. What is the quality of the bilingual education/ESL program offered?
    Specifically, what percent of LEP students by grade level have:
    a. Passed the state-mandated test in their first/native language? In their second language (e.g., English)?
    b. Evidenced sufficient mastery on criterion-referenced measures in their first/native language? In their second language (e.g., English)?
    c. Evidenced mastery of essential grade-level skills in their first/native language and in their second language (e.g., English) as measured by teacher-made tests?

Bilingual Education Exit Considerations

31. What criteria were used to exit the child from bilingual education/ESL program?
32. Does this criteria meet state guidelines on exiting students from bilingual education/ESL program?

*(continued)*

33. What language growth has the child evidenced at time of exit versus time of entry into bilingual education/ESL program in both his or her native language and English?

34. At the time of exit, was the noted language growth sufficient for the child to be academically successful in an English-only learning environment?

35. At the time of exit, how did this student's language growth compare with other second-language learner's language growth who had been in the same bilingual education/ESL program?

36. Did the language measures given at time of exit measure basic interpersonal communication skills (BICS) and/or cognitive academic language proficiency (CALP) types of language skills?

Proceed to Question 41.

Considerations to Review When No Bilingual Education/ESL Program Provided

37. What is the impact of not receiving bilingual education/ESL services on this student's language development and academic performance?

38. What alternatives and strategies have the school used to address the language needs of the student?

39. Does the team believe that the aforementioned alternatives and strategies listed in Question 38 are sufficient to provide educational conditions that will help the student display his or her optimal abilities?

40. What additional alternatives, strategies, and resources need to be utilized in order to assist the child to make progress?

Teacher Factors

41. If the child is currently in a general education classroom setting with no bilingual education/ESL program, what level of professional training and experience does the child's general education teacher have with second-language learners?

42. What is the child's current teacher track record on referring students to the prereferral team? In other words, does this teacher rarely refer students, or is this a teacher who refers a significant number of his or her students each year?

43. What specific instructional efforts has the teacher used to intervene with the child prior to bringing the child's situation to the attention of the prereferral team?

44. How long were these instructional efforts implemented?

45. What were the results of these efforts?

## EVALUATING STUDENT'S PERFORMANCE

46. How did/has the student perform(ed) across subjects and grade levels in bilingual education/ESL program instructional settings? Review grades provided on report card by subject area across grade levels. Note whether these grades are based on grade-level material.

47. Does the student's performance reviewed in Question 46 differ from that made by other second-language learners who have received the same bilingual education/ESL instructional

*(continued)*

program for approximately the same length of time? If yes, explain and review how the performances differ.

48. If student is no longer in, or has never been in, a bilingual education/ESL program, how has the student performed across subjects and grade levels in general education? Review grades provided on report card by subject area across grade levels.

49. Does the student's performance reviewed in Question 48 differ from that made by other second-language learners who received the same instructional bilingual education/ESL program and have been in the general education environment for approximately the same length of time? If yes, explain and review how they differ.

50. At what grade level does the child read in his or her first/native language and in English?

51. Does the student's reading ability in his or her first/native language and in English, noted in Question 50, differ from that of second-language learners who have received the same instructional bilingual education/ESL program and, if applicable, have been in a general education environment for approximately the same length of time? If yes, explain and review how they differ.

52. Has an academic portfolio (e.g., work samples) been obtained on this student across time? If it has, how does this student's portfolio compare with other second-language learners' portfolios?

53. If an academic portfolio has been obtained, has any progress been noted in academic content when instruction is provided in the child's first/native language and in English? How does this student's progress compare to that made by other second-language learners?

54. If the student has been in a bilingual education/ESL program, how does the child's current educational performance and overall trajectory in general education vary from that noted while the child was in a bilingual education/ESL program?

55. Does the child appear to need additional instructional support than is required by his/her English language learner peers?

## LANGUAGE CONSIDERATIONS

56. Is each of the suspected areas of difficulty noted in both the child's native language and in English?

57. Has the child obtained a cognitive academic language proficiency (CALP) level in his or her first/native language and in English?

58. If the answer to Question 57 is no in either the child's first/native language or in English, what is the child's current level of proficiency in both languages?

59. Does the student currently have sufficient English skills to be academically successful in an English-only general education instructional setting?

60. If the child has not attained cognitive academic language proficiency (CALP) in English and is at the basic interpersonal communication skills (BICS) level in English, is the general education teacher making inaccurate assumptions about the child's English skills not having an impact on his/her academic performance?

61. Does the child's performance improve when provided instructional assistance in his or her native language?

(*continued*)

62. Describe the student's affect while he or she participated in the bilingual education program and in general education? If applicable, describe the differences noted across these instructional settings. How does the child's affect differ from that of other second-language learners across both instructional environments?

63. How well does the child communicate in his or her first/native language and in English across different settings (e.g., home, classroom, playground, neighborhood, community)?

64. Does the child evidence the common language patterns, differences, and characteristics frequently noted in second-language learners?

65. How does the child feel about acquiring English?

## FAMILY AND CULTURAL FACTORS

66. Where were the child's parents born? If both parents were born in the United States, and the child is not a migrant student, proceed to Question 83.

### If Family Immigrated to the United States

67. What is the family's native country?

68. Why did the family immigrate to the United States?

69. Did the entire family immigrate together? If they did not, specify the order and date each family member came to the United States and who, if any, remain in the native country.

70. What was each parent's occupation in his or her native country? What job does each parent have in the United States?

71. What was the parents' socioeconomic status level in their native country? How does it compare to that in the United States?

72. What social support systems, if any, did the family have in the United States prior to their arrival? What social support systems do they have now?

73. If student was not born in the United States, how is life different in the United States as compared to his or her native country? Ask parent to describe a typical day at home for the child in his or her native country and in the United States.

74. How many times has the family moved since arriving in the United States? How long did the family stay at each location?

75. Has the family returned to their home country? If so, how often and for how long?

### For Migrant Families

If the child is not a migrant student, proceed to Question 83.

76. For how many years has the family migrated within a state or across state lines to find employment?

77. Does the family migrate between two specific locations? If so, from where to where, and how long is the family at each location?

78. Does the family migrate to several locations? If so, name the different locations and the amount of time spent at each.

*(continued)*

89

79. On average, how many days does the student not attend school per year due to traveling between locations?

80. Across his or her educational career, how many different schools has the child attended? What was the length of stay at each of the schools?

81. How many of the schools attended provided bilingual education/ESL programs for the student?

82. How does the curriculum vary across the different schools that the student has attended (especially across state lines)?

All Families from Culturally and Linguistically Diverse Backgrounds

83. Who lives in the student's home?

84. What is each parent's educational level?

85. What literacy skills does the parent have in his or her native language and in English?

86. What language(s) does each person in the home use to communicate with the child? If more than one language is used, specify the percent of time English and the native language is used for each person in the home.

87. What is the acculturational level of the student's family?

88. Is the child's level of acculturation different from that of his or her parents? If it is, does this result in added stress or additional responsibilities for the child?

89. What difficulties has the family experienced in adapting to U.S. culture? Do parents believe that this adaptation has had an impact of their child?

90. What thoughts, comments, or feelings has the child expressed about his or her school in relation to cultural and linguistic factors?

91. In what ways is the child's home culture different from that of the school culture?

92. If available, does the family watch television programs and listen to radio stations in their native/first language? To what extent does the family watch television and listen to the radio in English?

93. How does the child's family/culture view education and educators?

94. Is there anyone in the home or neighborhood who can assist the child with schoolwork in his or her native/first language and in English?

95. How does this student compare to his or her siblings with regard to developmental milestones?

96. Do parents have any concerns about their child's development as compared to their other offspring?

97. How does the pupil's academic performance compare to that of his/her siblings who are closest in age?

98. Has the student had any significant illnesses or injuries? If so, how were these addressed?

99. How does the student's culture view disabilities and illnesses? Is their conceptualization similar to that of the U.S. mainstream, which is based on the Western medical model? What stigma is associated with disabilities?

100. Other than academic factors, are there any behaviors that are a cause for concern? How are these behaviors interpreted by teacher/school versus child's family/culture?

# 6

# The Use of Interpreters in the Assessment Process and School-Based Practice

Ideally, there would be no need for a chapter on the use of interpreters in this book. In a perfect assessment world, all school-based practitioners would be perfectly in sync culturally and linguistically with the parents and students whom they serve. Any error or inaccuracy occurring during the assessment process would be limited to the built-in standard error of measurement that we are able to calculate and report. No other external variables would influence the accuracy of our assessment and interpretation.

Fortunately or unfortunately, as practitioners we will never be perfectly in sync with the remarkably heterogeneous population that we serve (see Chapter 1). Instead, we must recognize our individual cultural and linguistic limitations and seek appropriate assistance, as needed. This necessity is true for both monolingual and bilingual practitioners. The expertise of a bilingual practitioner is extremely valuable, but the scope of effective independent practice is unavoidably limited to the students and parents who share the same general culture and language background. Both monolingual and bilingual practitioners who serve a diversity of students often require the assistance of interpreters during day-to-day activities.

Very little information is available, however, regarding how to best incorporate interpreters into daily practice. In the absence of legal and ethical specifications and research-based best practice guidelines, many practitioners seek the assistance of an interpreter with little understanding of the associated assets, limitations, and liabilities. Ochoa, Gonzalez, Galarza, and Guillemard (1996), in the most comprehensive survey of school-based interpreter usage to date, found that the majority of school psychologists who reported using interpreters had received no, or very little, training to do so. Less than half (37%) reported that the individual providing interpretation services had received formal training. In only a handful of cases (7%) were both the school psychologist and the interpreter trained in the interpretation process.

This chapter is by Robert L. Rhodes.

The purpose of this chapter is to provide step-by-step guidelines and recommendations regarding who can best serve as an interpreter, the skills and training an interpreter should have, the legal and ethical responsibilities of interpreters, issues that arise during the interpretation process, and steps that practitioners and interpreters can take to make the process better. A checklist for interpreter selection and training is also provided. We begin by defining three essential terms: *native language*, *interpreter*, and *translator*.

## DEFINITIONS

### Native Language

When used with reference to an LEP individual, the term *native language* means the language normally used by the individual, or in the case of a child, the language normally used by the parents of the child (Individuals with Disabilities Education Act, Revisions of 1997).

### Interpreter and Translator

The terms *interpreter* and *translator* are often used by professionals interchangeably, although they have different meanings and functions. An interpreter conveys information from one language to the other in the oral modality; a translator conveys information in the written modality (Weber, 1990). It is an interpreter upon whom school-based practitioners most often rely during day-to-day practice.

## WHO CAN SERVE AS AN INTERPRETER?

Although the native language of students and parents must be used in testing assessment and communication procedures (see Chapter 3), there are minimal legal specifications regarding who is eligible to serve as an interpreter. From a strict legal perspective, the ability to speak the native language of the child and/or parent in addition to English may be the sole requirement of serving as an interpreter. As a result, the path of least resistance is all too often taken in the selection and use of an interpreter. A bilingual second-grade teacher, school secretary, or family member of the student or parent may be spontaneously called upon to serve as an interpreter in a given situation. This haphazard selection of interpreters has the potential to greatly limit the effectiveness of the interpretation process and ultimately the overall quality of service provision. The following criteria should be considered in the selection of an interpreter:

• At a minimum, the interpreter should be equally fluent in English and the native language of the student or parent. Helpful individuals who speak "a little Spanish" or "a little Japanese" or who "understand most of what they hear" in a second language may be of assistance in unplanned/impromptu conversations with a student or parent, but *under no circumstances* should be used in any formal capacity as an interpreter. The risk of error within the interpretation process is great even when the interpreter is fluent in both languages. This risk is increased exponentially if the person struggles for command of either language. It is important to note that this limitation holds true for command of both the first or native language (L1) and the second language (L2). If a potential interpreter has apparent command of the targeted second language but struggles in English, he or she faces the same limitations as our helpful individual who "speaks a little Spanish."

• Langdon (1994) suggests that interpreters should have a minimum of a high school diploma and communication skills that are adequate for the tasks assigned by the professional, including (1) an ability to accurately convey meaning from one language to another; (2) sensitivity to the style of the speaker; (3) ability to adjust to linguistic variations within different communities; (4) knowledge about the cultures of the people who speak the languages; (5) familiarity with the specific terminology used in the educational field; (6) understanding of the function and role of the interpreter in the multidisciplinary team process; and (7) flexibility (see the following section).

• Friends and family members of the student or parent should not be used as interpreters. The breech of student and parent confidentiality, likelihood of the manipulation of information to save the family from difficult news, and the role reversal that occurs when utilizing students and friends of the family as interpreters preclude this as an appropriate procedure (Lynch & Hanson, 1996). Friends of the family and family members who are not ordinarily involved in the special education process do not have privileged access to the confidential information requiring interpretation. Parent permission, via informed consent, to have a friend or family member serve as an interpreter is highly questionable in that it is impossible for a parent to know what information they are giving permission to be shared until it is actually interpreted.

• The relationship that develops between the interpreter and the student or parent can be useful in maintaining parent participation throughout the evaluation process. When possible, an interpreter who will be able to work with the student or parents on an ongoing basis should be selected (Rhodes, 1996). It is not uncommon for a student or parent to view the interpreter as a key member of the multidisciplinary team rather than a neutral conduit of information. The interpreter is typically the individual who hears the information from the student or parent first and the last person to speak to the student or parent on behalf of the school. Because of this unique relationship, it is not uncommon for the person receiving interpretive assistance to feel it is important to bring a new interpreter "up to speed" so that they have the whole picture of what was previously discussed (Rhodes, 1996).

## WHAT SKILLS/TRAINING SHOULD AN INTERPRETER HAVE?

Because of difficulties inherent in the use of interpreters, school districts are strongly encouraged to exhaust all means of obtaining professional personnel who are bilingual before seeking the assistance of interpreters (Council for Exceptional Children, 1996). Guajardo Alvarado (2003) recommends the following hierarchy of evaluation for personnel who work with culturally and linguistically diverse students: (1) trained bilingual evaluation specialist(s) fluent in the student's native language using evaluation measures in the student's two languages; (2) bilingual evaluation specialist(s) fluent in the student's native language using modified evaluation measures, translated tests, or tests with norming populations not representative of the student's background, etc., if it is clearly not feasible to use evaluation measures in the student's two languages; (3) English speaking evaluation specialist(s) assisted by a trained bilingual ancillary examiner using standardized evaluation measures; (4) English speaking evaluation specialist(s) assisted by a trained interpreter and using modified evaluation measures, translated tests, or tests with norming populations not representative of the student's background, etc.; and (5) evaluation specialist(s) using only nonverbal or performance intelligence evaluation measures for languages other than English or Spanish. The decision to use an interpreter should be made only after reviewing all possible options. When an interpreter must be used, it is obvious that individuals with unique skills and training are required. The following discussion provides an extensive overview of requisite skills and recommendations for skill-development training.

## Neutrality and Confidentiality

The role of the interpreter requires an ability to stay emotionally uninvolved with the content of discussions and to maintain neutrality and confidentiality (Langdon, 1994). The Family Educational Rights and Privacy Act of 1974, the Individuals with Disabilities Education Act, Revisions of 1997, and the National Association of School Psychologists (2000) Principles for Professional Ethics require that confidentiality of student and parent information be maintained (see Chapter 3). Individuals serving as interpreters must have an understanding of confidentiality requirements and must be informed of the extent and limitations of confidentiality.

## Adherence to Ethical Guidelines

The National Registry of Interpreters for the Deaf (RID; 2002) Code of Ethics provides useful guidelines for all individuals serving as interpreters within a school setting. The following are established by RID's Code of Ethics:

- *Interpreters shall keep all assignment-related information strictly confidential.* No information regarding any assignment shall be revealed, including the fact that the service is being performed, unless the service is being provided for a general audience and anyone being informed about the service can attend the event.

- *Interpreters shall render the message faithfully, always conveying the content and spirit of the speaker, using language most readily understood by the person(s) whom they serve.* Interpreters are not editors and must transmit everything that is said in exactly the same way it was intended. This may be especially difficult when the interpreter disagrees with what is being said or has to interpret profane language. Interpreters must remember that they are not at all responsible for what is said, only for conveying it accurately. If the interpreter's own feelings interfere with rendering the message accurately, he or she shall withdraw from the situation.

- *Interpreters shall not counsel, advise, or interject personal opinions.* Interpreters are to refrain from adding anything to the situation, even when they are asked to by other parties involved. They shall remain personally uninvolved because in doing so, they leave the responsibility of the outcome to those for whom they are facilitating the communication and do not assume this responsibility themselves.

- *Service providers shall accept assignments using discretion with regard to skill, setting, and the consumers involved.* Interpreters shall accept assignments for which they are qualified.

- *Interpreters shall request compensation for services in a professional and judicious manner.* Interpreters shall be knowledgeable about fees that are appropriate to the profession and shall be informed about the current suggested fee schedule of the national interpreter organization.

- *Interpreters shall function in a manner appropriate to the situation.* Interpreters shall conduct themselves in such a manner that brings respect to themselves, the consumers, the institution, and the national RID organization.
- *Interpreters shall strive to further knowledge and skills through participation in workshops, professional meetings, interactions with professional colleagues, and reading of current literature in the field.*

## Understanding Terms, Procedures, and Rationale of the Assessment Process

Numerous authors (e.g., Hallberg, 1996; Omark & Watson, 1981) have suggested that the interpreter receive training in the terms, procedures, and rationale of the assessment process and evaluation instruments. Knowledge of these factors enables the interpreter to monitor the appropriateness of the interpretation process and maintain standardization, as necessary. The terms used during informed consent procedures, interviews, assessment, and multidisciplinary team meetings need to be previewed and discussed prior to "live" interpretation. Likewise, the ability to exchange a word in one language for a word in another does not mean that the person interpreting understands the process in which he or she is participating. The concept of standardization and strict assessment procedures must be clearly communicated and understood.

Form 6.1 at the end of the chapter lists basic terms and concepts in both English (Form 6.1a) and Spanish (Form 6.1b) that should be reviewed with, and understood by, anyone providing school-based interpretation services.

## Cultural and Linguistic Expertise

Because the unique aspects of language, both verbal and nonverbal, vary from culture to culture, it is important that the interpreter have cultural expertise as well as linguistic expertise. Randall-David (1989) states that interpreters with cultural knowledge are ideal because they not only translate the interaction but also bridge the cultural gap. There are many terms and phrases that must be viewed within a cultural framework to be able to gain a full understanding of meaning during the interpretation process.

## Knowledge of Critical Issues

The individual serving as an interpreter must be familiar with issues that often arise when interpreting from one language into another (e.g., code switching on the part of the student; Rhodes, Kayser, & Hess, 2000). It is not unusual, for example, for a second-language learner to switch back and forth between two languages during a conversation. Sometimes this code switching or mixture of languages takes place within the same sentence. Kayser (1993) notes that when an individual untrained in these issues serves as an interpreter, there may be omitted, misinterpreted, or misunderstood information relayed to the family or professional.

A summary checklist for interpreter selection and training is provided at the end of the chapter in Form 6.2.

## WHAT RESOURCES ARE AVAILABLE
## OUTSIDE OF THE SCHOOL SETTING?

There are often resources outside of the school setting that provide interpretation services on a routine basis in the native language of the parent or student. Before concluding that interpretation services are not available for a student or parent, school personnel should first make certain that they have exhausted all appropriate means of interpretation assistance within and outside of the school setting. Although caution must be exercised to protect confidentiality and rights to privacy, these services may be of great assistance when working with parents or students who speak a language that is unfamiliar to school personnel. Recommended resources outside of the school setting include:

- *Court interpreters.* The judicial system routinely uses interpreters for a variety of languages and situations. These individuals are often highly trained, follow strict codes of confidentiality, and may be available for paid consultation with a school district on a case-by-case basis.
- *Embassy and consulate personnel.* Interpretive assistance may also be available through the appropriate embassy or consulate, whose personnel may be able to recommend a knowledgeable person in the local area or provide assistance via a phone conference.
- *Phone company resources.* Many phone companies employee individuals to provide customer service in a variety of languages. An international operator or other customer service representative may be able to provide interpretation services via a phone conference.
- *Professional association resources.* The National Association of School Psychologists, American Speech and Hearing Association, and other professional associations maintain and publish directories of bilingual professionals. These directories provide the names and contact information for persons by language and state.

## WHAT CAN BE DONE WHEN AN INTERPRETER IS NOT AVAILABLE?

What happens when it is clearly not feasible to conduct procedures in the student's native language or through the use of an interpreter (e.g., in the case of a low-incidence language or lack of available interpreters in a rural community)? In situations for which a bilingual practitioner or interpreter is truly not available, the Assistance to States for the Education of Children with Disabilities; Final Regulations (U.S. Department of Education, 1999a) recommends that other evaluation procedures (e.g., nonverbal measures of ability) be emphasized. Section 300.531 of the Final Regulations, however, emphasizes that alternate or altered methods of evaluation should be held to the same standard as verbally based procedures, including the following specifications:

- Materials and procedures are selected and administered to ensure that they measure the extent to which a child has a disability and needs special education, rather than measuring the child's English-language skills.
- A variety of assessment tools and strategies is used to gather relevant functional and developmental information about the child.
- Any standardized tests that are given to a child have been validated for the specific pur-

pose for which they are used and are administered by trained and knowledgeable personnel, in accordance with any instructions provided by the producer of the tests.

- No single procedure is used as the sole criterion for determining whether a child is a child with a disability.

## WHAT CAN BE DONE
## TO MAKE THE INTERPRETATION PROCESS BETTER?

Armed with the knowledge that appropriate interpretation is a formidable task requiring specific skills and training, mental health and educational professionals can offer specific support to make the interpretation process better. Lopez (1995), in a review of literature (Figueroa, 1990b; Langdon, 1985; Lopez, 1992), suggests the following best practices when using an interpreter:

- Allow time before the testing session for the interpreter to ask questions about test procedures and details related to the student's background (e.g., place of birth).
- Encourage interpreters to ask questions as the testing session or meeting is occurring.
- Throughout the interpretation process (1) speak in short, simple sentences; (2) avoid idioms, metaphors, or colloquialisms; (3) use specific terms and avoid jargon; and (4) allow the interpreter time to translate all messages.

Hallberg (1996) offers additional suggestions for making the interpretation process better:

- Preinterpretation practice and review of materials.
- Frequent checks during the interpretation process to ensure student or parent understanding.
- Supervision of all interpreter activities; it is recommended that all interpretation procedures be supervised and that the mental health or educational professional be present throughout the entire interpretation process.

In addition to the previous recommendations, school-based practitioners receiving interpretative assistance during the assessment process should consider the following suggestions:

- Speak naturally and clearly in brief but complete statements. Do not expect the interpreter to be able to accurately convey lengthy statements. Likewise, do not expect the interpreter to finish your thoughts or ideas for you.
- Look at and speak to the student or parent(s), not the interpreter.
- Monitor the facial expressions of the interpreter and student or parent(s) for apparent confusion or concern.
- Monitor the body language of the interpreter and student or parent(s) for possible discomfort or resistance.
- Feel free to ask the interpreter, student, or parent(s) if he or she has any questions or needs clarification.
- Allow extra time for interpretation and clarification; interpreted procedures *will* take longer.
- Maintain a physical presence during the entire assessment process; do not expect the

interpreter to monitor the student during the more tedious portions of the assessment process, while you follow up on another task.

- Encourage breaks for the interpreter throughout the process; interpretation is a mentally and physically tiring task.
- Meet with the interpreter after the session to debrief and discuss any issues that arose during the process.

Individuals serving as an interpreter during the assessment process should:

- Develop an understanding of the purpose of the session and the materials and procedures that will be used.
- Clarify any areas of concern or uncertainty prior to the start of the session.
- Provide a self-introduction to the student or parent and explain the interpreter's role in the assessment process.
- Interpret everything that is said to the student or parent; do not make assumptions regarding the importance or relevance of the information requiring interpretation—it is not the interpreter's role to act as a filter or censor of information.
- Reflect the pace, tone, and inflection of the speaker.
- Maintain neutrality throughout the process and monitor any emotional reaction to the events that are discussed and the decisions that are reached.
- Inquire about any words, terms, or statements that are unclear or unknown while the process is taking place; *accurate* interpretation is more important than seamless interpretation.
- Maintain the confidentiality of all aspects of the assessment process.

During group or multidisciplinary meetings, it is recommended that each member:

- Introduce him- or herself with the assistance of the interpreter.
- Look at, and speak to, the parent or student rather than to the interpreter.
- Listen while the parent or student is speaking, even if he or she is speaking directly to the interpreter. This focused attention displays an interest in the parent's or student's feedback and minimizes distractions for the interpreter.
- *Not* hold side conversations while the interpreter is talking; the parent has the legal right to be involved in each aspect of the multidisciplinary team meeting and is not able to be a full participant if part of the meeting is taking place without his or her input or knowledge.

## SUMMARY

School-based interpretation is a significant and complex process that is the vehicle for communication and collaboration for a growing number of parents and students—and often the only method through which assessment procedures and meetings can take place. Although deceptively simple to an outside observer, the provision of appropriate interpretation services is the culmination of thoughtful preparation and careful implementation. The guidelines and recommendations provided in this chapter should be carefully considered and, if appropriate, should serve as the impetus for new and more appropriate practice.

**FORM 6.1a.  Basic Terms and Concepts Necessary for School-Based Interpretation**

ability

annual review

assessment

attention-deficit disorder

autism

average

blind

case manager

ceiling

confidentiality

counselor

curriculum-based measurement

deaf

developmental delay

disability

due process

educational diagnostician

emotional disturbance

evaluation

expressive language

federal law

floor

goals

hearing impairment

IEP

inclusion

independent evaluation

intellectual disability

intelligence quotient (IQ)

interview

language disorder

language impairment

least restrictive environment

manifestation determination

mean

multidisciplinary team

multiple disabilities

normative group

norm-referenced

objectives

observation

occupational therapist

orthopedic impairment

other health impaired

percentage

percentile

performance

range

receptive language

reevaluation

reliability

scaled score

school psychologist

special education

specific learning disability

speech impairment

speech–language pathologist

standard score

standardization

traumatic brain injury

validity

verbal

visual impairment

z-score

## FORM 6.1b. Términos y Conceptos Básicos Necesarios para Llevar Acabo Traducciones en las Escuelas

habilidad

revisión anual

evaluación

trastorno de déficit de atención

autismo

promedio

ciego

director del caso

límite tope

confidencialidad

consejero(a)

basado en el currículo medición

sordo

demora del desarrollo

discapacidad

debido procedimiento legal

diagnosticador educativo

disturbio emocional

lenguaje expresivo

ley federal

límite suelo

metas

impedimento auditivo

Programa Educativo Individualizado (PEI)

inclusión

evaluación independiente

discapacidad intelectual

coeficiente intelectual (CI)

entrevista

trastorno de lenguaje

impedimento lingüístico entorno menos restrictivo

manifestación de determinación

media

equipo multidisciplinario

discapacidades múltiples

grupo normativo

referenciado con normas

objetivos

observación

terapeuta ocupacional

impedimento ortopédico

otros impedimentos de salud

porcentaje

percentil

desempeño

rango

lenguaje receptivo

revaluación

confiabilidad

puntuación escalar

psicólogo escolar

educación especial

impedimento de aprendizaje específico

impedimento del habla

patólogo del habla y lenguaje

puntuación estándar

estandarización

lesión cerebral traumática

validez

verbal

impedimento visual

puntuación z

FORM 6.2. Checklist for Interpreter Selection and Training

## CRITERIA FOR INTERPRETER SELECTION

1. Does interpreter have a minimum of a high school education? _____ Yes _____ No

2. Language(s) in which interpreter was educated?

   _____

   _____

3. Is the interpreter equally fluent/literate in English and target language?

   _____ Speaking _____ Reading _____ Writing

4. How was fluency/literacy determined?

   _____ Self-report

   _____ Controlled observation

   _____ Formal measure   Name of measure(s) _____

5. Has the interpreter received formal training as an interpreter? If yes, for what setting?

   _____ School _____ Legal/Court _____ Medical _____ Other

6. Does the interpreter have formal experience as an interpreter? _____ Yes _____ No

   If yes, in what setting?

   _____ School _____ Legal/Court _____ Medical _____ Other

7. In what situations has the interpreter provided interpretation services in a school setting?

   _____ Student interview

   _____ Parent interview

   _____ Informal assessment

   _____ Formal/standardized assessment

   _____ Multidisciplinary team meetings

   _____ IEP _____ Manifestation determination

8. Length of experience (in years) serving as an interpreter? _____

9. Self-reported comfort interpreting in various settings/situations?

   | 1—Very comfortable | _____ Student interview |
   | 2—Comfortable | _____ Parent interview |
   | 3—Unsure | _____ Informal assessment |
   | 4—Uncomfortable | _____ Formal/standardized assessment |
   | 5—Very uncomfortable | _____ Multidisciplinary team meetings |
   | | _____ IEP |
   | | _____ Manifestation determination |

*(continued)*

**Training Checklist**

The following terms, concepts, and procedures should be reviewed with prospective interpreters:

1. ___ Basic terms and concepts for school-based interpretation
   ___ Copy provided to interpreter?                 Date _____
2. ___ Ethical guidelines for interpreters
   ___ Copy provided to interpreter?                 Date _____
3. ___ Rights and limitations of confidentiality
   ___ Copy provided to interpreter?                 Date _____
4. ___ Student/parent interview format
5. ___ Purpose and restrictions of standardized testing
6. ___ All materials and instruments used in the assessment process
7. ___ Purpose and restrictions of multidisciplinary team meetings
8. ___ Etiquette of multidisciplinary team meetings

# 7

# The Interview Process

## *Practical Guidelines*

### PURPOSE OF THE INTERVIEW PROCESS

The purpose of the interview process is to develop a better understanding of a student's developmental, environmental, educational, and family history in relation to the referral question or concern. The information gained through a comprehensive interview can provide an invaluable glimpse into the life of a student and place into context the school-based referral information that we have at hand. This contextual frame of reference is essential for all students participating in the assessment process, and it is particularly necessary for an accurate assessment of students whose cultural and linguistic differences may otherwise obscure their true skills and ability.

### ADVANTAGES OF THE INTERVIEW PROCESS

The interview process offers numerous advantages. It is, for example, a tremendous way to gain child-specific, individualized information across countless areas of inquiry. Although often structured in format, it is not standardized, nor is the purpose of the interview to provide a normative comparison to other students. During a thorough and thoughtful interview, school-based practitioners have the opportunity to gain unique insight into the life and abilities of a student. This opportunity to step into students' experiential worlds is of great benefit when working with individuals who are culturally and linguistically diverse. The frame of reference that is provided enables practitioners to more clearly understand the challenges students face on a daily basis, the support that they are provided, and often the startling resiliency they have developed in adapting to the demands of their unique situation. No other method utilized during the evaluation process allows direct access to such valuable information. Additional advantages of the interview process include:

---

This chapter is by Robert L. Rhodes.

- Firsthand knowledge of the student's developmental, experiential, and academic history from a variety of sources across a variety of settings.
- Unique insight into the familial, cultural, and educational perspectives of the referral concern; the student, parent, and teacher interview allows for an analysis of the referral concern from the individual perspective of the various participants.
- Information regarding previous educational or community-based interventions that have been attempted in addressing the referral concern and the perceived success of these attempts.
- A description of the student's interactions with peers, teachers, and family members and the impact of the referral concern on the student's day-to-day activities.
- An early opportunity to provide parents with an overview of the entire assessment process and remind them of their legal rights during each phase of the process.

## LIMITATIONS OF THE INTERVIEW PROCESS

In spite of the very real advantages of the interview process, it is not without certain limitations that require careful consideration. The interview process alone, for example, is insufficient for eligibility determination purposes. Information gathered during the interview process must be balanced with other data, including formal and informal assessment results and observations across settings. Two common limitations of the interview process are:

- *The subjective nature of the process.* The personal account provided during an interview is, by definition, a subjective and singular perspective. Although on one hand it is precisely such a perspective that is sought during the process, the information provided must be balanced by other accounts and information.
- *Exaggeration or withholding of information on the part of the parent or teacher because of misunderstanding the purpose of the interview.* The parent or teacher may choose to overemphasize the student's concerns for fear that he or she will not receive much needed assistance otherwise. There are also times that a parent or teacher unintentionally leaves out critical information because it was not thought to be relevant or because he or she was not specifically questioned about the topic or concern.

As school psychologists, we are routinely reminded of the unique perceptions and concerns that may arise during an interview. One incident, in particular, characterizes the dilemmas many parents face during the interview process, often unbeknownst to the interviewer. Several years ago, one of us (R.L.R.) learned a valuable lesson on the dangers of making assumptions during the interview process. During an interview with the parent of a fourth-grade student who had recently moved to the United States from Mexico, the mother described normal academic progress during her child's schooling in Mexico and expressed surprise that he appeared to be struggling in a Spanish-language classroom. Following extensive evaluation procedures and various interventions in the classroom, the mother of the student stopped by to further discuss her child's concerns. During the course of this conversation, she revealed that her child had, in fact, been retained in the first grade three times while attending school in Mexico. She understandably stated that she was fearful that he would, once again, be placed in first grade upon school enrollment in the United States and would continue to fall further and further behind academically. Once informed of her legal rights and her child's educational rights, she expressed great relief and was actively involved in the remainder of the assessment process (for a thorough discussion of school psychology and special education services in Mexico, see Rhodes, 2000).

The purpose of this chapter is to provide practical guidelines for addressing frequently asked questions regarding the interview process with students who are culturally and linguistically diverse. Although there are many factors to consider when conducting an interview, several key areas require specific discussion. Guidelines and helpful tips are provided for the following topics:

- Preparing for the interview
- Issues to consider before conducting the interview
- Selecting an interview format
- Determining the relevancy of questions
- Asking difficult questions
- Determining who should be involved in the interview
- What to do if the parent isn't available for a face-to-face interview
- Limitations of conducting the interview by telephone
- Necessary conditions for a successful interview
- Consideration of cultural factors
- What to do after the interview

A topical listing of potential questions for parents, students, and teachers and a recommended flowchart for the interview process are also provided.


## PRACTICAL GUIDELINES AND FREQUENTLY ASKED QUESTIONS

The following section answers frequently asked questions regarding interviews with parents and students who are culturally and linguistically diverse. Practical guidelines are provided in response to each question.


### What Should Be Done to Prepare for the Interview?

Several preparatory steps are recommended prior to conducting an interview with a student, parent, or teacher. Although it is tempting to interview a parent following a chance meeting in the hallway or school office, a poorly planned interview typically generates disappointing results. Form 7.1 at the end of the chapter presents a preinterview checklist of 10 steps to consider in preparation for an interview.


### What Issues Should Be Considered before Conducting the Interview?

It is important to examine the presuppositions or beliefs that school-based practitioners may hold prior to the interview about the role, interest, and involvement of the parent in the interview process, specifically, and the assessment process, generally. Unless *proven* otherwise, it is recommended that practitioners begin the process with the belief that:

- *The parent is equally or more concerned than the practitioner about the problem or difficulty his or her child is facing.* If the parent does not appear to be as concerned as expected, it is recommended that the impact of culture specific beliefs regarding disability (see Rhodes & Páez, 2000) be examined, or the possibility that the parent has not been sufficiently informed of the various aspects of the concern.

- *The parent desires to be involved in each step of the assessment process.* The number of parents and children immigrating from other countries (see Chapter 1) and the number of parents with limited or different educational experiences may necessitate additional procedures to familiarize parents with the various steps in the assessment process. Additional factors such as transportation and child care may also need to be addressed.

- *The parent has information that is critical for an accurate assessment of his or her child.* The language(s) spoken by a parent should never be allowed to interfere with his or her participation in the interview process. School-based practitioners have both a legal and ethical responsibility to safeguard a parent's opportunity for full participation.

- *The parent has already worked to address the areas of concern or difficulty at home or through other resources.* Practitioners should ask what has and has not worked and what the parent would recommend in regard to school-based interventions. Without inquiry, many parents may not volunteer their experiences and insight. Among some members of the Hispanic culture, for example, teachers and other school personnel are held in such high esteem that the parent may hesitate to offer any information that appears to place the parent in a more knowledgeable or superior role.

## Should a Specific Format Be Used for the Interview?

In order to gain as much information as possible during the interview process, it is recommended that school-based practitioners establish a structured format for use with parents, teachers, and other individuals that have unique knowledge of the student. It is important to note that there is no specific format required for student, parent, and teacher interviews. Generally, any approach that allows the practitioner to address the referral concern and the multiplicity of related areas is acceptable. However, practitioners should not be so tied to a single format that it limits the natural flow of conversation and the sometimes circuitous route that is followed as parents and others discuss complex and sensitive issues.

A structured format, in addition to serving as a tool for addressing difficult topics (see "Asking Difficult Questions" later in this chapter), allows practitioners to follow a logical sequence during the interview, enables individuals providing interpretation services to preview the interview format and anticipate upcoming questions, and ensures that important topics and areas of inquiry are not overlooked.

A structured interview format also enables a translated version to be presented to parents in their native language in order for them to follow throughout the process. Without a structured format, it is very easy to spend an extended period of time discussing an important topic and forget to ask key questions on a separate and equally important topic. For school-based practitioners who have little experience working with students and parents who are culturally and linguistically diverse, it also provides a template for questions that may not be part of their usual repertoire and may be omitted otherwise.

Forms 7.2 (a and b), 7.3 (a and b), and 7.4 at the end of the chapter present a list of questions for parents, students, and teachers that could be included in a structured format.

## How Is the Relevancy of Questions Determined?

The scope of questioning in parent, student, and teacher interviews is typically quite broad. Numerous events and experiences in a student's life have the potential to impact his or her academic and behavioral performance. This may be particularly true for students who have learned English as a second language or who have attended school outside of the United States. There are so many possible events and experiences of importance, in fact, that it is sometimes difficult to know which questions are relevant to the situation. The following are general guidelines to consider regarding the appropriateness of potential questions:

- *Is the question related to the referral concern?* The information that is sought through a line of inquiry should be related to the referral concern and should be intended to either confirm existing information or provide new and relevant knowledge.
- *Will the question assist in the identification of a disability or area of needed intervention?* Questions that are intended to assist in eligibility determination, rule out other possible areas of disability, or identify additional areas of needed intervention are appropriate and should be incorporated into the interview.
- *Is the question related to a possible exclusionary factor?* It is critical that we establish a thorough understanding of the student's developmental and experiential history in relation to possible exclusionary factors. Questions related to this area should address all possible exclusionary factors (see Chapter 3).

If the answer is "yes" to any of the above questions, then the line of inquiry is most likely relevant and appropriate for inclusion. If specific or intrusive questions are not purposeful and do not address these questions, they should not be asked.

## How Are Difficult Questions Asked?

There are times when a question or line of inquiry is both relevant and appropriate yet difficult to ask. It is often helpful to begin the interview process by informing participants that a variety of questions will be asked and that each one is intended to give the practitioner a better understanding of the child and his or her experiences in order to better assist the child at school. It should also be stated that the participant has the right to not answer any question he or she deems inappropriate or would prefer not to answer. It is the responsibility of the school-based practitioner to exercise wisdom and good judgment in selecting suitable questions. It is often helpful to have participants follow along with a structured interview format. Presenting the questions in this fashion seems to ease the awkward introduction of sensitive subjects and minimize the likelihood that the participant will feel that the question is targeted toward him or her because of family-specific concerns or allegations.

## Who Should Be Involved in the Interview?

It is important that family members or other individuals with the best knowledge of the student in relation to the referral concern be invited to participate in the interview process. The person possessing the most complete and accurate knowledge of the student is typically, but not always, the parent. A grandparent, aunt, uncle, foster parent, or other individual may be a key participant, depending on the situation. In some families, for example, a grandparent may provide after-school care for the student while the parent works. In other families, an aunt or uncle may be the educational guardian for a child while the parent is working or living elsewhere. These and other situations should be taken into consideration when scheduling the interview in order to obtain an accurate picture of the child's developmental history, academic experiences, and day-to-day activities. School-based practitioners working with students who are culturally and linguistically diverse should be mindful of the following situations:

- Even if the parent of a student is predominantly English-speaking, the student's grandparents or other family members may require the assistance of an interpreter. It is important to provide this service for a grandparent or other extended family member rather than having the parent interpret for them (see Chapter 6).

- Interview participants may need the emotional support of a friend or family member during the interview process. Participants should be informed of the nature and purpose of the interview and should be encouraged to have anyone they desire present throughout the process. It is not the prerogative of the interviewer to determine the relevancy of the person chosen by the parent to accompany him or her during the interview. In some families and cultures, for example, it may be appropriate or expected that the matriarch or patriarch of the family be present during the interview. In other situations, it may be important for the child's father to be present in order to cultivate his involvement, interest, and approval of the evaluation process. Although less common, it is also possible that the parent may desire that a family advocate, spiritual leader, or community representative be involved in the interview process. Likewise, the parent may choose to have an acquaintance present who is knowledgeable about the special education process, such as a friend who has children receiving special education services. Overall, practitioners should work with the parent to identify the most appropriate persons to involve in the interview process, according to familial and cultural expectations and needs. It is important to remember that the more comfortable the parent or person participating in the interview process is, the more accurate the information provided.

## What If the Parent Is Not Available for a Face-to-Face Interview?

At times, the parent may not be able to be physically present for an interview because of employment or personal circumstances. Parents who work as migrant or seasonal laborers, for example, may have made the decision to have their child stay with a family member during the school year to avoid the educational disruption that is a characteristic of this type of employment. The family member charged with caring for the child may be generally unfamiliar with the child's previous developmental and educational history. In such situations it is recommended that the educational guardianship of the child be determined prior to discussing confidential aspects of the evaluation process with the family member caring for the child. If the family member in question has educational guardianship but limited long-term experience with the child, it is recommended that the guardian be interviewed in reference to current functioning, but that every effort be made to interview the parent—even if by phone or through the assistance of an interpreter by phone. Direct contact with the parent or relevant person is necessary in order to gain an accurate historical perspective and confirm information provided by the caregiver/educational guardian.

## What about Conducting the Interview by Telephone?

Although cited as an example in the preceding section, conducting an interview by telephone is a method that should only be used in extreme circumstances. The impersonal nature of a telephone interview is antithetical to the conditions necessary to establish a successful interview. A telephone interview invariably creates emotional distance between the two parties and severely limits the secondary benefits of the interview process (e.g., rapport building, personal contact). Likewise, under such circumstances the practitioner is unable to monitor facial expressions or physical reactions and is not cognizant of other persons who may be party to the conversation and potentially limiting the participant's response. A telephone interview also minimizes the opportunity for full parent participation and potentially places parents in the limited role of information provider rather than as a full partner in the assessment process.

## What Conditions Are Necessary for a Successful Interview?

A successful interview is dependent upon numerous circumstances and conditions. Some variables are within the control of the interviewer and some are not. Conditions that are within the control of the interviewer include:

- The selection of a comfortable location for the parent or participant. Whenever possible, the parent should be given a choice regarding whether to meet at home or school for the interview. For parents unfamiliar with the educational system in the United States, meeting at home may provide a more comfortable venue for the personal nature of the interview process. If conducting the interview at the home of a parent (a practice especially common for early childhood practitioners), it is always recommended that school-based practitioners go with a partner, never alone. It is also important that the safety of each individual situation be carefully evaluated and that plans are made accordingly.
- Parents' understanding of their legal rights and the decisive factor those rights play in the entire evaluation process.
- Parental understanding of the purpose of the interview process and the specific ways in which the information provided during the interview will, and will not, be used. This is an extremely important aspect of the interview process and will severely curtail the flow of information unless addressed.
- Sufficient time on the part of both parties to comfortably participate in the interview and not feel rushed or limited by other appointments or activities.

- An environment free from distractions, to the greatest extent possible. Child care or other forms of assistance should be considered if the interview is conducted somewhere other than the parent's home.
- Practitioner understanding of prereferral activities, the referral concern, and existing records and documentation.
- Information regarding cultural priorities and protocol obtained prior to scheduling the interview.
- The need for an interpreter determined and confirmation of his or her availability secured.
- Permission obtained from the parent to contact him or her following the interview to clarify any points of confusion or to ask any questions that were overlooked during the initial interview.
- Any other relevant sources of information that are referenced during the interview process (e.g., previous teacher, community-based therapist or counselor) should be contacted. When appropriate, a release of information should be requested from the parent or guardian at the conclusion of the interview for this purpose.

## What Steps Should Be Followed during the Interview Process?

It is sometimes difficult to know where to begin or what steps to take during the interview process. Figure 7.1 provides a flowchart of recommended steps to follow during the interview process.

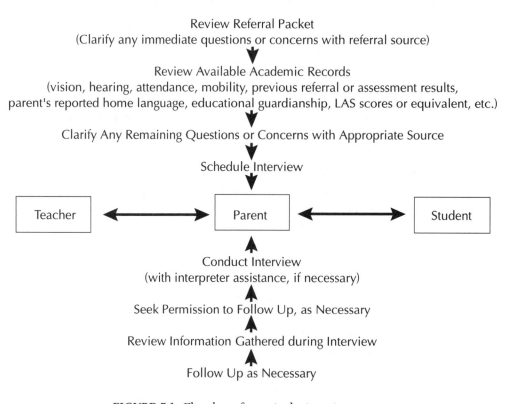

FIGURE 7.1. Flowchart of steps in the interview process.

## What Should Be Done after the Interview?

The steps taken after the interview is over are perhaps as important as those taken prior to the interview. At the conclusion of the interview, it is recommended that practitioners:

- Return to the referral source to clarify any new or contradictory information.
- Review the information gathered during the interview and cross-check for any topical areas that were not addressed.
- Follow up with any newly introduced sources of information, being certain to obtain signed permission on a release-of-information form, when appropriate.
- Acquire information regarding any cultural issues or other considerations that arise during the interview process.

# DANGER OF ASSUMPTIONS

The following example provides a final thought on the danger of making assumptions. Early in our careers, one of us (R.L.R.) was interviewing the parent of a preschool-age child who had been referred for evaluation because of significant difficulties interacting with peers and teachers and developing a relationship or rapport with others. During the interview, which was conducted in a structured format, the biological mother described her labor and delivery experience with the child in great detail. The next question in the structured format asked if the child was adopted and was quickly skipped over in order to move on to other "more relevant" questions. The mother was also following along with a copy of the interview format and noted that the question related to adoption had been skipped. She was confidently informed that she was correct, it had been skipped, and she, in turn, confidently stated that her child had been adopted. Based on superficial knowledge, this did not make sense. From a review of records and previous conversations, it was understood that the child had lived with her continuously and that she was indeed the biological mother. In a notably less confident manner, she was asked to provide more information about the situation. She stated that she had been living in a distant state and that her baby had been immediately placed with a planned adoptive family at birth. She added that by state law she had up to 6 months to rescind the adoption and that she did so during the sixth and final month. This information was previously unknown, provided potentially relevant insight into the bonding and attachment experiences of the child, and would never have been discovered if "logical" assumption had not been interrupted by a parent carefully following the structured interview format.

# SUMMARY

The information provided in this chapter establishes practical guidelines for addressing frequently asked questions regarding interviews for students who are culturally and linguistically diverse. The steps and strategies recommended are designed to enhance preinterview preparation, interview procedures, and postinterview follow-up, while, at the same time, minimizing extraneous factors that might curtail the flow of information. Approached with an open mind, cultural awareness, and careful preparation, parent, student, and teacher interviews can be a key component of the overall assessment process.

## FORM 7.1. Preinterview Checklist

1. Determine exact referral concerns through careful review of the referral packet.

2. Clarify any immediate questions or concerns with referral source.

3. Organize existing paperwork and review available records, including vision and hearing screening, attendance record, mobility, previous referral history, previous assessment results, previous special education placement, language assessment scores, and reported home language.

4. Determine educational guardianship, if unclear, from referral packet and record review.

5. Document necessary information that is unclear, contradictory, or missing from records.

6. Contact the parent or guardian to discuss the purpose of the interview, preferred location, and possible times.

7. If not previously determined, evaluate the need for interpretation assistance during the initial conversation with the parent or guardian.

8. Schedule a convenient time for all parties (including interpreter, if necessary) to participate in the interview.

9. Provide courtesy reminder for parent or guardian and interpreter prior to meeting.

10. Examine any presuppositions or beliefs that you may hold as the examiner prior to the interview (see section in this chapter titled "What Issues Should Be Considered Before Conducting the Interview?").

FORM 7.2a. Questions for Parents during the Interview Process

**Birth History**

1. How was your pregnancy with _____?
2. Were you able to have prenatal care and checkups with a physician throughout your pregnancy?
3. Was the pregnancy full term?
4. Were there any complications during labor or delivery?
5. Did the delivery take place at home or in a hospital?
6. Were there any complications after _____ was born?
7. How much did s/he weigh at birth?
8. How long did you and s/he have to stay in the hospital?
9. Were any follow-up visits to the hospital or doctor's office recommended? If so, were you able to attend these follow-up visits?
10. Where was _____ born (country/city)?

**Family History**

11. Who is in _____'s family?
12. Who does s/he live with at home?
13. Does s/he have any brothers or sisters? What are their names and ages?
14. How does s/he get along with family members?
15. Have there been any changes in the number of family members who live at home with her/him? What was the reason for this change?
16. Does s/he have a stepparent or other person with whom s/he also spends time?
17. Has s/he ever lived away from you? If yes, for what period of time?
18. Has anyone in her/his family had any similar difficulties?
19. What was your (parent's) school experience like?
20. What do _____'s family members think about her/his difficulties?

**Developmental History**

21. How old was _____ when s/he first began to crawl?
22. How old was s/he when s/he first began to walk?
23. How old was s/he when s/he first began to talk?
24. When did s/he first speak in complete sentences?
25. How did s/he develop in comparison to his/her brother(s) or sister(s)?
26. Did anything about _____'s development surprise you?
27. Does s/he usually do things quickly or slowly?
28. Would s/he rather watch or participate in activities?
29. Would you say _____ has matured more physically, emotionally, or intellectually over the past few years?
30. What concerns did you have as s/he was growing up?

*(continued)*

**Language History**

31. What language(s) did your child first speak?

32. What language(s) does s/he prefer to speak now?

33. What language(s) do parents, grandparents, siblings, other family members, family friends, and their friends speak at home?

34. What language(s) do you usually use at home when you speak to _____?

35. Is s/he able to hold a conversation in your home language?

36. Does _____ speak to persons outside of the family in your home language?

37. Does s/he ever help interpret for other family members?

38. In what language is s/he usually disciplined?

39. In what language does s/he speak to you when s/he is hurt or upset?

40. In what language does s/he speak to her/his brother(s) or sister(s)?

**Health History**

41. What illnesses or injuries has _____ experienced?

42. Has s/he ever experienced a head injury, lost consciousness, or been "knocked out"?

43. Has s/he had high fevers? How frequently?

44. Has s/he had ear infections? How frequently?

45. Is s/he currently taking any medication?

46. What kind of medication has s/he needed in the past?

47. Has s/he had her/his hearing and vision checked recently?

48. Does s/he need glasses? Does s/he wear glasses?

49. Does s/he see a dentist?

50. What other health problems or concerns does s/he have?

51. Is there anything you would like to find out about from a doctor, but have not been able to ask yet?

**Behavioral History**

52. How would you describe _____'s behavior as an infant, toddler, young child, and now?

53. How has her/his behavior changed over time?

54. Have you been concerned about these changes in behavior?

55. How does _____ respond to household rules?

56. Is s/he able to follow instructions?

57. What responsibilities does s/he have at home?

58. What seems to motivate her/him?

59. What does s/he complain about most often?

60. What does s/he prefer to do in her/his free time?

61. Would you describe her/him as active or relaxed? How else would you describe her/him?

62. How well does s/he sleep at night?

*(continued)*

114

**Acculturational Status**

63. What are _____'s favorite television shows and movies?

64. In what language?

65. What kind of music does s/he enjoy listening to?

66. In what language?

67. Where has s/he child lived?

68. What holidays do you celebrate as a family?

**Educational History**

69. Did _____ go to preschool or Head Start? Where?

70. When did s/he first learn the alphabet?

71. Did s/he enjoy being read to?

72. When did s/he first learn to read?

73. Did s/he go to kindergarten? Where?

74. What schools has s/he attended?

75. Has her/his attendance been regular or irregular?

76. In what countries has s/he attended school?

77. In what language(s) has s/he been instructed?

78. Has s/he repeated any grades? If so, why?

79. Has s/he needed extra help with her/his schoolwork?

80. Has s/he received special education services before? If yes, for what reason? If no, has s/he previously been referred for testing?

81. What does s/he seem to enjoy most about school?

82. What is the most frustrating thing about school for her/him?

**Concerns and Aspirations**

83. What is _____ best at?

84. What does s/he struggle with the most?

85. What are you most proud of about her/him?

86. What concerns you the most?

87. What are your hopes and dreams for her/him?

88. What do you think needs to be done at school to help her/him?

89. What else do you think could help?

90. Is there anything that was not asked about that you think is important to know about her/him?

FORM 7.2b. Preguntas Realizadas a los Padres de Familia en el Proceso de una Entrevista

### Historial de Nacimiento

1. ¿Cómo fue su parto con _____?
2. ¿Pudo obtener cuidados prenatales y chequeos con un doctor durante su embarazo?
3. ¿Fue de término completo su embarazo?
4. ¿Hubo alguna complicación durante la labor de parto o nacimiento?
5. ¿El nacimiento tomó lugar en su casa o en el hospital?
6. ¿Hubo alguna complicación después de _____ nació?
7. ¿Cuánto pesó el/ella cuando el/ella nació?
8. (Si la respuesta a la pregunta cinco fue un hospital) ¿Cuánto tanto tiempo estuvo usted y el/ella en el hospital?
9. ¿Fueron recomendadas visitas consiguientes al hospital o al consultorio del doctor? Si es así, ¿Pudo asistir a estas visitas consiguientes?
10. ¿Donde nació _____ (país/ciudad)?

### Historial Familiar

11. ¿Quiénes forman parte en la familia de su hijo(a)?
12. ¿Con quién vive el/ella en casa?
13. ¿Tiene el/ella hermanos o hermanas? ¿Cuáles son sus nombres y edades?
14. ¿Cómo se lleva el/ella con los demás miembros de la familia?
15. ¿Ha habido cambios de miembros de familia que viven en casa con el/ella? ¿Cuál fue la razón de ese cambio?
16. ¿Tiene el/ella un padrastro/madrastra o alguna otra persona con quien también pasen tiempo?
17. ¿Ha vivido el/ella lejos de usted? Si es así, ¿Cuál fue el periodo de tiempo?
18. ¿Ha tenido alguien dificultades similares en la familia de el/ella?
19. ¿Cómo fue su experiencia escolar?
20. ¿Qué piensan los miembros de la familia de _____ acerca de sus dificultades?

### Historical del Desarrollo

21. ¿Qué edad tenía _____ cuando el/ella empezó a gatear?
22. ¿Qué edad tenía el/ella cuando el/ella empezó a caminar?
23. ¿Qué edad tenía el/ella cuando el/ella empezó a hablar?
24. ¿Cuándo empezó a hablar el/ella en oraciones completas?
25. ¿Cómo se desarrollo el/ella en comparación con su(s) hermano(s) o hermana(s)?
26. ¿Le sorprendió algo acerca de su desarrollo?
27. ¿Usualmente el/ella hace las cosas rápidamente o lentamente?
28. ¿Prefiere el/ella observar o participar en las actividades?

*(continued)*

29. ¿Diría usted que ha madurado más físicamente, emocionalmente, o intelectualmente durante estos últimos años?

30. ¿Qué preocupaciones tuvo usted conforme el/ella estaba creciendo?

## Historial de Idioma

31. ¿Qué idioma(s) habló su hijo(a) primero?

32. ¿Qué idioma(s) prefiere el/ella hablar ahora?

33. ¿Qué idioma(s) son hablados en casa por los padres de familia, abuelos, hermanos, otros miembros de la familia, amigos de la familia y sus amigos?

34. ¿Qué idioma(s) habla usted usualmente en casa cuando se dirige a _____?

35. ¿Es el/ella capaz de sostener una conversación en el idioma que se habla en casa?

36. ¿Hablan ellos a personas fuera de su familia en el idioma que se habla en casa?

37. ¿Alguna vez ha ayudado a traducir a otros miembros de la familia?

38. ¿En qué idioma se le disciplina usualmente?

39. ¿En qué idioma le hablan a usted cuando ellos están lastimados o enojados?

40. ¿En qué idioma le(s) habla a su(s) hermano(s) o hermana(s)?

## Historial de Salud

41. ¿Qué enfermedades o lesiones a padecido _____?

42. ¿Ha tenido el/ella una lesión en la cabeza, ha perdido el conocimiento, o se ha quedado "sin sentido"?

43. ¿Ha tenido el/ella fiebres elevadas? ¿Con qué frecuencia?

44. ¿Ha tenido el/ella infecciones en el oído? ¿Con qué frecuencia?

45. ¿Actualmente están tomando algún medicamento?

46. ¿Qué tipo de medicamento ha necesitado en el pasado?

47. ¿Le han revisado su vista y su audición recientemente?

48. ¿Necesitan lentes? ¿Se ponen los lentes?

49. ¿Tienen la posibilidad de ver a un dentista?

50. ¿Qué otros problemas o dificultades de salud tienes el/ella?

51. ¿Hay alguna cosa que quisiera saber de un doctor pero que aún no haya tenido oportunidad de preguntar?

## Historial de Comportamiento

52. ¿Cómo describiría usted comportamiento de _____ como infante, niño(a) pequeño(a), joven y ahora?

53. ¿Ha cambiado el/ella comportamiento a través del tiempo?

54. ¿Le han preocupado estos cambios en su comportamiento?

55. ¿Cómo reaccionan a las reglas de la casa?

56. ¿Son capaces de seguir instrucciones?

57. ¿Qué responsabilidades tienen en la casa?

58. ¿Qué parece motivarlo a el/ella?

*(continued)*

59. ¿De qué el/ella quejan más a menudo?
60. ¿Qué prefieren hacer en su tiempo libre?
61. ¿Los describiría usted como activos o relajados? ¿De qué otra manera los describiría?
62. ¿Qué tan bien duerme el/ella en la noche?

### Estatus Aculturativo
63. ¿Cuáles son películas y programas de televisión favoritos de _____?
64. ¿En qué idioma son?
65. ¿Qué tipo de música le gusta escuchar a el/ella?
66. ¿En qué idioma es?
67. ¿Dónde ha vivido el/ella?
68. ¿Qué días festivos celebran como familia?

### Historial Educativo
69. ¿Tuvo educación preescolar o asistió a Head Start? ¿Dónde?
70. ¿Cuándo aprendió el alfabeto por primera vez?
71. ¿Disfrutaban cuando el/ella les leía?
72. ¿Cuándo aprendieron a leer por primera vez?
73. ¿Asistieron al kindergarten (kinder)? ¿Dónde?
74. ¿A qué escuelas han asistido?
75. ¿Asisten escuela regular o irregular?
76. ¿En qué países han asistido a la escuela?
77. ¿En que idioma(s) ha sido el/ella instrucción?
78. ¿Han reprobado algún año? Si es así, ¿Por qué?
79. ¿Han necesitado ayuda extra con el/ella trabajo escolar?
80. ¿Han recibido servicios de educación especial en el pasado? Si es así, ¿Por qué razón? Si no es así, ¿han sido referidos previamente para ser evaluados?
81. ¿Qué parecen disfrutar más de la escuela?
82. ¿Qué es lo más frustrante de la escuela para el/ella?

### Preocupaciones y Aspiraciones
83. ¿Qué es lo que mejor hace _____?
84. ¿Con qué batalla más el/ella?
85. ¿Qué le enorgullece más de el/ella?
86. ¿Qué es lo que más le preocupa?
87. ¿Cuáles son sus anhelos y esperanzas para el/ella?
88. ¿Qué cree usted que se necesite hacer en la escuela para ayudarlo(a) a el/ella?
89. ¿De qué otra manera cree usted que se le pueda ayudar?
90. ¿Hay algo que no le fue preguntado que crea usted que sea importante saber acerca de el/ella?

## FORM 7.3a. Questions for Students during the Interview Process

Many questions typically asked of parents can also be asked of students, depending upon their age. In addition, it is also recommended that the following questions be considered.

### Language Use

1. What languages do you speak?
2. What language are you most comfortable speaking?
3. What language do you prefer to read in?
4. What language do you prefer to write in?
5. When you think to yourself, what language do you usually use?

### Acculturational Status

6. What language(s) do your friends speak?
7. What are some of your favorite television shows?
8. What are some of your favorite movies?
9. What types of books do you like to read?
10. What language do you read best in?
11. What kind of music do you like to listen to?

### Education

12. What is your favorite subject in school?
13. What is your least favorite subject in school?
14. What language does your teacher usually speak?
15. Have you ever had a teacher who spoke to you in [insert student's native language]?
16. What kinds of difficulties do you have in school?
17. When did you first notice that you were having difficulties?
18. What kind of extra help have you been given in school?
19. What seems to have helped you the most?
20. What have you done to try to make your difficulties at school better?
21. Has this seemed to help?
22. What else do you think would help?
23. What could your teacher(s) do differently to help you?
24. Who else could help you?
25. What would you change about school?
26. What was your favorite grade in school? Why?

### Family/Home

27. What responsibilities do you have at home?
28. What do you usually do after school?

*(continued)*

29. What do you like to do in your free time?
30. What do you wish you had time to do?
31. How do you get along with your brothers and sisters?
32. How do you get along with your friends?
33. Do you have a best friend? Tell me about him or her.
34. Do you seem to have trouble keeping the same friends?
35. What do your parents think of your friends?
36. Do you have a job outside of school?

**Health**

37. How well do you sleep at night?
38. Do you ever have trouble seeing things clearly?
39. Do you ever have difficulty hearing things?
40. When was the last time you visited the doctor?
41. Are you worried that something might be wrong with you physically?

**Social–Emotional Functioning**

42. What types of things are you good at?
43. What things do you worry about the most?
44. How have you gotten along with your teachers?
45. What do you want to be when you grow up? (elementary)
46. What do you want to do when you finish school? (secondary)
47. What is something that would surprise people to know about you?
48. What was one of the best days of your life?
49. What was one of the worst days of your life?
50. What else is important to know about you?

## FORM 7.3b. Preguntas Realizadas a los Estudiantes en el Proceso de una Entrevista

Muchas de las preguntas que se les hacen típicamente a los padres de familia también se les pueden hacer a los estudiantes dependiendo de su edad. Además de esas preguntas, es también recomendable que las siguientes preguntas sean consideradas.

### Uso de Idioma

1. ¿Qué idiomas hablas?
2. ¿En qué idioma te sientes más cómodo cuando hablas?
3. ¿En qué idioma prefieres leer?
4. ¿En qué idioma prefieres escribir?
5. ¿Cuándo estas pensando que idioma usas usualmente?

### Estatus Aculturativo

6. ¿En qué idioma(s) hablan tus amigos(as)?
7. ¿Cuáles son algunos de tus programas de televisión favoritos?
8. ¿Cuáles son algunas de tus películas favoritas?
9. ¿Qué tipo de libros te gusta leer?
10. ¿En qué idioma lees mejor?
11. ¿Qué tipo de música te gusta escuchar?

### Educación

12. ¿Cuál es tu materia favorita en la escuela?
13. ¿Cuál es tu materia menos favorita en la escuela?
14. ¿En que idioma habla tu maestra(o) usualmente?
15. ¿Has tenido alguna vez a un maestro que te hable en [entre la idioma nativo de el/ella]?
16. ¿Qué dificultades tienes en la escuela?
17. ¿Cuándo fue que te diste cuenta por primera vez que estabas teniendo dificultades?
18. ¿Qué tipo de ayuda adicional se te ha dado en la escuela?
19. ¿Qué es lo que más parece haberte ayudado?
20. ¿Qué has hecho para tratar de mejorar tus dificultades en la escuela?
21. ¿Esto parece haber ayudado?
22. ¿De qué otra manera piensas que se te puede ayudar?
23. ¿Qué pueden hacer tus maestro(s) diferente para ayudarte?
24. ¿Quién más te puede ayudar?
25. ¿Qué más cambiarías de tu escuela?
26. ¿Cuál fue tu año favorito en la escuela? ¿Por qué?

### Familia/Hogar

27. ¿Qué responsabilidades tienes en casa?
28. ¿Qué haces usualmente después de la escuela?

*(continued)*

29. ¿Qué te gusta hacer en tu tiempo libre?
30. ¿Qué desearías que tuvieras tiempo de hacer?
31. ¿Cómo te llevas con tus hermanos y hermanas?
32. ¿Cómo te llevas con tus amigos(as)?
33. ¿Tienes un mejor amigo(a)? Platícame acerca de el o ella.
34. ¿Te parece como si tuvieras problemas para mantener los mismos amigos?
35. ¿Qué piensan tus papás de tus amigos?
36. ¿Tienes un trabajo fuera de la escuela?

**Salud**

37. ¿Qué tan bien duermes por las noches?
38. ¿Alguna vez has tenido problemas para ver algo claramente?
39. ¿Alguna vez has tenido dificultad para escuchar las cosas?
40. ¿Cuándo fue la última vez que visitaste al doctor?
41. ¿Estás preocupado de que algo esté mal contigo físicamente?

**Funcionamiento Social–Emocional**

42. ¿Para qué tipo de cosas eres bueno?
43. ¿Cuáles son las cosas que más te preocupan?
44. ¿Cómo te has llevado con tus maestros(as)?
45. ¿Qué quieres ser cuando crezcas? (primaria)
46. ¿Qué quieres hacer cuando termines tus estudios escolares? (secundaria)
47. ¿Qué es algo que le sorprendería a la gente saber de ti?
48. ¿Cuál fue uno de tus mejores días de tu vida?
49. ¿Cuál fue uno de tus peores días de tu vida?
50. ¿Qué más es importante saber de ti?

### FORM 7.4. Questions for Teachers during the Interview Process

**Educational History**

1. How long have you known _____?
2. How long has s/he been in your class?
3. What type of reading instruction has s/he received?
4. What type of math instruction has s/he received?
5. What grade level is s/he at across subjects?
6. What work samples are representative of her/his academic concerns?
7. What is her/his best subject?
8. What is the subject s/he struggle with the most?
9. What time of the day does s/he seem to do best?
10. What type of progress or decline have you seen in her/him?

**Intervention History**

11. What classroom-based interventions have been attempted? What were the results?
12. What school-based interventions have been attempted? What were the results?
13. What community-based interventions have been attempted? What were the results?
14. What was done to help _____ before s/he started in your classroom?
15. What other things have you tried in order to help her/him?
16. What seems to have helped the most?
17. What other accommodations have been made for her/him in the classroom?

**Language Use**

18. What languages does _____ speak?
19. What language(s) does s/he speak in the classroom?
20. What language(s) does s/he speak with her/his friends?
21. Is s/he able to communicate thoughts and needs with you?
22. How does s/he react if s/he is unable to communicate clearly?
23. What language(s) does s/he speak on the playground and during free time?
24. Do you feel the student's ability to speak English interferes with her/his academic progress?

**Social–Emotional Functioning**

25. What do you most enjoy about _____ as a student?
26. What seems to serve as a motivator for her/him?
27. What were her/his previous school experiences?
28. Has s/he been suspended, expelled, or experienced other disciplinary action?
29. Does s/he take any type of medication at school?
30. What else is important to know about her/him?

# 8

# Acculturational Factors
# in Psychoeducational Assessment

Of the many factors that influence the manner or process by which psychoeducational assessment is carried out, perhaps the two most important relate to language development and acculturation. Language, or more precisely, lack of English-language proficiency, is an obvious variable that naturally commands immediate attention within the scope of evaluation. After all, failure to communicate with the examinee effectively precludes valid assessment. The issues related to how language might impact the design or execution of a particular evaluation are relatively well known and form the focus of Chapter 10. The present chapter discusses issues relevant to acculturation—specifically, the process of becoming acculturated to the U.S. mainstream—and how they affect many of the decisions and procedures used in evaluation. Unlike language, acculturation is not a variable that is as readily or intuitively understood by school psychologists and other school personnel. Indeed, the exact nature of acculturative influences are often misunderstood and frequently ignored altogether. The purpose of this chapter is to provide school-based practitioners with a clear discussion regarding the potential mitigating and attenuating effects of acculturation on school and test performance as well as a systematic method for evaluating the relative influence of acculturation and its impact on drawing valid inferences and making accurate interpretations.

## THE EMERGENCE OF ACCULTURATIONAL FACTORS IN TESTING

Over the preceding several decades, an awareness regarding acculturational factors and their impact on the psychoeducational assessment of culturally and linguistically diverse individuals has grown steadily. Many point to both litigation and legislation as two of the main forces that drove acculturation into the limelight and brought it squarely to the attention of practitioners (Oakland, 1977; Oakland & Laosa, 1977; Reschly, 1981; Valdés & Figueroa, 1996). For example, in 1973 the settlement in *Diana v. State Board of Education* required that testing, particularly for the purposes of special education placement, must be conducted in the student's primary language

This chapter is by Samuel O. Ortiz.

124

and that culturally biased items had to be dropped from tests. This ruling gave formal recognition to the importance of the influence of English-language proficiency on testing as well as factors related to acculturation. The California Department of Education later reinforced this connection and made it abundantly clear in the following excerpt, drawn from the California Education Code, Part 30, Chapter 1, Article 2, Section 56324(a): "Any psychological assessment of pupils shall be made in accordance with Section 56320 and shall be conducted by a credentialed school psychologist who is trained and prepared to assess *cultural* and ethnic factors appropriate to the pupil being assessed" (emphasis added).

By the time Public Law 94-142 (the Education for All Handicapped Children Act) was passed in 1975, there was a clear recognition that testing had the potential of being discriminatory in relation to a number of factors, not just acculturation, and that such assessment needed to be modified to prevent misdiagnosis, misclassification, or other such negative consequences. The most recently authorized version of the original Public Law 94-142 (now known as the Individuals with Disabilities Education Improvement Act, or IDEIA), Section 300.532, states that "each public agency shall ensure, at a minimum, that—(a) Tests and other evaluation materials used to assess a child under Part B of the Act—(1) are selected and administered so as not to be discriminatory on a racial or *cultural* basis . . . " (emphasis added).

Although language and culture were clearly identified as important factors to consider in the course of evaluation, the fact that the term *culture* or *cultural* was used, and often interchanged with *ethnic* or *race*, has resulted in a poor understanding of this factor.

## CULTURE, BIAS, AND ACCULTURATION

### Misconceptions of Culture

There is an unfortunate tendency identified in both theory and practice to equate the term *culture* with a person's race or ethnic heritage (Flanagan & Ortiz, 2001). There is no question that those to whom the label "culturally different" is applied are frequently from different racial or ethnic backgrounds. But to assume that culture and race are equivalent is dangerous and often wrong. From the inception of ability and intelligence tests, there has been considerable attention given to establishing fairness by examining and eliminating psychometric forms of bias (Gould, 1996; Kamphaus, 1993). It is important to note that bias was defined primarily, if not exclusively, as a function of a systematic difference that might result in test performance between one group or another that is not due to measured ability but rather some defect in the test. Because the early developers of ability and intelligence tests possessed views consonant with the prevailing societal and scientific zeitgeist, systematic differences that were not identifiable within the structure of the test were not seen as evidence of bias but rather as support for preconceived ideas of reality—namely, that there was a racial hierarchy in ability and intelligence and that whites were at the top of the pyramid (Gould, 1996). Assumptions related primarily to construct validity went unquestioned except by a very insightful few.

Even in the midst of what must have been enormous pressures, a few researchers began to question whether or not factors such as language and culture might influence test performance with linguistically or culturally diverse groups more so than the accepted notions of genetically and racially based differences in intelligence and ability. With regard to testing, George Sanchez (1934), a Mexican American psychologist, expressed this sentiment eloquently: "As long as tests do not at least sample in equal degree a state of saturation [assimilation of fundamental experiences and activities] that is equal for the 'norm children' and the particular bilingual child it cannot be assumed that the test is a valid one for the child" (p. 770; text in brackets added for clarification).

In time, it became clear that all tests, particularly those purporting to measure intelligence or cognitive ability, were reflections of the culture of their creators. By the very definition of psychometric tests, their creation and invention in the United States and elsewhere *had* to be based on the culturally bound values and beliefs of their authors. In a landmark article on intelligence, Neisser and colleagues (1996) stressed that "it is obvious that the cultural environment—how people live, what they value, what they do—has a significant effect on the intellectual skills developed by individuals" (p. 86). What has often seemed to be a question of race or ethnicity is in reality an issue of culture. If the goal is to evaluate individuals from diverse cultures in a nondiscriminatory manner, then it must be understood that "intelligence cannot be tested independently of the culture that gives rise to the test" (Cole & Cole, 1993, p. 502). Indeed, Scarr (1978) asserts that "intelligence tests are not tests of intelligence in some abstract, culture-free way. They are measures of the ability to function intellectually by virtue of knowledge and skills in the culture of which they sample" (p. 339).

That culture is an important issue in evaluation has become accepted and acknowledged in the field of psychological assessment (Matsumoto, 1994). Yet it is not culture itself that is central to evaluation procedures but *differences* in culture. As noted previously, tests sample the culture from which they spring. Individuals who do not come from the culture of the test may be at a disadvantage in terms of performance. Thus, it is not so much that an individual is from a different culture that creates the problem, but that the individual lacks knowledge of the culture that underlies the test. In this sense culture is much like language in that it is not simply that an individual speaks another language that is a problem; rather, it is the individual's lack of English-language proficiency that presents the obstacle to valid measurement of ability, skill, or knowledge. Likewise, it is not simply that an individual is from another culture that is a problem but that the individual's lack of cultural knowledge presents an obstacle to valid measurement. This lack of cultural knowledge, or the process of acquiring it, is called *acculturation*. And it is to acculturation that we must look when we seek to test individuals whose own cultural backgrounds differ from that which is expected on tests that may be administered in the course of an evaluation.

## Cultural Bias in Testing

Decades of research on the psychometric bias of standardized tests has resulted in one largely undisputed conclusion: Well-designed, well-constructed, and appropriately normed tests show no bias (Sattler, 1992; Valdés & Figueroa, 1996). Examination of item content, sequence, structure, difficulty, factor solutions, and prediction have all failed to find any real evidence of bias, particularly any that might threaten reliability (Niesser et al., 1996; Sattler, 1992). Of course, little empirical attention has been given to the idea that perhaps it is not reliability that is at issue but validity. Is the test measuring what we believe it should be measuring? Despite the seemingly obvious answer when dealing with individuals who cannot speak the language of the test or who have not been raised in the culture from which the test samples, adherence to claims of validity regarding these tests persists.

In order for a test to measure validly what it was designed to measure, the individual being evaluated must meet certain assumptions—the same assumptions that underlie the test. Put simply, 5 year-olds are compared to 5-year-olds, 11th graders are compared to 11th graders, and so forth. That is, we recognize the developmental nature of cognitive and academic abilities, skills, and knowledge. Development is invariant in every sense, and what we call acculturation, or the process of acquiring culture, is as invariant as language development, cognitive development, and so forth. With regard to acculturation, as with other forms of development, it is the simple, basic foundations that are learned in the first stages (e.g., the more common elements of the culture). Intermediate and advanced stages of development follow, wherein the more complex elements of the culture are acquired in relatively predictable and measurable ways. According to Salvia and Ysseldyke (1991), recognition of the process of acculturation and its developmental nature, much like that of age, grade, or English-language proficiency, is as integral to test development as the "assumption of comparability." The assumption of comparability is described by these researchers in the following manner:

> When we test students using a standardized device and compare them to a set of norms to gain an index of their relative standing, we assume that the students we test are similar to those on whom the test was standardized; that is, we assume their acculturation is comparable, but not necessarily identical, to that of the students who made up the normative sample for the test. (Salvia & Ysseldyke, 1991, p. 18)

Two points are significant here: (1) that comparability of acculturation is crucial in determining whether a test is valid for an individual, and (2) that acculturation differences can be based on any experiential differences, not just those attributable to culture. What is most important is that a relatively equivalent level of acculturation exist between the examinee and the individual to whom the test is being given. Whenever this assumption is not met, the validity of obtained results is highly suspect. Individuals who are not being raised in the U.S. mainstream by parents who themselves are not fully acculturated into the mainstream will not, by definition, meet the assumption of comparability. Salvia and Ysseldyke (1991) provide further comment on this point: "When a child's general background experiences differ from those of the children on whom a test was standardized, then the use of the norms of that test as an index for evaluating that child's current performance or for predicting future performances may be inappropriate" (p. 18).

As such, bias in testing will occur whenever a test of intelligence, ability, or achievement that was developed and normed in the United States is given to an individual whose cultural background, experiences, or exposure is not comparable to the individuals who comprised the normative group against whom performance will be compared. In short, validity of results will always be suspect for any individual who is "culturally different" or "culturally diverse." Bias will occur not due to any defect in the test itself but because the test will measure a lower range of ability, skill, or knowledge in culturally different and culturally diverse individuals; in short, it will assess well the level of development currently attained. Acculturation, like all other forms of development, is invariant, and the test will sample only the degree of cultural content acquired by the individual to that point, irrespective of age or grade. However, because the individual's performance will be compared to others of the same age or grade, he or she will likely perform less well because he or she began the acculturation process at a point different (i.e., some time after birth) from that of the individuals in the normative group. Standardized tests measure quite well the degree to which an individual has become acculturated, much as they measure quite well the degree of English-language proficiency obtained by an individual. They are both developmental processes that remain invariant, regardless of the age at which they begin. Typically, these processes begin at birth, but in the case of individuals who are culturally different, they may begin much later.

The potential bias that operates in testing culturally diverse populations is therefore more a function of validity than reliability and should not be viewed as a deficit within the test itself but rather recognition that the test is culturally loaded—that it contains culturally specific elements and expects examinees to possess a given level of acculturation commensurate with a given age or grade. Defining bias in this manner—that it involves cultural *loading* versus cultural bias—is an inherently different definition than those that traditionally have been the focus of previous research. Culture is manifested in test performance through the process of acculturation and its developmental nature. Culture is not a unitary or monolithic variable that should somehow inter-act with the psychometric properties of a test and result in systematically disrupted performance. As noted by Flanagan and Ortiz (2001), "although there is considerable research evidence suggesting that many intelligence and cognitive ability tests are technically sound, appropriately normed, and are not culturally *biased*, they are, nevertheless, culturally *loaded*" (p. 220; emphasis in original).

## EVALUATION OF ACCULTURATION

For practitioners faced with the task of fairly and equitably evaluating the abilities of culturally and linguistically diverse individuals, knowledge of their level of acculturation becomes crucial. Without a clear picture of acculturational factors unique to each individual being evaluated, it is difficult, if not impossible, to arrive at accurate or defensible estimates of his or her true ability, skill, or knowledge. To the extent that an individual's acculturation differs from that of the main-stream, performance in the classroom or on standardized tests will likely be attenuated to the same proportion. Acculturation, as with language (discussed in the next chapter), forms the context within which all data and information must be evaluated.

As is evident throughout this book, and in keeping with guidelines for best practices (Ortiz, 2002), the collection of data in the course of any assessment should not be predicated upon a single test, method, or procedure. Evaluating an individual's level of acculturation is no different. It is likely that some form of scale or questionnaire may be the most efficient manner in which to approach the task, but such instruments are not the only, or necessarily even the preferred, method of evaluating acculturation. Interviewing and observation are also valuable procedures for ascertaining an accurate picture of acculturation.

The measurement of acculturation is a rather broad field within the domain of psychology (Chun, Organista, & Marín, 2003). There has long been an interest in acculturation as a factor in many aspects of psychological functioning, including learning and development (the two most central to this book). Likewise, acculturation has been a topic of study in and of itself (Berry, 2003). In the attempt to evaluate the cognitive and academic abilities of individuals from cultur-ally diverse backgrounds, there is perhaps a bit of both of these traditions involved in the process, because individuals can vary along a spectrum from absolutely not acculturated to fully or com-pletely acculturated and everything in between. This continuum is very similar to, and shares a great deal of variance with, dimensions of bilingualism and the process of acquiring English as a second language. Valdés and Figueroa (1996) outlined the nature and process of bilingualism as a function of generational differences. An adaptation of their outline is presented in Table 8.1, which shows a distinct progression through four familial generations.

The pattern of linguistic and bilingual evolution from the first to the fourth generation is parallel to that which would be expected for acculturation. For first-generation individuals—those not born in the United States—acculturation would be expected to be quite low, whereas for fourth-generation individuals, who have grandparents who were born in the United States, acculturation would be expected to be quite high, if not comparable to that of other individuals reared in the U.S. mainstream. In essence, many, if not most, fourth-generation individuals and beyond (barring other factors) could be considered highly or fully acculturated.

One of the more important considerations in evaluating acculturation is recognition of this process of change. Whether by intention or circumstance, the majority of individuals who are culturally different in the United States are essentially on a path toward ultimate assimilation. Whether movement toward assimilation is seen as desirable or undesirable, there are predictable and often negative outcomes associated with it. For example, second-generation individuals often find themselves caught between cultures that compete for their identification and loyalty—belonging in part to both but fully to neither. Second-generation children encounter this dilemma and are subject to its effects upon entering the United States public school system, and its relevance to understanding an individual's acculturation cannot be underestimated (Ortiz, 1999). Similarly, individuals who are third or even fourth generation may consider themselves, and appear to be quite, acculturated to the mainstream, but that does not mean they have lost significant parts of their identification with their cultural heritage (Marín & Gamba, 1996). As such, evaluation of acculturation is not captured merely by evaluating proximity to the mainstream or acquired mainstream knowledge but also by evaluating distance, if any, from the native culture and the extent to which that culture remains embedded in aspects of the individual's life.

## Evaluating Acculturation via Interview

Perhaps the most direct and simple method for evaluating an individual's level of acculturation is through the process of interview. In general, an interview that is designed to examine acculturation should be focused and directed. An open-ended style of interview is unlikely to lead quickly to relevant information and is not the most efficient manner for gathering the necessary data. Use of a semistructured interview is quite helpful in maintaining focus on the relevant questions and can be readily developed from a variety of sources, including the questions to be outlined later in this section. Sometimes the problem with an interview format for evaluating acculturation is not so much what questions need to be asked as it is *of whom* should the questions be asked. If the individual is an adult, it is a straightforward matter to conduct the interview. However, if the individual is a child or young adolescent, the matter is more complicated. In such cases, it may be most helpful to interview the individual's parents in addition to, or in cases of very young children, instead of, the individual.

In determining what should be asked, practitioners should remain aware of the nature of the information they wish to collect and its relevance to the evaluation. Basically, enough data should be collected to allow for a determination or judgment regarding level of acculturation—specifically, the distance between the individual's own acculturation and that of the mainstream (typically, the U.S. mainstream for evaluations conducted in the United States). When it can be

TABLE 8.1. Dimensions of Bilingualism and Relationship to Generations

| Type[a] | Stage | Language use |
|---|---|---|
| | | First generation—foreign born |
| A | Newly arrived | Understands little English; learns a few words and phrases. |
| Ab | After several years of residence—Type 1 | Understands enough English to take care of essential everyday needs; speaks enough English to make self understood. |
| Ab | Type 2 | Is able to function capably in the work domain where English is required. May still experience frustration in expressing self fully in English. Uses immigrant language in all other contexts where English is not needed. |
| | | Second generation—U.S. born |
| Ab | Preschool age | Acquires immigrant language first; may be spoken to in English by relatives or friends. Will normally be exposed to English-language TV. |
| Ab | School age | Acquires English and uses it increasingly to talk to peers and siblings. Views English-language TV extensively. May be literate only in English if schooled exclusively in this language. |
| AB | Adulthood—Type 1 | At work (in the community) uses language to suit proficiency of other speakers. Has greater functional ease in his or her first language in spite of frequent use of second. |
| AB | Adulthood—Type 2 | Uses English for most everyday activities; uses immigrant language to interact with parents or others who do not speak English. Is aware of vocabulary gaps in his first language. |
| | | Third generation—U.S. born |
| AB | Preschool age | Acquires both English and immigrant language simultaneously. Hears both in the home, although English tends to predominate. |
| aB | School age | Uses English almost exclusively; is aware of limitations in the immigrant language and uses it only when forced to do so by circumstances. Is literate only in English. |
| aB | Adulthood | Uses English almost exclusively; has few opportunities for speaking immigrant language. Retains good receptive competence in this language. |
| | | Fourth generation—U.S. born |
| Ba | Preschool age | Is spoken to only in English. May hear immigrant language spoken by grandparents and other relatives, but is not expected to understand immigrant language. |
| Ba | School age | Uses English exclusively. May have picked up some of the immigrant language from peers, but has limited receptive competence in this language. |
| B | Adulthood | Is almost totally English monolingual, though may retain some receptive competence in some domains. |

*Note.* Adapted from Valdés and Figueroa (1996, p. 16). Copyright 1996 by Ablex Publishing. Adapted by permission.
[a] "A" refers to the native language; "B" refers to the second language (e.g., English); uppercase letters indicate a higher level of proficiency than lowercase letters; bold letters indicate the dominant language (sometimes equal).

determined that an individual's level of acculturation is very close to the mainstream, then expectations regarding classroom or test performance need not vary much from that expected typically from others of the same age or grade. Conversely, when it is determined that an individual's level of acculturation is far from that of the mainstream, then expectations regarding performance must be adjusted accordingly in order to arrive at fair and equitable conclusions. Thus, the measurement of acculturation is fundamentally an effort to establish the degree to which the individual has, or has not, acquired the level of acculturation that might otherwise be expected for his or her age or grade. Questions that remain focused on this topic will prove most useful in the course of evaluation.

Because the questions that might be asked regarding acculturational levels could be of a sensitive and personal nature, it is important to remember to be forthright and clear about their intended purpose but to do so with the necessary cultural sensitivity (for more information regarding appropriate practices when working with culturally and linguistically diverse children and families, see Ortiz & Flanagan, 2002). An individual who is informed of the reasons why such information is necessary will be more likely to respond honestly and without suspicion or fear of judgment. Table 8.2 lists some of the types of questions that may be used with older adolescents or adults who possess the necessary level of insight to offer valid information. These questions are not exhaustive, and school-based practitioners should evaluate the appropriateness of any question that might be asked and ensure that the final collection of questions is unique and appropriate for the particular evaluation being conducted.

As can be seen, the questions revolve around aspects that reflect, to one degree or another, the individual's identification, participation, comfort, familiarity, knowledge, or affiliation with the customs, values, language, and beliefs of the mainstream culture. It is important, however, to recognize that simply because an individual may identify, or even prefer to be identified, with mainstream culture does not mean that he or she actually possesses full knowledge of the culture. This is one reason why evaluation of acculturation should not be based solely on an interview or any other single method or procedure.

Evaluation of acculturation in young or school-age children generally cannot be accomplished via direct interview. Not only might a particular child lack the necessary insight required to properly respond to certain questions, he or she may also lack the development needed to fully comprehend the questions. In such cases, it may be more advantageous to interview the child's parents to obtain the necessary information. The questions to be asked remain quite similar, if not identical in nature, to those asked of adults: however, the subject in question is the child, not the adult answering the question. In very young children, it may even be feasible to simply assess the parents' level of acculturation and use it as an estimate of the acculturation of the child, because the child's exposure to mainstream culture will be primarily a function of the parents' experience with it and thus relatively equal. As children enter the public school system, particularly if they were born in the United States, their experiences with, and acquisition of, mainstream culture and cultural knowledge will rapidly surpass that of their parents and should be carefully evaluated separately. But make no mistake: The experiences of children in the home are, in large measure, a function of the acculturation level of the parents, despite individual preferences or personal identification to the contrary. Just as language development is heavily predicated upon what an individual is taught in the home, so too is acculturation primarily a product of the environment created and managed by a child's parents.

**TABLE 8.2. Sample Interview Questions for Evaluation of Acculturation**

| Domain | Example questions |
|---|---|
| Language use or language preference | • What language do you use most frequently during your day?<br>• What language do you feel most comfortable using in social situations?<br>• In what language do you speak to your children most frequently? |
| Social affiliation | • Do you tend to seek out relationships with people who share your native culture?<br>• Are most of your friends people who have a similar background as you have?<br>• Does your child seek out friends with similar or different cultural backgrounds? |
| Daily living habits | • What kinds of food do you cook most often in your household?<br>• How are the responsibilities of maintaining the home managed and decided?<br>• What kind of chores or responsibilities does your child have at home? |
| Cultural traditions | • Do you currently observe any traditions from your native culture?<br>• Have you begun to engage in any new or different traditions here in the United States?<br>• Are you teaching your children any of the same traditions with which you grew up? |
| Communication style | • Do you feel you express yourself better in your native language or English?<br>• Do you feel your style of communication with others has changed?<br>• Has your children's manner of speaking with you changed in any way? |
| Cultural identity or cultural pride | • Is your cultural identity more in line with your native culture or the United States?<br>• Do you participate in any cultural activities that show your pride in your culture?<br>• Do you feel your child takes pride in his or her native culture and heritage? |
| Perceived prejudice or discrimination | • Have you ever felt put down or ridiculed because of your heritage or practices?<br>• Do you think people from your culture are discriminated against in any way?<br>• Has your child had any problems in school because he or she is culturally different? |
| Generational status | • Were you born in the United States, and if not, when did you come to the United States?<br>• Were your parents born in the United States, and if not, when did they come to the United States?<br>• Was your child born in the United States, and if not, at what age did he or she come to the United States? |
| Family socialization | • Does your family participate in any cultural traditions or celebrations with others?<br>• To what extent is your native culture or heritage a part of your daily family life?<br>• Are you teaching your children about their native culture and heritage? |
| Cultural values | • Are your personal beliefs and values still consistent with your cultural heritage?<br>• What are your current religious beliefs and practices?<br>• Does your child's behavior seem consistent with or different from your culture? |

## Evaluating Acculturation via Observation

Attempts to measure acculturation through observational methods can be difficult and are probably the least efficient procedures for such evaluation. Observation is a powerful tool because there is little evidence more convincing than that which can be seen in direct action. Whereas observation is an excellent data gathering method for such areas as language use or preference, specific learning problems, skill difficulties, and so forth, acculturation is more of a latent process that is not always directly observable.

Due to the inherent limitations concerning evaluation of a variable that is more latent than manifest, observation of acculturation revolves around patterns of preference, identification, participation, and affiliation with the practices, customs, values, and beliefs of the mainstream culture. For example, an individual may be observed to the extent that he or she interacts with members of the mainstream culture or society. Likewise, an individual can be observed for patterns of language usage that may indicate a preference for, as well as knowledge of, the mainstream language (i.e., English). Other observable areas include manner and style of dress; participation in, or celebration of, holidays; and overt expressions of cultural knowledge or familiarity. Again, these variables represent only a fraction of the types of cues that could be observed.

It is crucial that practitioners remember that identification with one culture does not mean lack of identification with the native culture. Although the intent of evaluation is to uncover an individual's relative distance from the mainstream, it should not be assumed that such distance reflects the inverse distance from the native culture. As such, observations that reveal what may appear to be high levels of acculturation may be misleading. For such reasons, multiple observations should be made across multiple settings. In adults, this may be quite difficult to do—which speaks to the inefficiency of this approach. In children, however, there is often ample opportunity to observe at school during classroom instruction, recess, and lunch as well as at home. As noted previously, the home environment is a particularly rich source of information regarding acculturation, and any opportunity to observe in that setting should be taken seriously.

As was discussed with regard to evaluating acculturation via interview, observations should be systematic and structured. Practitioners may wish to establish the parameters for the observation with a specific focus on what shall be observed and to what extent. The goal of observation is no different from that which guides other forms of data collection. The fundamental purpose is to assess the degree of cultural knowledge acquired by an individual and the extent to which that cultural knowledge represents the level ordinarily expected of individuals of the same age or grade. It is only in this manner that fair and equitable inferences regarding ability or functioning can be drawn.

## Evaluating Acculturation via Questionnaire

Without question, the most efficient and perhaps most popular method for assessing acculturation is through the use of questionnaires or scales developed expressly for this purpose. Chun and colleagues (2003) list no less than 22 different scales of acculturation. Not all of these scales, however, are suitable for use with all populations. Many of the scales are specific to Latino groups (Mexican Amercian, Puerto Rican, etc.), African Americans, Native Americans, and Asian American groups. Marín and Gamba (1996) cited 16 different acculturation scales prior to proposing their own (the

Bidimensional Acculturation Scale for Hispanics [BAS]). In her attempt to create a less discriminatory method for evaluating the intelligence of individuals with diverse cultural and linguistic backgrounds, Mercer (1979) included an acculturation scale in the System of Multicultural Pluralistic Assessment (SOMPA). So there is no paucity of acculturation scales from which to choose for the practitioner who is interested in this manner of evaluation.

## Selection

The first consideration in using a scale or questionnaire to evaluate acculturation relates to selecting one that is appropriate for use with the individual or target population in question. Despite the availability of scales for various cultural groups, there are potential problems that may arise. It was discussed previously that culture is not the same as race or ethnicity. An excellent example can be seen in Puerto Rican culture, where the racial composition of the people has a blended heritage that includes Western Europeans (from Spain and France), Africans (brought to the island via the slave trade), and native peoples (the Taino, who originally inhabited the island). To characterize Puerto Ricans in terms of race does not provide an accurate representation of what Puerto Rican culture involves. If a practitioner fails to recognize this issue, a scale designed for Mexican Americans may erroneously be used on individuals from Colombia, and invalid results would be obtained. Practitioners therefore should carefully evaluate the suitability of a particular scale for use with a particular individual to ensure that the culture of the scale matches the culture of the individual.

## Acculturational Domains

It has been noted that acculturation is far from a unitary or monolithic construct. Indeed, it is multifaceted and can be evaluated in a number of different ways and along a wide variety of dimensions. Chun and colleagues (2003) identified 10 distinct domains that are assessed by existing acculturation scales. These domains include language use/preference, social affiliation, daily living habits, cultural traditions, communication style, cultural identity/pride, perceived prejudice/discrimination, generational status, family socialization, and cultural values. No scale exists that measures every one of these domains, which means that practitioners will need to decide which domains are most relevant to the evaluation. In addition, many of these scales are unidimensional, in that they are based on the assumption that as acculturation progresses, individuals move from one end (full native culture) of the acculturational spectrum to the other end (full mainstream culture). This assumption carries with it the implication that acquisition of cultural knowledge or habits in one direction (usually toward the mainstream culture) is accompanied by concomitant decrements in the other direction (away from the native culture). The BAS (Marín & Gamba, 1996) was designed to address this shortcoming in the evaluation of acculturation for Hispanics.

## Psychometric Issues

In general, scales that have more items tend to be more reliable. When scales measure more than one construct, the reliability of each of the constructs being assessed is also a function of the number of items that comprise it. Practitioners should take note of this and other psychometric issues when selecting an appropriate scale. Consider, for example, that some scales have as little as one item for a particular dimension, whereas others have as many as 100. Simply because a scale has been published does not automatically imbue it with desirable psychometric characteristics. According to Marín and Gamba (1996):

> Other problems with current acculturation scales include the fact that authors have seldom measured various areas of acculturative change and, more important, few have utilized data-reduction techniques to psychometrically derive their acculturation scales. A common procedure has been the writing of items that a priori are assumed to measure a given acculturative dimension (e.g., language use, patterns of media use), and the score derived from these items is utilized as if the items actually formed a psychometric scale. In many of these cases, there is no information available on the internal consistency of the prior "scale," and validity indicators, other than possibly face validity, are often missing. (p. 298)

Practitioners need to pay careful attention to issues of reliability and validity in scale construction. Not only do such factors affect the degree of confidence in results, but they may also limit the generalizability of the scale in the first place.

## Interpretive Issues

The nature and meaning of scores obtained from the use of acculturational scales varies from one instrument to another. Thus, what is measured by one scale and what the score means cannot be presumed to be the same as that measured by another scale. Different scales measure different domains, and inferences about results should be limited to only those domains that were actually assessed. Beyond the measurement of a particular domain, practitioners should also be cognizant of how the results are meaningful within the context of the broader assessment. Other than for researchers, acculturation by itself is rarely the ultimate target of psychological evaluations. Acculturation represents a powerful explanatory variable in psychological functioning. Whenever that functioning is measured in individuals who come from diverse cultural backgrounds, knowledge of acculturation becomes crucial because it dictates the manner in which all data can or should be viewed. This knowledge is particularly important when standardized tests of ability are used in an evaluation: How level of acculturation is considered within that realm will be determined by the practitioner's level of knowledge. For the current discussion, level of acculturation influences the meaning of collected data by providing the appropriate frame of reference within which that data can be understood. Whether it be expectations of performance, behavior, learning, or development, acculturation plays a prominent role in our ability to understand the individual in whatever psychological domain may be of interest (Sandoval, Frisby, Geisinger, Scheuneman, & Grenier, 1998).

## SUMMARY

Of all the factors that affect an individual's behavior or performance on a given task, none is more likely to exceed those of culture. Virtually everything that an individual knows, does, feels, thinks, believes, or says can be traced to the interaction between the cultural roots of the home, the community, and the society in which the individual is raised. In order to understand the functioning of an individual on a measured task, we must first understand the influences which caused the individual to perform in the manner observed. When we fail to account for such culturally based behavior, we run the greatest risk of identifying simple differences as serious deficits.

This chapter provided school-based practitioners with a discussion of the manner in which acculturation affects the psychological functioning of individuals and the various methods that can be employed in evaluating it. The importance of acculturation as a significant mitigating variable in psychological functioning has been widely recognized for several decades. Too often, however, acculturation has been confused with culture, which in turn has been confounded with race, ethnicity, or other demographic variables. What *is* known about acculturation is that it is one of the most influential factors operating within the context of any evaluation. This influence exists for any individual whose background experiences are not comparable to that of the U.S. mainstream. Moreover, acculturation is not always directly observable or measured in the same way by various scales. Practitioners who seek to improve their practice by investigating effects of acculturation will need to contend with the tasks of making informed decisions regarding manner of evaluation, domains to be assessed, quality of scales (if used), and the derivation of defensible inferences and interpretations. Acculturation is undoubtedly a complex variable, but with concerted effort and rehearsal, it can be easily accommodated into current practice.

# 9

# Language Proficiency Assessment

## The Foundation for Psychoeducational Assessment of Second-Language Learners

There are several key developmental components of language and language proficiency that should be included and considered in any framework that seeks to fairly and equitably evaluate the abilities of second-language learners. These components include general recommended practices in the area of language proficiency assessment and the formal and informal methods of assessment that should be utilized. An additional component is the interpretation of language proficiency data. Moreover, a discussion of the various language profiles that may be exhibited by second-language learners is discussed.

## RECOMMENDED PRACTICES FOR ASSESSING LANGUAGE PROFICIENCY

Four general methodologies for assessing language proficiency have been recommended in the literature. Despite the fact that language assessment cuts across several disciplines, there is a good deal of consensus about these practices in the fields of school psychology, special education, and speech and language pathology.

### Assessing Language Proficiency in Both Languages

As a function of compliance with best practices (Ortiz, 2002) as well as legal mandates (Individuals with Disabilities Education Act, 1997, 34CFR Sec. 300.534[b]; Ochoa, Galarza, & Gonzalez, 1996; see Chapter 3 for more information), school-based practitioners who assess second-language learners must obtain information about students' language abilities in both their native and English language. Without this information, practitioners are unable to ascertain: (1) if the

---

This chapter is by Salvador Hector Ochoa and Samuel O. Ortiz.

child's current classroom setting is appropriate, given his or her language abilities (Ochoa, Galarza, & Gonzalez, 1996); (2) if assessment of achievement and intelligence were conducted in the appropriate language(s) (Figueroa, 1990); (3) the degree to which language proficiency in both the first and second language influences or possibly explains test performance on cognitive and achievement measures; and (4) if the areas of concern are a result of a real disability or simply a reflection of the normal process of second-language acquisition (Chamberlain & Medinos-Landurand, 1991; Willig, 1986).

The primary reason that data on language proficiency in both languages are critical is obvious: How else would an evaluator know how best to proceed or which linguistic modality is more appropriate? Moreover, the manifestation of learning problems cannot be attributed to difficulties that are apparent in only one language. Thus, professionals who assess second-language learners will find it necessary to ensure that the reasons or concerns that prompted the referral are documented in both the child's native language and in English. According to Willig, "A true disability must be apparent in both languages. If there is no disability in the child's dominant language, there can be no disability. Any symptoms of disability must then be manifestations of the process of second language acquisition" (1986, p. 14). In other words, a second-language learner should not be identified as being, for example, LD, when the deficits exist in English but not in Spanish. Individuals only have one brain, not an English brain and a separate Spanish brain (Bialystok, 1991). If the second-language learner can successfully decode while reading in Spanish, but not in English, the child cannot be LD. Clearly, documenting whether there is a problem across both languages cannot be established without knowledge of the individual's language proficiency skills in both the child's first and second languages.

## Utilizing Both Formal and Informal Methods

It is important that both formal and informal measures be used to assess the language abilities of LEP students. This approach has long been recommended by many within the field of school psychology and special education (Figueroa, 1990a; Lopez 1995, 1997; Maldonado-Colon, 1986; Ochoa, 2003; Ochoa, Galarza, & Gonzalez, 1996). The use of both formal and informal methods allows for different aspects of language skills to be assessed—an important consideration, given Standard 9.10 of the 1999 Standards for Educational and Psychological Testing developed by the American Educational Research Association, American Psychological Association, and the National Council on Measurement in Education (1999). Standard 9.10 states that "inferences about test taker's general language proficiency should be based on tests that measure a range of language features, and not a single skill" (p. 99). Many formal measures examine students' language abilities by focusing on surface components that include one or more of the following linguistic components: phonology, morphology, syntax, grammar, and vocabulary (Damico, 1991). Informal measures examine how language is used in real-life situations, including the classroom. Ortiz and Kushner (1997) state: "In selecting language-assessment instruments and procedures, it is important to keep in mind that tests that emphasize accuracy of the surface structures of language . . . will overidentify language minority students as having language or learning disabilities" (pp. 670–671). Moreover, it is important to recognize that there are limitations to using both formal and informal methods (discussed in more detail later in this chapter). Given this rationale, school-based practitioners should seek to utilize both types of measures, as each provides important information related to either evaluation or intervention.

## Obtaining Information about the Student's Language Development (BICS and CALP)

As previously discussed in Chapter 2, there are two types of language proficiency: BICS (basic interpersonal communication skills) and CALP (cognitive academic language proficiency) (Cummins, 1984). Obtaining information about an LEP student's skills in both types of language proficiency has been recommended (Lopez, 1997; Ochoa, 2003; Ortiz, 1997, 2001, 2002; Roseberry-McKibbin, 2002). The developmental nature of language acquisition, as described by the interplay between BICS and CALP, is an important consideration in evaluating the progress of a student because it sets the stage for expected levels of performance. Moreover, to avoid making interpretive errors about a child's language abilities, it is important for evaluators to ascertain, as clearly as possible, which type of language proficiency skills (BICS vs. CALP) are being assessed by the formal measures they employ. Roseberry-McKibbin (2002) notes:

> Many English proficiency tests administered in school evaluate only BICS. . . . [M]any professionals administer English tests to "English Proficient" students, believing that a label of "English Proficient" based on English proficiency tests means that the students have the language skills necessary to perform adequately on tests standardized on monolingual, English-speaking children. A student who is identified as English Language Proficient on BICS-type language proficiency measures can easily be misdiagnosed as having a language learning disability if CALP has not been fully developed. (pp. 206 and 208)

## Assessing Both Receptive and Expressive Skills

Assessing language skills across both receptive and expressive domains has been recommended (Lopez, 1997; Ortiz, 1997). Many examiners do not question the need to assess the child's expressive skills because these skills are deemed critical, particularly in the classroom, for their considerable influence on a student's ability to communicate his or her thoughts and knowledge in both oral and written fashion. Nevertheless, it is important that receptive skills also be assessed as a necessary component of the learning process. Ortiz (1997) states that "receptive skills should be assessed, because so much school time is spent receiving messages from teachers and others, as for example, in class lectures, in reviews, or when directions for completing assignments are given" (p. 327).

## Using Current Language Proficiency Data

Because the early stages of language acquisition proceed at a rather rapid pace, it is important for school-based practitioners to obtain current language proficiency testing data. If such data are unavailable from another source (e.g., second-language department) or are considered to be unreliable for any reason, then the measurement of current language proficiency can best be accomplished by the practitioner him- or herself. Of course, in situations where the practitioner does not speak or does not possess sufficient skills in the native language of the child, this measurement can be difficult to accomplish. Thus, many school psychologists and other practitioners rely on language proficiency data obtained by external sources, usually bilingual education or ESL programs. For example, Ochoa, Galarza, and Gonzalez (1996) found that school psychologists did not conduct their own assessment of language proficiency in approximately 40% of the cases involving second-language learners. However, in these situations, Ochoa et al. (1996) also found that the data used in approximately 50% of the cases were outdated (i.e., more than 6 months old). Maldonado-Colon (1984, as cited in Maldonado-Colon, 1986) also found that language proficiency data used to make decisions about LEP students were frequently outdated. Ortiz and Polyzoi (1986) and Ortiz (2002) contend that language proficiency data that is older than 6 months should not be utilized to make a decision about the child's current performance. Rather than relying on outdated language proficiency data, it is necessary for monolingual practitioners to seek the assistance of another bilingual psychologist, speech–language pathologist, special education teacher, or trained interpreter (see Chapter 6) to secure the necessary data.

## FORMAL LANGUAGE PROFICIENCY TESTS

Although there are several commercially available language proficiency measures in English and Spanish, there are only a few measures available in low-incidence languages. One example is the Basic Inventory of Natural Language (BINL), which is available in many different languages. When the need to assess children from low-incidence language groups arises, examiners will have to use informal language proficiency measures primarily, if not exclusively.

It is beyond the scope of this chapter to review each of the commercially available formal language proficiency instruments. In selecting which formal language proficiency measure to use, school-based practitioners should consider several important factors, such as (1) norming properties; (2) psychometric factors, including reliability and validity; (3) skills assessed; (4) theoretical foundation used to develop the measure; and (5) the extent to which the instrument incorporates the four recommended language proficiency practices described previously. Additionally, practitioners should refrain from using only a single formal instrument that measures one particular language skill and should instead utilize multiple sources of corroborating information and data.

In light of the key components of language proficiency assessment specified at the outset of this chapter, we believe that one noteworthy test of language proficiency that merits discussion is the Woodcock–Muñoz Language Survey (WMLS; 1993, 2001). This measure is based in part on Cummins's (1984) theoretical model of language proficiency that includes the concepts of BICS and CALP. Unlike many instruments that only measure skills that are represented by BICS, the WMLS is one of the few measures available that provides specific information about a student's CALP development in his or her first language and in English. Students can obtain a CALP level in both English and Spanish that ranges from 1 to 5, where 1 = negligible, 2 = very limited, 3 = limited, 4 = fluent, and 5 = advanced. Students who obtain at least a level of 4 are deemed to have attained CALP in that language. CALP scores are provided in oral language, reading/writing, and broad language domains. The WMLS is comprised of four subtests (Picture Vocabulary, Verbal Analogies, Letter–Word Identification, and Dictation). The first two subtests provide information about oral language CALP, whereas the latter two subtests provide information about reading/writing CALP. All four subtests are used to obtain information about the student's broad language CALP. Moreover, a relative performance index (RPI) can be obtained for each of the domains. In general, the RPI indicates the percentage of the content that the student would be expected to master, as compared to other students who mastered 90% of the content. The WMLS was initially normed in 1993 and renormed in 2001.

## Limitations of Formal Language Measures

School-based pratitioners need to be aware that formal language measures have many limitations. First, many language measures have weak psychometric properties (Barona & Santos de Barona, 1987; Damico, 1991). Second, there is a lack of Spanish or other language norms for many language measures. Although a specific instrument may have been translated into another language, it does not ensure that the test was actually renormed with individuals who speak that language. In such cases, only monolingual English norms are available for use with individuals who are, in fact, bilingual, and thus such norms are hardly representative of the population with which they are used (Barona & Santos de Barona, 1987).

Third, when Spanish or other language norms are available, they are likewise primarily obtained from monolingual speakers in other countries. Monolingual speakers in other countries are very different from the circumstantial bilinguals born or raised in the United States who are learning a second language (Roseberry-McKibbin, 2002). Because of the failure to attend to the issue of developmental language differences, native-language norms are often no more appropriate than English-language norms for bilingual individuals living in the United States who are no longer monolingual in their native language (Mattes & Omark, 1991; Ortiz, 2001, 2002). Although norms based on a particular language would be appropriate to use if the student had immigrated very recently to the United States and still speaks that language, such norms cannot be considered adequate or truly representative of that same individual as he or she progresses invariably toward becoming bilingual, particularly in the case of school-age children. Thus, use of native-language norms does not ensure that inferences with regard to proficiency, performance, or ability will be fully valid or equitable (Flanagan & Ortiz, 2001; Ortiz, 2001, 2002).

Fourth, significant problems can occur when tests are translated from English to Spanish (Barona & Santos de Barona, 1987) because "translation . . . does not take into consideration differences in semantic, syntactic, and phonological complexity among languages" (Peña, Quinn, & Iglesias, 1992, p. 269). Moreover, there are some words in English that do not have an equivalent counterpart in another language (Mattes & Omark, 1991; Roseberry-McKibbin, 2002). Additionally, words can vary in their item difficulty across two languages.

Fifth, there are many dialects of Spanish and different Spanish terms used to convey the same concept in different Latin American countries. Moreover, there are dialectal differences between Spanish spoken within the United States by Cuban Americans in Florida and that spoken by Puerto Ricans in New York or Mexican Americans in the Southwest. The extent to which language measures include all these dialects as acceptable responses is highly suspect.

Sixth, formal language proficiency measures require that language be utilized in the same manner across cultures. For example, many language proficiency measures require that the student name an object, and many children in the United States are taught names for particular objects (Peña et al., 1992). Peña et al. (1992) found that "one-word labeling of objects is not emphasized in the same manner or frequency across all cultural/language groups" (p. 271). Instead, some cultures emphasize the "functions" of the object (Gutierrez-Clellen & Iglesias, 1987, as cited in Peña et al., 1992). As a result of this difference, LEP students from these cultures might appear to have weak vocabulary skills (Peña et al. 1992).

Seventh, as noted above, formal measures are discrete point language instruments that assess one, some, or all of the structural components of languages (i.e., phonology, morphology, syntax, grammar, and vocabulary; Damico, 1991). De Valenzuela and Cervantes (1998) note that "different tests give different proportional weights to the various components of language—pronunciation, comprehension, grammatical structure, vocabulary" (p. 156). Thus, the extent to which structural components are emphasized, while others are completely ignored, in a particular language measure can greatly impact the score that is obtained.

Eighth, formal language measures are said to lack "authencity" (Damico, 1991, p. 173) or "ecological validity" (Jitendra & Rohena-Diaz, 1996, p. 43). Damico (1991) states that assessing the structural components of language in a standardized manner with formal language proficiency measures does not accurately reflect how language is used in real-life situations. August and Hakuta (1998) note that "second language abilities should be assessed in relation to the uses of language the learner will require, rather than in isolation as an abstract competence" (p. 10).

Ninth, one use of language that is important for LEP students to obtain consists of those language skills that are required in learning activities in the classroom (i.e., CALP). As noted above, very few language measures assess CALP (Roseberry-McKibbin, 2002).

These limitations need to be considered by school-based practitioners when interpreting data obtained from formal language proficiency measures. Our point is not to suggest that these measures should be not be utilized to assess second-language learners; their *sole* use to assess language proficiency of LEP students, however, is not recommended. Rather, we see these limitations as providing a strong rationale for using informal measures to supplement formal measures. In this manner, practitioners can examine the extent (if any) to which these limitations had a bearing on the data obtained from the formal measures they employed. The use of informal measures also allows for an examination of the LEP child's language abilities across many different settings that are reflective of situations in which he or she will be expected to use both BICS and CALP.

## INFORMAL METHODS TO ASSESS LANGUAGE PROFICIENCY

Several informal methods have been recommended for the assessment of language proficiency. The use of informal methods to assess language proficiency is critical when assessing children from low-incidence languages, particularly because there do not exist many standardized instruments for this population. These methods include observations, questionnaires, teacher rating scales, storytelling, story retelling, cloze procedures, and language samples. Each of these methods is described.

### Observations

The informal method of observation has been recommended for use with English-language learners by professionals in school psychology (Lopez, 1997; Ochoa, Galarza, & Gonzalez, 1996; Ortiz, 2002), special education (Ortiz, 1997), and speech and language pathology (Kayser, 1989; Mattes & Omark, 1991). Observations of an LEP student while interacting in the classroom and in other settings can provide critical information about how well the child communicates. Observing the child's language usage during instructional activities in the classroom can provide an estimate of his or her CALP skills (Lopez, 1997).

A critical issue when conducting observations is how to evaluate the language-usage patterns displayed by English-language learners. One informal inventory in this area is the Bilingual Oral Language Development (BOLD) scale (Mattes & Omark, 1991). The BOLD requires that the evaluator note whether the LEP student has adequately performed 20 important communicative behaviors that are needed for a student to be an effective communicator. Mattes and Omark state that it is also acceptable to obtain information from the child's teacher, based on the teacher's observations. The researchers recommend that the evaluator follow up with parents to see if they have noted the difficulties at home observed by the evaluator or teacher on the BOLD. Importantly, Mattes and Omark caution that it is important for evaluators to ascertain whether the 20 communicative behaviors noted on the BOLD are culturally appropriate for the LEP student who is being assessed. If a given communicative behavior is not culturally appropriate for a given LEP student, a deficiency in this particular skill should not be interpreted as a problem.

## Questionnaires

Questionnaires can be quite helpful in obtaining valuable information from parents and have been recommended by Kayser (1989) and Lopez (1997). This information can provide a picture about how both the native and English language are used within the child's home. Moreover, questionnaires give parents an opportunity to contribute their perspective regarding their child's skills. One questionnaire that has been developed to obtain parent input is the Bilingual Language Proficiency Questionnaire by Mattes and Santiago (1985). This questionnaire was "developed specifically for use in assessing children's development of English and Spanish and their use of each language in their home environment" (Mattes & Omark, 1991, p. 67). The questionnaire consists of 30 questions, each of which is written in both English and Spanish. The Bilingual Language Proficiency Questionnaire is also available in Vietnamese.

## Teacher Rating Scales

The use of teacher rating scales to examine the language proficiency skills of LEP students has been recommended by Roseberry-McKibbin (2002) and de Valenzuela and Cervantes (1998). Obtaining teacher input is critical because they have had significant opportunity to observe the student's language and have communicated with the student in academic and interpersonal situations. One common teacher rating scale that is used to examine the language of second-language learners is the Student Oral Language Observation Matrix (SOLOM), which was initially developed by the San Jose Bay Area Consortium and subsequently revised under the direction of the Bilingual Education Office of the California Department of Education. The SOLOM, which has been placed in the public domain and can be downloaded from the Internet, examines the following five components of language: comprehension, fluency, vocabulary, pronunciation, and grammar. Each component is rated by the child's teacher on a 5-point Likert scale. Each point on the Likert scale has a detailed description to enable the teacher to easily rate his or her student's language on each of the five components. Thus, the highest score that a student can obtain on the SOLOM is 25 points. Students who obtain at least 19 points are deemed to be proficient in that language. Teachers can use the SOLOM to rate the child's language skills in both the native and English language.

## Storytelling

The use of storytelling to assess LEP students' language proficiency has been recommended by Ortiz (1997), Ortiz and Kushner (1997), and Roseberry-McKibbin (2002). This technique is used to evaluate the LEP student's expressive abilities (Ortiz, 1997). This technique "reveals information about a child's ability to organize information, sequence events, draw conclusions, and evaluate actions" (Ortiz, 1997, p. 327). Roseberry-McKibbin (2002) recommends that the evaluator use the following questions in order to determine the quality of the LEP student's story:

> Does the student organize the story in such a way that it can be easily understood? Is the information in the story comprehensible to the listener? Does the student give elaborated comments, opinions, and explanations that are relevant to the story? . . . Does the student include all the major details of the story? If questioned, can the student remember specific details from the story? (p. 257)

## Story Retelling

The use of story retelling to assess second-language learner's linguistic proficiency in both languages has been recommended by Mattes and Omark (1991), Ortiz (1997), Ortiz and Kushner (1997), and Roseberry-McKibbin (2002). This technique is used to evaluate the LEP pupil's receptive skills (Ortiz, 1997). When utilizing this informal method, students are told a story and then asked to retell the story to the evaluator. Mattes and Omark (1991) emphasize that the story given to the child to retell should be one that has cultural relevance for him or her.

## Cloze Techniques

The use of cloze techniques with second-language learners has been recommended by Mattes and Omark (1991), Ortiz (1997), and Ortiz and Kushner (1997). A cloze technique can be presented in a written or oral format. Although there are commercially available cloze procedures, use of this technique with the specific curriculum that is being taught is the most beneficial and authentic. The cloze technique consists of a text passage that has every $n$th word deleted. Students are required to provide a word for every deleted word in the passage. Mattes and Omark (1991) offer specific guidelines on how to construct and administer oral cloze techniques and note that "The cloze procedure is especially helpful in determining whether children from bilingual backgrounds have acquired the academic language proficiencies necessary for successful performance in classroom reading activities" (p. 114).

## Language Samples

Many professionals (Kayser, 1989; Lopez, 1997; Mattes & Omark, 1991; Ochoa, Galarza, & Gonzalez, 1996; Ortiz, 1997; Roseberry-McKibbin, 2002; de Valenzuela & Cervantes, 1998) recommend that language samples be used to assess the linguistic abilities of second-language learners. Language samples can be obtained in several ways. In one method the examiner carries on a conversation with the student on a topic that is of interest to the child. In another method the examiner observes the student while he or she is participating in oral dialogue with an instructor or classmates. Language samples can also be obtained by asking the child to perform certain tasks that require an extended oral response (Roseberry-McKibbin, 2002). For example, students can be asked to put a series of pictures in sequential order and then to verbally explain what occurred in the pictures (Roseberry-McKibbin, 2002). When collecting language samples, evaluators should make an audio recording of the student (Mattes & Omark, 1991; Roseberry-McKibbin, 2002).

Language samples can be analyzed for the presence of both structural mistakes and pragmatic features (Mattes & Omark, 1991; Roseberry & McKibbon, 2002). However, analyzing language samples can be a difficult process for many school-based practitioners. In particular, evaluating structural errors requires in-depth training about linguistics that is beyond the current level of competence possessed by most practitioners. As an alternative Damico (1991) stresses the need to analyze language samples by examining pragmatic features of language. His research used the following seven pragmatic features: "linguistic nonfluency," "revisions," "delays before responding," "nonspecific vocabulary," "inappropriate responses," "poor topic maintenance," and "need for repetition" (Damico & Oller, 1980, p. 88; Damico, Oller, & Storey, 1983). Damico and Oller (1980) found that teachers who were trained to look for pragmatic components of language, versus those trained to look for surface/structural mistakes, were significantly "more accurate in their referrals" to speech–language pathologists (p. 91). They concluded that "the pragmatic criteria for referrals seems to be superior for identifying language disordered children. Teachers were able to identify language disordered children more readily by using . . . pragmatic criteria than they can by using morphological/syntactic criteria" (Damico & Oller, 1980, p. 91). Damico et al. (1983) also found that the use of pragmatic features was "more effective . . . in identifying" (p. 392) bilingual students with language disabilities.

Jitendra and Rohena-Diaz (1996) provide an in-depth case study on how psychologists need to work collaboratively with bilingual speech–language pathologists to examine the pragmatic features of language. Practitioners who do not possess sufficient expertise in linguistics will need to evaluate language samples by judging the degree to which the LEP child is able to adequately convey and understand messages in each language across different settings. School-based practitioners should note if and how LEP students differ in conveying and understanding messages in both their native language and English.

## DEVELOPMENTAL INTERPRETATION OF LANGUAGE PROFICIENCY DATA

We have identified four critical factors to consider when reviewing and interpreting language proficiency data. Each of the factors discussed in this section will provide the school-based practitioner with important information to consider when reaching conclusions about a student's language proficiency in both the first and second language and its possible relationship to academic performance.

### Factor 1: Considering the Context of Previous Educational Services and Home Literacy Factors

One important factor is to interpret obtained scores and data in the context of the educational services provided to the child and the child's home literacy environment. Ascertaining this context can be accomplished in two ways. The first way is to interpret the data based on what is known about second-language acquisition. The WMLS allows the examiner to ascertain if the child has attained CALP in his or her first language (i.e., achieving at least a level of 4). A second-language learner who has obtained a CALP level of 4 in Spanish has a sufficient threshold level in his or her first language to facilitate the development of his or her English language skills and to subsequently foster adequate academic performance in English. This student can now be deemed as ready to be transitioned from a bilingual education setting. This student might want to be considered for participation in an ESL program or in a general education classroom setting. If, on the other hand, the second-language learner has not obtained a CALP level of 4, then he or she has not obtained a minimal threshold level in the first language and would be expected to experience academic difficulty on English academic tasks without bilingual and/or ESL instructional support. If this particular student is not in a bilingual education classroom setting and only receives instruction in English, he or she is likely to struggle. Insufficient development in his or her first language is likely to have negatively affected his or her English-language development and academic performance. In situations where second-language learners have not obtained CALP in their first language (i.e., level 4) and are required to attend English-only academic settings, it is imperative that school-based practitioners consider the degree to which the child's limited language abilities in both languages are contributing to their low academic performance.

The second way to interpret the data is to review them based on what is known about the effectiveness of the type of bilingual education program in which the child has participated. Several examples are provided to illustrate how this task can be accomplished.

In Scenario A we have a sixth-grade student who has been in a well-implemented two-way/dual bilingual program since kindergarten. We would expect that this student has been given a sufficient amount of time and the opportunity to develop his native language in order to obtain CALP in his first language. Moreover, we would expect that this student would be very close to developing, or already have developed, CALP in English. If this student has not obtained CALP in his first language or is at a very low CALP level in English on the WMLS, this could be a cause for concern because research (Thomas & Collier, 1997, 2002) indicates that second-language learners in this type of bilingual education program perform at, or near, the national average on English-reading achievement measures. Students need to obtain CALP in both languages in order to increase the likelihood of experiencing academic success in each of these languages.

In Scenario B we have a sixth-grade student who has been in an ESL pullout program since kindergarten. In this situation, we also need to examine the child's home literacy background. Did she receive any instructional assistance/services in her native language at home or church? At home, this assistance could come from an older sibling, parent, or relative. We have been told of many situations in which students from Hebrew, Greek, Arabic, African, Chinese, Japanese, and other Asian-language-speaking backgrounds receive formal instruction in their native language outside of their regular school experience (e.g., at church, synagogue, mosque, temple, after-school community programs, etc.) during the week and often on weekends as well. If this sixth-grade student in an ESL pullout program did not receive any additional instruction in her native language outside of school, we would *not* expect her to have received a sufficient amount of time and opportunity to develop her native language to the point of CALP. Subsequently, we would not expect this student to have developed CALP in English because she has yet to develop CALP in her first language. If this student has not obtained CALP in her first language or is at a very low CALP level in English on the WMLS, this would *not* automatically be a cause for concern because research (Thomas & Collier, 1997, 2002) indicates that second-language learners in ESL pullout programs perform approximately at the 35th NCE on English-reading achievement in sixth grade.

In Scenario C, we have a second-grade LEP student who has been in a transitional program since kindergarten. The ratios of L1 to L2 instruction in kindergarten through second grade were

80:20 in kindergarten, 60:40 in first grade, and 30:70 in second grade. This student has not obtained CALP in Spanish or English, but this finding would not automatically be a cause for concern because he has not received sufficient opportunity and time to develop his first language.

## Factor 2: Comparing the LEP Child's Language Abilities with Other Second-Language Learners

A second important factor to consider is the degree to which the LEP child's language abilities differ from those of other LEP children. This information can be obtained from both a formal measure (e.g., WMLS) and informal measures (e.g., observations, questionnaires, teacher rating scales). First, if the WMLS is used by your district's bilingual education program, this homogeneity enables the psychologist and other school personnel to compare the language growth progress or trajectory of the LEP student in question with other LEP students who have received the same, or very similar, bilingual education or ESL programs across grade levels. Some states require that students' language proficiency be assessed each year to ascertain if they are ready to be exited from bilingual education. (If the WMLS is not used by your school district, compare the student's language abilities with those of his or her second-language peers by using the measure that is employed by the bilingual education/ESL program in your district.) If the student's CALP scores do not differ significantly from, and evidence similar growth across grade levels with, those of his or her LEP peers in the same grade, then this finding might indicate that his or her language abilities are developing normally. If, however, the student's CALP scores do differ significantly from, and do not evidence the same degree of growth across grade levels with, those of his or her LEP peers in the same grade, then the normal second-language acquisition process might not be the cause of this student's academic or language difficulties.

It is also important to ascertain the degree to which the student's language abilities differ from those of other LEP students' language abilities on informal language measures. While conducting observations of the child in the classroom, it is important to simultaneously compare his or her language abilities with those of his or her LEP classmates. Moreover, if the BOLD is used, it is important to ask the student's teacher how the student's abilities on the 20 communicative behaviors differ with those of his or her LEP classmates. This same method of comparison can be made with teacher rating scales, such as the SOLOM. If questionnaires such as the Bilingual Language Proficiency Questionnaire are utilized, it is important to have parents compare the child being tested with his or her siblings.

## Factor 3: Consistency of Data across Formal and Informal Language Measures

Given the limitations of many formal language proficiency measures previously noted, it is important to ascertain if the data obtained across formal and informal measures are consistent. When the data are consistent across all types of data collected, the school-based practitioner can have a greater degree of confidence that he or she has obtained an accurate picture of the child's language proficiency in one or both languages. When the data collected are not consistent across formal and informal language measures, it is critical to ascertain why this divergence has occurred. In these situations, it is important for practitioners to decide which data are more reflective of the student's genuine language proficiency skills.

### Factor 4: Ascertaining Where the Student Is along the Second-Language Acquisition Continuum

Data from the WMLS, when collaborated with other data obtained from informal measures, help to identify where the second-language learner is along the second-language acquisition continuum. In other words, it helps the school-based practitioner ascertain what type (profile) of second-language learner he or she is assessing. In the last section of this chapter, the various language profiles of second-language learners are reviewed.

### Additional Caveats in the Developmental Interpretation of Language Proficiency Data

Two important issues are frequently misunderstood in regard to their significance in understanding and evaluating language proficiency. The first involves the concept of dominance. Although it is helpful to ascertain if the second-language learner is more dominant in various language skills (e.g., oral expression, reading ability, writing skills), patterns of dominance are most often a reflection of history and circumstance, not developmental problems. In addition, dominance indicates only that one language is better developed than the other but reveals nothing about overall proficiency in either language. For example, a student who is minimally proficient in both English and his or her native language may well be *dominant* in his or her native language, but the fact remains that his or her level of proficiency in both is still quite low. As such, dominance does not dictate the course of assessment; rather, it is the absolute level of proficiency in each language that governs the path for evaluation. A further explanation of this issue is provided in the following section, which describes various profiles of language proficiency.

The second issue revolves around speech and pronunciation, particularly whether or not an individual speaks English with an accent. When students appear to speak and pronounce English well (i.e., without an accent), there is a tendency to equate their language proficiency with that of their monolingual peers. This tendency is unfounded. An accent, or lack thereof, only indicates the point in time in which a language was acquired or learned—the earlier the exposure and experience with the language, the less likely an accent will be evident. Thus, the presence or absence of an accent is not an indicator of language proficiency and should not be used to make inferences regarding the actual linguistic abilities of any given individual.

## LANGUAGE PROFILES OF SECOND-LANGUAGE LEARNERS

With regard to evaluating language proficiency and development across both languages spoken by a student, there are various language profiles that school-based practitioners can expect to find within the LEP population. Of the nine profiles presented in Table 9.1, seven of the most relevant are described in this chapter. (Profiles 7 and 8 are not discussed in this chapter.) These seven language profiles serve to illustrate the most common variations along the continuum of second-language learners. To assist in explaining this continuum, three levels of proficiency are used: minimal, emergent, and fluent. Some of the language profiles occur considerably more frequently

**TABLE 9.1. Language Profiles of Second-Language Learners**

| Language profile | L1 proficiency level | L2 proficiency level | Description |
| --- | --- | --- | --- |
| Profile 1 | Minimal | Minimal | CALP levels in native language (L1) and English (L2) are both in the 1–2 range—individual has no significant dominant language, and proficiency and skills in both languages are extremely limited. |
| Profile 2 | Emergent | Minimal | CALP level in native language is in the 3 range and English is in the 1–2 range—individual is relatively more dominant in native language, and proficiency and skills are developing but limited; English proficiency and skills remain extremely limited. |
| Profile 3 | Fluent | Minimal | CALP level in native language is in the 4–5 range and English is in the 1–2 range—individual is highly dominant and very proficient in native language; English proficiency and skills remain extremely limited. |
| Profile 4 | Minimal | Emergent | CALP level in native language is in the 1–2 range and English is in the 3 range—individual is relatively more dominant in English, with developing but limited proficiency and skills; native language proficiency and skills are extremely limited. |
| Profile 5 | Emergent | Emergent | CALP level in native language is in the 3 range and English is in the 3 range—individual has no significant language dominance and is developing proficiency and skills in both but is still limited in both. |
| Profile 6 | Fluent | Emergent | CALP level in native language is in the 4–5 range and English is in the 3 range—individual is relatively more dominant in native language, with high proficiency and skills; English proficiency and skills are developing but still limited. |
| Profile 7 | Minimal | Fluent | CALP level in native language is in the 1–2 range and English is in the 4–5 range—individual is highly dominant and very proficient in English; native language proficiency and skills are extremely limited. |
| Profile 8 | Emergent | Fluent | CALP level in native language is in the 3 range and English is in the 4–5 range—individual is dominant and very proficient in English; native language proficiency and skills are developing but limited. |
| Profile 9 | Fluent | Fluent | CALP level in native language and English are both in the 4–5 range—individual has no significant dominant language and is very fluent and very proficient in both. |

than others. An understanding of each of the profiles will help guide school-based practitioners on how best to proceed with the academic and cognitive assessments outlined in the chapters that follow.

## Profile 1: Minimal Proficiency in Both Languages

Students who display this language profile are minimally proficient in both languages. These are students who are described by some teachers as being semilingual, because they appear to have no, or very limited, language skills in both English and their native language. Such a child could be a student who obtains a WMLS Broad CALP score of 1 or 2 in both Spanish and English. Information from informal measures should corroborate the data obtained from the WMLS before concluding that the student has deficient skills in both languages. Sequential second-language learners who are in English-only instructional settings, particularly those who were non-English speakers before entering school or who were not yet educated in their native language, may exhibit this profile. In addition, an important factor to consider in this situation is to ascertain if language loss in the student's native language has occurred (see Chapter 2), which would signify that the student has become minimally proficient as a function of educational circumstances.

## Profile 2: Emergent Proficiency in L1 and Minimal Proficiency in L2

Second-language learners who display this pattern will have stronger skills in their first language but have yet to obtain CALP in their first language. Such a child could be a student who has command of his or her conversational native language (i.e., BICS) and obtains WMLS Broad CALP scores of 3 in Spanish and 2 or 1 in English. Information from informal measures should corroborate the data obtained from the WMLS before concluding that the student displays this language profile. Students who display this pattern are on the verge of obtaining CALP in Spanish. It is important to recognize that these students in this profile need more L1 instructional time in order to meet a threshold level in this language. Although students who display this profile have stronger language abilities in their first language, they still have limited language skills that could significantly influence their performance on cognitive measures.

## Profile 3: Fluent Proficiency in L1 and Minimal Proficiency in L2

Students who display this profile have obtained CALP in their first language and have very low skill levels in the second language. Such a child could be a student who obtains WMLS Broad CALP scores of 4 or 5 in Spanish and 2 or 1 in English. Information from informal measures should corroborate the data obtained from the WMLS before concluding that the student displays this language profile. This student has developed a threshold level in his or her first language that will help to foster CALP in English. A student who displays this profile may have attended elementary school (e.g., up through grade 4 or 5) in their native country and has recently arrived in the United States and currently is in middle school. This profile may be noted among second-language learners in the United States who have been instructed in well-implemented maintenance or dual bilingual education programs. These students have sufficient language skills to be assessed in their first language.

## Profile 4: Minimal Proficiency in L1 and Emergent Proficiency in L2

Second-language learners who display this pattern will have stronger skills in their second language but have yet to obtain CALP in this language. Such a child could be a student who obtains WMLS Broad CALP scores of 1 or 2 in Spanish and 3 in English. Information from informal measures should corroborate the data obtained from the WMLS before concluding that the student displays this language profile. A variety of reasons could account for this language profile in second-language learners. First, LEP students whose parents have rejected bilingual education services will most likely have stronger skills in English, because this is the language in which they have been instructed. Second, LEP students who have received only ESL instructional services or who have been prematurely exited from bilingual education are likely to exhibit stronger English skills. Third, this profile could be found in LEP pupils who are in a transitional program that has switched, too soon, to providing instruction in English for the majority or entirety of the time. Although such a student might have stronger skills in English, practitioners should exercise caution not to assume that this student has sufficient English skills to be given cognitive measures in English only.

## Profile 5: Emergent Proficiency in Both L1 and L2

Students who display this profile are able to converse socially in both languages but have yet to attain a CALP level in either language. Such a student could be a student who obtains a WMLS Broad CALP score of 3 in both Spanish and English. Information from informal measures should corroborate the data obtained from the WMLS before concluding that the student displays this language profile. This profile may be found among simultaneous second-language learners—for example, students from homes where the parents can fully support language development in English and another language. This profile could also reflect the pattern that might be found in students who received native-language instruction up to about the third grade before coming to the United States and who were subsequently instructed in English from that point. While their English advances to the emergent level, their native language remains at the emergent level or deteriorates (language loss) from a slightly higher level. As noted previously in this volume, it is important that school psychologists and other education personnel recognize that although they can converse quite well with this child in English, this apparent facility does not mean that the student has sufficient English-language skills to be given cognitive measures in English only. The "visible" portion of social language (i.e., BICS) is too often mistaken for a level of proficiency that is, in fact, higher than the reality.

## Profile 6: Fluent Proficiency in L1 and Emergent Proficiency in L2

This profile depicts those second-language learners who have obtained CALP in their first language and who have emergent skills in English. Such a child could be a student who obtains WMLS Broad CALP scores of 4 or 5 in Spanish and 3 in English. Information from informal measures should corroborate the data obtained from the WMLS before concluding that the student displays this language profile. This student has developed a threshold level in his or her first language that will help to foster CALP in English; indeed, the student is on the verge of obtaining

CALP in English. This profile may be found among second-language learners in the United States who have been given sufficient time to develop their first language in well-implemented maintenance or dual bilingual education programs (i.e., grades K–6).

### Profile 9: Fluent Proficiency in L1 and L2

Students who display this profile have obtained CALP in both their first and second language. Such a child could be a student who obtains WMLS Broad CALP scores of 4 or 5 in Spanish and English. Information from informal measures should corroborate the data obtained from the WMLS before concluding that the student displays this language profile. Examples of students who might exhibit this profile include those who have graduated from dual-language programs or successfully transitioned from well-implemented maintenance programs, and students from other countries who received a strong education in their native language (up through 7th or 8th grade) prior to coming to the United States and who have since learned and mastered English. Such a student has sufficient language skills to be assessed in both languages.

### SUMMARY

The information provided in this chapter clearly underscores the importance of assessing the language proficiency in both of the languages spoken by a student. Utilizing the recommended language proficiency practices culled from the literature and summarized in this chapter will elicit information that is essential for reaching appropriate conclusions about LEP students' linguistic abilities as well as making important decisions about how to proceed with testing. Success in these two endeavors—drawing inferences and decision making—will also depend, in large part, on a recognition of the issues that bear upon fair and equitable interpretation of formal and informal data. Understanding the limitations of standardized instruments, particularly in regard to the lack of attention paid to bilingual versus monolingual language development, is an example of a particularly important consideration in this regard. As will become evident in the chapters that follow, a clear understanding and evaluation of an individual's language proficiency in both the native language and English are critical because they serve as the foundation for a defensible— and *fair*—assessment and interpretation of cognitive and academic abilities.

# 10

# Conceptual Measurement and Methodological Issues in Cognitive Assessment of Culturally and Linguistically Diverse Individuals

The changing demographic patterns of the United States provide a strong indication that practitioners of all kinds will encounter situations requiring evaluation of culturally and linguistically diverse individuals with increasing frequency. Most practitioners recognize readily that multicultural or multilingual evaluations present unique challenges not ordinarily encountered when working with ostensibly monolingual and monocultural individuals from the U.S. mainstream. Driven by either legal prescriptions or a lack of training, practitioners often distilled these challenges in practice simply as efforts to overcome the linguistic barrier to communication—an unfortunately narrow and erroneous distillation. Although linguistic factors are perhaps the most obvious concern facing practitioners, the nature and influence of cultural factors on test performance are in no way less of a concern. Too often, culture is confounded with race or ethnicity and remains largely ignored in most assessment practices and in the very tests commonly employed in such endeavors. This significant error/oversight occurs despite the fact that nondiscriminatory assessment requires that considerable attention be paid to the profound and dynamic influences of both language and culture as they define behavior and affect performance on tests or other procedures. Indeed, the very validity of any data collected in a multicultural or multilingual assessment is inextricably linked to the degree to which the methods and procedures used for evaluation and interpretation have reduced any potential biasing influences as a function of both linguistic and cultural differences.

The purpose of this chapter is to describe the relevant conceptual and measurement issues associated with the cognitive assessment of culturally and linguistically diverse students. It is important that practitioners first have a clear understanding of how multilingual–multicultural assessment differs from general assessment.

---

This chapter is by Samuel O. Ortiz and Salvador Hector Ochoa.

153

## CONCEPTUAL, MEASUREMENT, AND METHODOLOGICAL ISSUES
## IN ASSESSMENT

According to Ochoa, Powell, and Robles-Piña (1996), the most commonly used instruments with diverse individuals include a Wechsler Intelligence Scale (generally administered completely in English), the Bender Visual–Motor Gestalt test, the Draw-A-Person test, and the Leiter. Generally speaking, given the inadequate psychometric properties, inappropriate norms and comparison groups, unidimensional assessments, linguistic and cultural confounds, and so forth, that characterize many of these tests, such a combination (or battery) is problematic. Moreover, the problems associated with the use of such tests with diverse populations are not entirely solved when native-language tests are used or when interpreters are used for the process of administration (Lopez, 1997; McCallum & Bracken, 1997). But perhaps the greatest problem associated with the use of any set of tests or test battery lies in the fact that these tests are often selected, administered, and then interpreted in a manner that is not guided by the literature on how culture or language influence test performance of individuals from various cultures or with various linguistic backgrounds. As such, decisions and conclusions based on such data are haphazard and largely indefensible because they do not address the known patterns of bias that can arise when standardized, norm-referenced tests are incorporated within the assessment process. Among others, bias in testing may stem from any one of three characteristics of the tests themselves, including (1) the cultural content embedded in any given test; (2) the linguistic demands inherent in any given test; and (3) lack of representation within norm samples of individuals from diverse backgrounds in any given test. In addition, potential bias may exist related to the concept and process of assessment: for example, the belief that use of interpreters or language-reduced tests alone is sufficient to overcome bias and communication barriers, and that as long as results are interpreted "with extreme caution," valid conclusions may still be drawn from essentially invalid data. Such beliefs must be reevaluated in light of the technical and psychometric properties of tests, particularly issues involving validity and generalizability.

### Cultural Bias versus Cultural Loading

Understanding the manner in which standardized tests may produce biased results requires recognition of the fact that the very construct of intelligence and the instruments developed to assess it are both inventions of U.S. and Western European culture. According to Kamphaus (1993), "the traditions of Galton, Binet, Wechsler, Cattell, and others underlie all modern tests of intelligence. These tests emanated from French, British, German, North American, and other similarly European cultures" (p. 441). In describing his work with David Wechsler on the revision of the WISC, Kaufman (1994) provides a poignant description regarding the degree to which test content, at the most fundamental level, is often a very real reflection of the attitudes and beliefs of the individuals who create them. Wechsler's words, as quoted by Kaufman (1994), that "Chivalry may be dying. Chivalry may be dead. *But it will not die on the WISC*" (p. x; emphasis in original) clearly illustrates the degree to which subjective cultural experience is deeply embedded in the instruments often upheld as objective measures of universal constructs.

Unquestionably, *all* tests of intelligence and cognitive ability reflect the culture (values, beliefs, ideals, etc.) from which they emanated. Neisser et al. (1996) stress that "it is obvious that the cultural environment—how people live, what they value, what they do—has a significant effect on the intellectual skills developed by individuals" (p. 86). In order to assess fairly individuals from diverse linguistic and cultural backgrounds, practitioners need to come to terms with the fact that "intelligence cannot be tested independently of the culture that gives rise to the test" (Cole & Cole, 1993, p. 502) and that "intelligence tests are not tests of intelligence in some abstract, culture-free way. They are measures of the ability to function intellectually by virtue of knowledge and skills in the culture of which they sample" (Scarr, 1978, p. 339).

Despite recognition of the pervasive influence of culture, the vast majority of research into the nature of bias in intelligence tests has failed to find much evidence of it. Numerous studies have examined potential bias as a product of test items (including content and novelty), test structure (sequence, order, difficulty), test reliability (measurement error or accuracy), factor structure (theoretical structure, cluster or composite scores), and prediction (academic success or achievement) without producing any consistent significant findings (Cummins, 1984; Figueroa, 1983, 1990a; Jensen, 1980; Valdés & Figueroa, 1996). However, the reasons underlying the failure to identify bias appear to be related to the manner in which it is defined. Culture (and, in effect, cultural bias) has historically been viewed as a unitary, monolithic construct that is expected to influence an individual's performance on a test in some manner such that the individuals' measured performance fails to maintain the same relationship as that found in the measured performance of other individuals. For example, a score that does not predict as well, or does not correlate as well, as it does for other people, in general, would be evidence that bias exists (Figueroa, 1990a, 1990b; Valdés & Figueroa, 1996). Thus, bias has been defined primarily as a psychometric issue (or an inherent defect in the test) that somehow results in systematic differences in performance between groups that cannot attributed to the ability being measured.

With the advent of sophisticated test construction methods and more precise norming procedures, the psychometric view of bias has become largely a "straw man." The obvious influence of culture or language has long been addressed, but the definition remains unchanged. A purely psychometric definition of bias is inaccurate and unrealistic because intelligence tests and tests of cognitive ability measure quite well the degree to which *anyone*, irrespective of cultural background, has acquired and can access the culturally bound information inherent in their design. It is not differences in culture, per se, that act as a biasing factor; rather it is an individual's exposure (or lack thereof) to the test's underlying cultural content that affects performance on such tests (Cummins, 1984; Figueroa, 1990a; Matsumoto, 1994; Valdés & Figueroa, 1996). In short, culture dictates which responses are right and which are wrong on tests of intelligence and cognitive ability every bit as much as it sets the norms and expectations for proper behavior in society. Performance is, therefore, partly dependent on learning what the rules are in any given society, and failure to follow those rules leads to the exact same negative consequences, irrespective of the reasons why they were not followed (i.e., intentional disregard vs. lack of knowledge).

Acquisition of the cultural content of the dominant society is known as *acculturation*. The process of acquiring culture (i.e., acculturation) is developmentally invariant, predictable, and easily measured. As with other developmental patterns, the simpler, commoner elements of culture are learned first, and the more complex elements are learned later. Standardized tests are based directly on this principle, known as the "assumption of comparability." According to Salvia and Ysseldyke:

> When we test students using a standardized device and compare them to a set of norms to gain an
> index of their relative standing, we assume that the students we test are similar to those on whom the

test was standardized; that is, we assume their acculturation is comparable, but not necessarily identical, to that of the students who made up the normative sample for the test. (1991, p. 18)

For comparisons of performance to be valid, a relatively equivalent level of acculturation must exist between the individuals on whom the test was standardized and on whom the test is used. Clearly, this assumption is often distant from the reality that exists when working with individuals from diverse cultural or linguistic backgrounds. Salvia and Ysseldyke (1991) also comment on this point: "When a child's general background experiences differ from those of the children on whom a test was standardized, then the use of the norms of that test as an index for evaluating that child's current performance or for predicting future performances may be inappropriate" (p. 18).

Cultural bias in testing thus occurs whenever tests (developed and normed in the United States) are given to individuals whose cultural background, experiences, and exposure are not comparable to that of the individuals comprising the norm group. Thus, results may be biased with regard to construct validity because the test measures level of acculturation more so than actual cognitive ability. For example, a practice of basing a test on what the average 10-year-old is expected to have internalized in terms of incidental exposure to culture works well only if the individual has had the full 10 years of exposure to that culture. An immigrant to the United States who comes to this country at the age of 5 is, when 10, held to the same standard as other 10-year-olds who have been here their entire lives, even though the immigrant has experienced only *half* of the incidental cultural exposure and learning. The comparison is inherently unfair, and performance—or rather poor performance—is thus a question of validity. Given that individuals from diverse cultural backgrounds come from multitudinous circumstances, from being descendants of multigenerational, U.S.-born ancestors to first-generation immigrants who recently arrived in the country, such tests and their norms simply cannot be applied to render valid conclusions regarding true performance in every case. Those who have not had sufficient opportunity to become acculturated to the same level as their peers are likely to score lower because they do not possess the knowledge and content, not because their ability is actually lower (Valdés & Figueroa, 1996).

As such, bias related to culture is best construed as involving *cultural loading* and distinct from definitions that are based solely on psychometric characteristics that either ignore or cannot account for differences that arise as a function of developmentally embedded cultural content. Measures of reliability (e.g., item difficulty, prediction, factor structure) are not altered by cultural content as long as that content covaries developmentally with the measurement of ability—which it does quite well. Thus, it is more accurate to say that although cognitive ability tests are not culturally *biased*, per se, they *are* culturally *loaded* (Sattler, 1992; Valdés & Figueroa, 1996). The validity of results obtained in the assessment of diverse individuals may therefore be improved if two important and interrelated pieces of information can be obtained: (1) the individual's level of acculturation as compared to age-related peers, and (2) the degree to which performance on a stand-alone test or a test from a battery is contingent upon possession of culture-specific knowledge. Level of acculturation and issues related to methods for its measurement were discussed previously in Chapter 8. Methods for addressing the relative impact of embedded cultural content of tests on the performance of diverse individuals have been outlined in the cultural and linguistic extensions of the Cattell–Horn–Carroll (CHC) cross-battery approach (Flanagan, McGrew, &

Ortiz, 2000; Flanagan & Ortiz, 2001; McGrew & Flanagan, 1998) and are presented later in this chapter.

## Language Bias versus Linguistic Demand

The effect that language differences have on test performance is quite similar to that described for cultural differences. Valdés and Figueroa (1996) note that "empirically established difficulty levels in psychometric tests are not altered by cultural differences. Neither are they because of proficiencies in the societal language" (p. 101). Language development is experientially based and follows an invariant, predictable, and measurable developmental course, much like acculturation. Because the sequence of items on standardized tests is developmentally arranged, the attenuating effect of language development, or language proficiency, is not revealed in comparisons of performance within any single test. Cummins (1984) and Valdés and Figueroa (1996), among others, have noted that it is the lack of concurrence between constructs measured through different channels (i.e., a set of verbal subtests vs. a set of nonverbal subtests) that begins to expose bias in tests. The few studies that have examined linguistic bias using such a comparative approach have been extremely consistent in their findings that tasks that are primarily language based do not measure incidental learning equally well compared to tasks that are more visual or perceptual in nature (Cummins, 1984; Jensen, 1974, 1976). In other words, individuals who are limited in their English proficiency may learn just as quickly as native English-speaking individuals in situations where neither language system is favored. However, when learning is measured on tasks that favor English-language proficiency skills, such as those found on tests of intelligence and cognitive abilities, individuals with limited or no English proficiency will not fare as well.

All tests of intelligence or cognitive ability are intentionally constructed in ways that require or presume a level of language proficiency sufficient to comprehend instructions, understand basic concepts, formulate and verbalize responses, or otherwise complete a given task or provide an appropriate response (Cummins, 1984; Figueroa, Delgado, & Ruiz, 1984). This presumption is based on age and grade-related expectations of development in language and other abilities. In cases where the focus is on evaluating language-related abilities of monolingual English-speaking individuals, there is no problem because such individuals will score lower if they are limited in language ability, as compared to their monolingual age- and grade-related peers. However, in the case of a non-native English speaker, the likelihood that the expected level of language development and proficiency for that individual is commensurate with the age- and grade-related expectations of the test is rather small. When an individual is limited in English proficiency, age and grade often do not provide a suitable basis for comparison of performance, because English-language acquisition or learning (1) will have begun at different points in time for the bilingual individual as compared to the monolingual individual (at a later age, such as entry to kindergarten vs. from birth); (2) will result in differences in language exposure in terms of number of languages (two instead of one); and (3) will result in differences in terms of number of hours of experience with English (significantly less for non-native English speakers). In the case of the dual-language learner, the test begins to measure the current level of language proficiency (which will continue to develop over time) more so than actual language or language-related ability (or disability). Thus, tests are linguistically biased not because of any inherent psychometric defect, but simply because of the expectations and assumptions regarding the comparability of language proficiency that are rarely met when working with diverse individuals.

In sum, use of tests without knowledge of their linguistic demands creates a situation in which the tests tend to "degenerate in unknown degrees into tests of English language proficiency" when used with non-native English speakers (Figueroa, 1990a, p. 93). Equitable assessment thus requires information regarding the individual's level of proficiency in English and any other language he or she has acquired or has been exposed to (no matter how little the exposure may be), and the degree or level of language required by any test or tests that will be used for the purposes of evaluation. Obtaining information regarding language proficiency is often accomplished through use of one of the many English-language proficiency tests available on the market today (see also Chapter 9), whereas information regarding the linguistic characteristics of tests can be found via the cultural and linguistic extensions of the CHC Cross-Battery approach discussed later in this chapter.

## Norm Sample Inclusion versus Representation

At the most fundamental level, standardized norm-referenced tests are designed to provide information that allows comparison of individual performance against the performance of a group of individuals with similar characteristics when all other relevant factors are controlled. The notions and rationale behind standardization, mainly the concept of generalizability, go hand-in-hand with the use of norms in achieving this purpose. Naturally, norm samples over the years have become increasingly more representative with regard to issues of age, gender, race, education level, socioeconomic status, geographic location, etc. The difficulty with norms in the assessment of culturally and linguistically different individuals lies in the question regarding exactly what constitutes adequate representation. In order to draw valid comparisons of true performance, the underlying assumption of comparability regarding experiential background must hold true. The importance of this assumption is revealed in comments by Salvia and Ysseldyke (1991), in which they emphasize the danger in drawing conclusions in situations where the assumption is not met:

> Incorrect educational decisions may well be made. It must be pointed out that acculturation is a matter of experiential background rather than of gender, skin color, race, or ethnic background. When we say that a child's acculturation differs from that of the group used as a norm, we are saying that the *experiential background* differs, not simply that the child is of different ethnic origin, for example, from the children on whom the test was standardized. (p. 18)

Salvia and Ysseldyke's comments make it clear that skin color, race, or ethnicity should not be equated with cultural differences—or more accurately, acculturational differences—and that it is the difference in experiential background (which may or may not be related to differences in cultural background) that adversely affects test performance. Because these differences in experiences occur as a function of cultural differences, not racial or ethnic differences, test "fairness" rests not so much on the inclusion of racially or ethnically diverse individuals (e.g., in accordance with their frequency in the general population) as it does on controls for variation in cultural experiences (Valdés & Figueroa, 1996). It cannot be overstated that *stratification in the norm sample on the basis of race is not equivalent to stratification on the basis of culture*. Indeed, there are no tests currently available that have norm samples in which differences in experiential background (i.e., acculturation) have been systematically controlled. Despite its importance in establishing a defensible and fair basis for comparisons of performance, adequate representation of culturally diverse individuals within any norm sample simply has not been achieved (Cummins, 1984; Figueroa, 1990a; Samuda, Kong, Cummins, Pascual-Leone, & Lewis, 1991; Valdés & Figueroa, 1996). In recognition of the difficulty of such an accomplishment, it seems likely that test developers will continue to permit the illusion and promote the fallacy that racial inclusion in the norm sample is equivalent to cultural fairness in the test when clearly, it is not.

In similar fashion, differences in English-language proficiency between individuals is a variable that also remains uncontrolled in the norm samples of present-day tests of all kinds. LEP individuals do not differ from the mainstream simply because they lack English proficiency (although that is an important distinction) but also because they are *bilingual*—they possess two or more linguistic histories and developmental patterns that are distinct from their monolingual English-speaking counterparts. The dimensions of bilingualism and its evolution within individuals and across generations are well known and predictable (Hakuta, 1986; Valdés & Figueroa, 1996). Nowhere is the issue of bilingualism more salient or more controversial than in U.S. public schools. Because the fundamental goal of the U.S. educational system is English literacy, irrespective of the manner or specific program used to achieve this goal, every pupil who enters the system as a non-English or limited-English speaker is invariably set upon a path toward circumstantial bilingualism (Krashen, 1985). Although language proficiency is a major factor in attenuating performance on standardized tests, test developers have not often recognized, or have largely ignored, the significance of creating norm samples that stratify groups on the basis of dual-language ability or bilingualism. Instead, the testing industry, as have many professionals, seems to view the issue rather superficially—as one that relates to overcoming the language "barrier." The result has been the development of native-language tests with monolingual native-language norms that are no more appropriate for bilingual individuals living in the United States than are the English-language norms.

For example, the Batería–R: Pruebas de habilidad cognitiva (Batería-R COG; Woodcock & Muñoz-Sandoval, 1993) is an extremely well-designed and sophisticated native-language cognitive ability test, yet its norm sample is comprised primarily of monolingual Spanish speakers, just as the norm samples of its English-language counterparts, the Woodcock–Johnson Revised (WJ-R) and Woodcock–Johnson III (WJ III), are comprised of monolingual English speakers. Because it is the experience of dual-language or *bilingual* development that is the crucial factor in establishing comparability, norm samples comprised of monolingual Spanish speakers cannot be said to offer the implied representative comparison group for U.S. bilingual people. Although some bilingual individuals are undoubtedly included in the norm samples of various native-language tests, their inclusion remains largely perfunctory and does little to to provide an adequate basis for comparison to other individuals of varying acculturation and bilingualism residing in the United States. In the absence of appropriate norms, measuring the cognitive or intellectual performance of diverse individuals, whether in English or the native language, becomes a question of validity. Such tests amount to a measure of language proficiency and acculturation more than of actual cognitive ability (Cummins, 1984; Valdés & Figueroa, 1996). This conclusion is shared by a number of researchers (e.g., Bialystok, 1991; Figueroa, 1990b; Samuda et al., 1991), all of whom endorse the contention that "tests developed without accounting for language differences are limited in their validity and on how they can be interpreted" (Figueroa, 1990a, p. 94).

## Nonverbal Assessment

In working with dual-language learners, there is a common misconception that use of "nonverbal" or "performance" tests of cognitive ability or intelligence effectively addresses issues related to language bias or linguistic demand, and even cultural loading, to some extent. For example, an impressive, mass-mailing advertisement for the Leiter International Performance Scale—Revised (Leiter-R; Roid & Miller, 1997) once proclaimed in bold letters on the front page that it contained "no cultural or language bias" and that it was "fair for all cultural and ethnic backgrounds." The reality, however, is that reducing the oral or spoken language requirements in any given test does not, in fact, eliminate all the potential linguistic bias and does little, if anything, to reduce bias related to acculturation (Flanagan & Ortiz, 2001; Ortiz, 2001). Administering tests that utilize less oral-language demands can certainly assist in generating less discriminatory results for individuals whose English proficiency is not commensurate with their same-age peers (McCallum & Bracken, 1997). Yet apparent "fairness" of these tests is often illusory, particularly with regard to the issues described above: norm sample representation and cultural loading (Figueroa, 1990a).

There seems to be an unwritten rule in assessment that when working with linguistically diverse individuals, tests that are nonverbal (i.e., that do not require verbal responses) are inherently preferable to those that are verbal (i.e., require spoken responses). However, although nonverbal tests may not require any oral or expressive language ability, per se, they often require of the examinee a high level of nonverbal receptive language skill in order to comprehend the examiner's instructions and expectations (e.g., Wechsler Block Design). In other words, tests that are often seen as representing verbally reduced functioning may contain lengthy and possibly confusing verbal directions that can affect an individual's ability to comprehend what is expected or to provide an appropriate response. Test performance, even with tests administered entirely with gestures or in pantomime, continues to remain dependent upon the level of communication, albeit nonverbal, between the examiner and examinee, and both individuals' ability to interact effectively in a nonverbal manner. In addition, the type of nonverbal communication that may be required for administration in such tests often carries as much or more culturally based implications than verbal communication (Ehrman, 1996).

The presence or absence of physical gestures, facial nuances, and subtle body movements and their meanings are very culturally bound elements of any attempts at communication and significantly affect the interaction. In sum, nonverbal tests may well carry less language demands, as compared to verbally oriented tests, and as such, do represent, in general, better alternatives for English-language learners who might otherwise have significant difficulty with high language demands. But they are by no means the "answer" to the issues being addressed here, because they continue to have many of the same problems that plague verbal tests (e.g., inadequate norm sample representation, cultural loading, narrow range of measured abilities).

## BILINGUAL ASSESSMENT VERSUS ASSESSMENT OF BILINGUAL INDIVIDUALS

The zeal for the development of native-language tests (i.e., tests in languages other than English) has resulted in the availability of a wide range of tests and batteries in other languages. Having a choice of tests that may be available in two or more languages raises interesting issues regarding the appropriate methods and procedures that should be employed in assessment. The basic question is whether to attempt "bilingual assessment" or "assessment of bilingual individuals." Practitioners who engage in the assessment of diverse individuals need to understand clearly the difference between the two, what each approach entails, and which one falls within the scope of their competency, training, and ability.

## Bilingual Assessment

Use of tests in which the language of administration is other than English requires either that the examiner possess the linguistic competency to administer the test in the individual's native language or the use of an interpreter/translator (Lopez, 1997, 2002). In the case of diverse individuals, questions about the language(s) of assessment often arise, especially in light of legal mandates regarding evaluation in the primary language. It is often believed that native-language testing constitutes bilingual assessment, but this is incorrect. Bilingual assessment is rightfully defined as evaluation of a bilingual individual, by a bilingual examiner, in a bilingual manner. That is, both the examiner and the examinee are free to use both languages (English and the native language) as may be necessary or desired throughout the testing process. As noted, the bilingual mind is not merely two monolingual minds in one (Bialystok, 1991; Grosjean, 1989; Hakuta, 1986). Bilingual individuals freely code switch (i.e., shift from one language to another) as the need or situation might indicate (Bialystock, 1991; Cole & Cole, 1993; Grosjean, 1989; Hamayan & Damico, 1991a). Bilingual assessment also requires a practitioner (1) who is knowledgeable about, and familiar with, the examinee's culture; (2) who has the prerequisite training and education in nondiscriminatory assessment, including knowledge about how culture and language differences affect test performance; (3) who speaks the examinee's language fluently enough to evaluate functioning properly (Ochoa, Powell, & Robles-Piña, 1996; Ortiz, 2002). Given the small fraction of practitioners who possesses all of these skills and training, it is safe to say that such evaluation is quite rare (Ochoa, Powell, & Robles-Piña, 1996).

By the definition just outlined, there is little doubt that the vast majority of current evaluative practices conducted under the moniker of *bilingual assessment* are not, in fact, bilingual but rather monolingual (in the native language) or bilingual only in the sense that evaluation was conducted in two different languages (which is, perhaps, more accurately described as *multilingual* in nature). Interpreters are sometimes employed to assist in the process of evaluation, but even in these cases, the process cannot be considered truly bilingual in nature. In fact, use of an interpreter may result in additional confusion regarding the nature and meaning of test results, primarily because there is a tendency to discount the influence of native-language proficiency on performance on native-language tests. It is important to recognize that "mere possession of the capacity to communicate in an individual's native language does not ensure appropriate, nondiscriminatory assessment of that individual. Traditional assessment practices and their inherent biases can be easily replicated in any number of languages" (Flanagan et al., 2000, p. 291). That which meets the definition for true bilingual assessment is an entirely new endeavor in assessment for which there is virtually no research to guide the process of evaluation or interpretation. As such, efforts in this regard should be undertaken only by individuals who possess the specific competencies noted above and with recognition of the fact that such evaluation is not guided by any currently accepted standards of practice. As is discussed later, the lack of any literature base to use as a foundation and guide for assessment means that bilingual assessment, as defined here, is difficult to defend because it may not be accomplished in a systematic manner or based on established psychometric principles.

### Bilingual Assessment and the Bilingual Verbal Ability Test

The Bilingual Verbal Ability Test (BVAT; Muñoz-Sandoval, Cummins, Alvarado, & Ruef, 1998) deserves particular mention because it is perhaps the very first test ever developed that attempts to examine the bilingual abilities of the bilingual individual. The BVAT is comprised of three tests drawn from the WJ-R COG (Picture Vocabulary, Oral Vocabulary, and Verbal Analogies) with an approximate administration time of 30 minutes. Administration of the three subtests is done first in English and any missed items are subsequently readministered in the native language. Items that the individual was able to answer correctly in the native language are then added to the score for correct items obtained in English to get a total score for the subtest. The resulting composite score is seen as a reflection of the individual's combined knowledge in both languages and referred to as bilingual verbal ability, or BVA. The BVAT also provides a measure of cognitive academic language proficiency (CALP; Cummins, 1984) in English and generates an aptitude score that could presumably be used to predict or compare performance on the Woodcock–Johnson—Revised Tests of Achievement (WJ-R ACH; Woodcock & Johnson, 1989).

The developers of the BVAT are to be commended for pioneering this new research arena. Their test represents an important advance in construction compared to existing native-language tests and a significant departure from the way in which abilities of bilingual individuals have traditionally been conceptualized (as possessing independent language abilities). However, many of the cautions outlined previously regarding standardized tests have not been fully addressed by the BVAT. For example, although the norm sample of the BVAT includes some bilingual individuals, it has no actual systematic control for issues related to acculturation, language proficiency (either in English or the native language), or type of bilingual education program that such bilingual individuals have received or are receiving. People who are raised in their native culture, with native-language-speaking parents, and educated in their native language are largely monolingual and do not represent the types of individuals encountered in the United States—who, by definition and policy, are in the process of becoming bilingual immediately upon entrance into the public school system. Therefore, not only are the backgrounds of U.S. bilingual individuals not comparable to monolingual English speakers in the United States, they are also no longer comparable to the monolingual individuals of the culture from whence they came. Additionally, the linguistic ability of the individual is still measured in a consecutive, monolingual fashion, not a truly bilingual fashion. As discussed previously, bilingual individuals do not divide their communication into separate, disconnected strings of discourse. Bilingual communication is fluid and dynamic, alternating effortlessly between languages at the whim of the speaker. Indeed, bilingual communication is only possible between bilingual individuals and cannot be captured adequately merely by stitching together separate tasks. Other concerns with the BVAT pertain to the true nature and utility of the BVA composite, which at times is purported to be a measure of general intellectual ability, whereas at other times it is upheld as an indicator of language proficiency. These shortcomings notwithstanding, future refinements of the BVAT and information culled from the small but emerging research on the nature of bilingual assessment will no doubt continue to improve the BVAT and advance the research trend it has begun.

## Bilingual Assessment and the Broad Cognitive Ability—Bilingual Scale

Alvarado (1999) developed a method for evaluating the broad cognitive ability of bilingual individuals in a manner that relies on language-reduced tests in English and, where available, results from native-language testing to form the Broad Cognitive Ability—Bilingual Scale (BCA-Bil). In general, the BCA-Bil is comprised of selected tests drawn from a specific combination of the BVAT, the WJ-R COG, and the Batería-R COG (see Table 10.1). The BCA-Bil attempts to measure a broad range of cognitive functioning in keeping with the notion of a general or broad ability measure, by incorporating at least one test of the various CHC broad abilities that are commonly measured in evaluation (i.e., Crystallized Intelligence [Gc], Fluid Intelligence [Gf], Auditory Processing [Ga], Visual Processing [Gv], Processing Speed [Gs], Short-Term Memory [Gsm], and Long-Term Storage and Retrieval [Glr]). As can be seen in Table 10.1, Gc is measured by the BVA composite from the BVAT, and tests 1, 3, 7, 12, 17, and 18 are drawn from the WJ-R COG or Batería-R COG. Because the Batería-R COG provides parallel, Spanish-language assessment of the same abilities as the WJ-R COG, the subtests that comprise the BCA-Bil for Spanish speakers are taken from the native-language battery rather than the WJ-R COG and provide mostly a native-language measure of all abilities. However, for any language other than Spanish, the BCA-Bil is represented by the BVA composite from the BVAT, plus the six additional tests given in English and pulled from the WJ-R COG.

Much as with the BVAT, the BCA-Bil is an approach that pioneers the attempt to validly measure the cognitive abilities of bilingual individuals in a manner that is more consistent with modern conceptualizations of bilingual functioning. The BCA-Bil represents a balance between measurement of a broad range of cognitive abilities (as opposed to nonverbal assessments that tend to measure primarily Gv or Gf and little else) and linguistic concerns regarding issues of dominance and accommodations for native-language ability. The BCA-Bil represents a sophisticated and systematic adaptation of available tests that may well provide a more accurate estimate of the global functioning of individuals from diverse backgrounds. Yet some cautionary concerns regarding its utility and validity, much like that with the BVAT, are necessary. For example, the BCA-Bil contains only one measure of each of the broad abilities (with the exception of Gc, because the BVA composite from the BVAT is comprised of three tests). Thus, actual deficits in ability, as might be

TABLE 10.1. Composition of the BCA-Bil

| Cognitive factor | English- or other-language dominant: WJ-R COG and BCA (Bil) | Spanish-language dominant: Batería-R COG and BCA (Bil) |
| --- | --- | --- |
| Verbal Ability (Gc) | BVAT BVA | BVAT BVA |
| Long-Term Retrieval (Glr) | Test 1: Memory for Names | Test 1: Memoria para nombres |
| Short-Term Memory (Gsm) | Test 17: Numbers Reversed | Test 17: Inversión de números |
| Processing Speed (Gs) | Test 3: Visual Matching | Test 3: Pareo visual |
| Auditory Processing (Ga) | Test 18: Sound Patterns | Test 18: Configuración de sonidos |
| Visual Processing (Gv) | Test 12: Picture Recognition | Test 12: Reconocimiento de dibujos |
| Fluid Reasoning (Gf) | Test 7: Analysis–Synthesis | Test 7: Análisis–Síntesis |

*Note.* Adapted from Alvarado (1999, p. 1). Copyright 1999 by Riverside Publishing Company. Adapted by permission.

expected in the case of individuals with a true disability (e.g., LD), or even spuriously low scores on any one of these abilities might attenuate the overall score. Moreover, the lack of at least two measures for each broad ability precludes reliable interpretation of functioning in those areas (again, with the exception of *Gc*).

The psychometric issues of the BCA-Bil are relatively unimportant in light of the larger issue of validity. As with the scores from all other standardized tests, the BCA-Bil composite is derived from norm samples that remain based primarily upon monolingual populations (approximately 6,359 English speakers for the WJ-R COG and 2,000 Spanish speakers for the Batería-R COG). Likewise, the norm samples are constructed without any systematic control for level of acculturation. Whether testing in English or the subject's native language, it cannot be overlooked that what is being measured in bilingual examinees is not necessarily true ability but rather English- or native-language proficiency as well as level of acculturation to the U.S. mainstream. These criticisms should not mask the fact that Alvarado (1999) offered perhaps the very first attempt to provide an estimate of the entire repertoire of ability and knowledge available to the bilingual mind and has advanced the standards to which future methods for evaluating bilingual individuals should strive to reach.

Alvarado (1999) also attempted to evaluate the broad range of differences in linguistic ability and the impact of those differences on performance. In examining the correlations between two estimates of the BVA composite for reliability (one in which the subtests were administered first in English, and another in which the subtests were administered first in Spanish), Alvarado categorized the subjects in terms of language dominance and created five categories: monolingual Spanish dominant, bilingual but Spanish dominant, bilingual with equal dominance in Spanish and English, bilingual but English dominant, and monolingual English. Although not the main purpose of the BCA-Bil, this study exemplifies the type of research that is emerging and which is desperately needed within the nascent field of bilingual assessment.

### Bilingual Assessment and the General Intellectual Ability—Bilingual Scale

The release of the Woodcock–Johnson III Tests of Achievement (WJ III) (Woodcock, McGrew, & Mather, 2001a) necessitated realignment of the BCA-Bil components based on the WJ-R. The new incarnation of this composite is now called the General Intellectual Ability—Bilingual Scale (GIA-Bil). Contained within the framework of the Diagnostic Supplement to the WJ III, the GIA-Bil is both conceptually and structurally similar to the old BCA-Bil. Indeed, the changes are rather cosmetic. For example, the GIA-Bil maintains the practice of including at least one measure of each of the seven broad CHC abilities, and many of the tests included remain unchanged. For example, Long-Term Retrieval (*Glr*), Short-Term Memory (*Gsm*), Processing Speed (*Gs*), and Auditory Processing (*Ga*) are measured by the very same tests used for the BCA-Bil (and taken from the WJ-R) and which now appear in the WJ III. The two changes made in the composition of the GIA-Bil related to Visual Processing (*Gv*), which is now measured by Spatial Relations instead of Picture Recognition, and Fluid Reasoning (*Gf*), which is now measured by Concept Formation instead of Analysis–Synthesis. The specific tests that comprise the GIA-Bil are noted in Table 10.2 alongside the tests from the BCA-Bil for comparative purposes.

According to the information contained in the manual of the Diagnostic Supplement, it is intended to expand the applicability of the WJ III to bilingual populations. The GIA-Bil is built

TABLE 10.2. Comparison of the Composition of the GIA-Bil and BCA-Bil

| Cognitive factor/cluster | GIA-Bil tests (2003) | BCA-Bil tests (1998) |
|---|---|---|
| Verbal Ability | | |
| Comprehension and Knowledge (*Gc*)—for English/Spanish speakers | **Test 1: Verbal Comprehension** **Test 31: Bilingual Verbal Comprehension** | BVAT BVA |
| Comprehension and Knowledge (*Gc*)—for English- and other-language speakers | BVAT BVA | BVAT BVA |
| Thinking Abilities | | |
| Long-Term Retrieval (*Glr*) | Test 21: Memory for Names | Test 1: Memory for Names |
| Auditory Processing (*Ga*) | Test 23: Sound Patterns | Test 18: Sound Patterns |
| Visual Processing (*Gv*) | **Test 3: Spatial Relations** | Test 12: Picture Recognition |
| Fluid Reasoning (*Gf*) | **Test 5: Concept Formation** | Test 7: Analysis–Synthesis |
| Cognitive Efficiency | | |
| Processing Speed (*Gs*) | Test 6: Visual Matching | Test 3: Visual Matching |
| Short-Term Memory (*Gsm*) | Test 7: Numbers Reversed | Test 17: Numbers Reversed |

*Note.* Tests in **bold** were added or changed in the construction of the GIA-Bil from the BCA-Bil. Data from Alvarado (1999) and Woodcock, McGrew, Mather, and Schrank (2003).

upon a language-reduced bilingual thinking ability cluster and a procedure borrowed from the BVAT for assessing the verbal ability of bilingual English/Spanish subjects. As can be seen in Table 10.2, Test 1, Verbal Comprehension, and Test 31, Bilingual Verbal Comprehension, form the pair of tests drawn from the BVAT that are combined to yield an overall verbal ability score. These tests are appropriate only for Spanish/English bilingual individuals; however, examiners may use the BVAT to obtain a measure of verbal comprehension in any of the languages available. The Bilingual Verbal Ability (BVA) may be substituted for the verbal comprehension composite, which will then be used in the derivation of the GIA-Bil.

One of the stated goals in the development of the GIA-Bil was to provide a language-reduced format throughout the testing. The attempt to provide a language-reduced format for the tests comprising the GIA-Bil represents an accommodation consistent with the longstanding practice of using less verbally laden or linguistically demanding tests. Indeed, a systematic method for selection of tests with reduced language and cultural demands has been developed to assist practitioners in this regard (Ortiz & Flanagan, 1998; Flanagan et al., 2000; Flanagan & Ortiz, 2001). Yet, it seems rather curious that only two of the six tests were actually changed from the original BCA-Bil in developing the GIA-Bil and that one of those tests, Concept Formation, is one in which the respondent is asked to make fine semantic distinctions in the use of the conjunctions "and" and "or" as well as to express an abstract relationship in linguistic terms. Conversely, the change from Picture Recognition to Spatial Relations in the measurement of *Gv* seems much more logical.

Unlike the BCA-Bil, the GIA-Bil also specifies clinical clusters that may be evaluated in addition to the broad CHC abilities being measured. These clinical clusters include Verbal Ability (essentially the *Gc* factor), Thinking Abilities (comprised of *Gv*, *Gf*, *Glr*, and *Ga*), and Cognitive Efficiency (measured by *Gs* and *Gsm*). Although these clusters do not represent theoretically specified constructs, they are helpful in understanding patterns of performance in some cases.

Apart from these minor organizational and structural changes, the GIA-Bil remains much the same as its predecessor and is thus subject to many of the same criticisms and limitations (which need not be repeated here). Practitioners should remain cognizant of the difficulties related to instruments and procedures used in bilingual assessment. For as desirable as practitioners may wish it to be, neither the BVAT, BCA-Bil, nor the GIA-Bil can be viewed as substantive solutions to the intricacies involved in bilingual assessment. The sophistication of psychometric methods often impresses, but until there is an appropriate accounting of the two variables that most significantly and directly influence the resultant validity—developmental differences in dual-language proficiency and acculturation—fair and equitable bilingual assessment will remain quite problematic. Nonetheless, although by no means perfect, the methods described herein are the only guidelines and procedures available to practitioners for engaging in bilingual assessment, and they have begun to set the standard for what will surely follow.

## Assessment of Bilinguals

Assessment of bilingual individuals is defined as the practice of giving monolingual tests in monolingual fashion to bilingual individuals, without specific regard to their bilingual ability, and in a manner that does not actually involve bilingual interchange between the examiner and the examinee. As described previously, repeated testing in one language and then another, even if one of the languages is the individual's native language, may seem to be bilingual, but it is not, and therefore should remain rightly a practice couched under the general rubric of assessment of bilingual individuals. According to Ortiz (2002), "assessment of bilinguals is the line of inquiry where the vast majority of research and practice exists and it has been conducted almost exclusively with tests given in English to people with varying levels of English language proficiency but rarely in a systematic way" (p. 7). Thus, compared to bilingual assessment, which is an emerging field, a great deal more is known about how people who are non-native English speakers will perform on standardized tests given in English than is known about how they perform on tests given bilingually or in their native language. This larger knowledge base is perhaps the one area that makes assessment of bilingual individuals much more practical and defensible than bilingual assessment—and, more importantly, which brings the practice within the professional reach of the vast majority of practitioners who are not bilingual.

Bilingual assessment, as described in the previous section, requires possession of linguistic competency, not to mention education and training in nondiscriminatory assessment methods and procedures. Assessment of bilingual individuals only requires the latter. Given the fact that the vast majority of evaluations to be conducted on individuals from diverse backgrounds will not be conducted by evaluators who possess both the linguistic proficiency and the evaluative competency necessary to conduct a fair and equitable evaluation, it is perhaps fortuitous that systematic and practical methods for nondiscriminatory assessment do exist and are available to the largest segment of the practitioner population. These methods and procedures comprise the content of the next chapter, where they are discussed at length.

## SUMMARY

It is no doubt apparent at this point that assessment of culturally and linguistically diverse individuals is far more complicated than it may seem on the surface and certainly involves a great deal more than the misguided search for the "right" test. The manner in which tests are constructed and the psychometric principles that underlie their development inevitably lead to problems when carried over to populations for whom many of the basic assumptions do not hold true (e.g., comparable levels of language development as a function of age). Although these tests have been shown to have little psychometric bias, as traditionally defined, it cannot be disputed that they remain culturally loaded and linguistically demanding—that is, they continue to require some type of communication, verbal or nonverbal, in order to be administered. Even in cases where the difficulties in communicating with the examinee are managed, the resulting increase in "fairness" does little to establish a defensible basis for the validity of any obtained results, let alone for the generalizability of any particular findings, because norm samples do not account for the varying levels of proficiency in two different languages that mark bilingual individuals as distinct from native-language or English-only speakers.

Bilingual individuals are simply not the same as monolingual individuals and they cannot be treated as such or evaluated as if they were (Bialystok, 1991). Because they differ in significant ways with regard to language development, they may also differ with regard to cognitive development and acquisition of academic skills. Moreover, linguistic differences are very often accompanied by cultural differences, which have the same potential to influence cognitive and academic development (and hence test performance) in ways that are not common or comparable to monolingual age- or grade-related peers of the mainstream culture. These differences are developmentally based, invariant, and must be clearly understood in relation to the structural and psychometric properties of tests in order to reveal the reasons that may underlie poor performance.

Unfortunately, how to accommodate all of the relevant variables in the process of assessment remains a rather daunting task, particularly for practitioners with either little background in these issues or little training and experience in working with individuals from diverse backgrounds. It is precisely from this need to find a way to allow practitioners the opportunity to more easily and systematically integrate these many variables that several new approaches to the assessment of culturally and linguistically diverse individuals have been born. These new approaches are discussed in the next chapter.

# 11

# Cognitive Assessment of Culturally and Linguistically Diverse Individuals

## An Integrated Approach

In the preceding chapter, issues related to conceptual, methodological, and measurement problems were presented and discussed. In attempting to provide some type of nondiscriminatory assessment of culturally and linguistically diverse individuals, practitioners must become well acquainted with such issues as they establish the context within which evaluation must occur and upon which its validity must rest. Indeed, any approach to the cognitive assessment of diverse individuals will need to consider, manage, and ultimately integrate these issues successfully, if it is to represent a viable and defensible option for evaluation.

In general, there are two basic questions that confront practitioners from the outset in the assessment of culturally and linguistically diverse individuals. The first question revolves primarily around the type and nature of the assessment to be conducted. On the surface it would appear that this decision is a rather straightforward matter that often involves an assessment of language dominance (i.e., the individual's preferred and better developed language) and then evaluating accordingly. There are several problems with this approach that are best summarized by the fact that bilingual speakers do not cease to be bilingual by virtue of having become English (or other-language) dominant. Consider first that few tests are available in languages other than Spanish. More importantly, such an approach fails to accommodate the student's varying levels of development in both languages, as influenced by formal education and acculturational experience that differentially influence expectations regarding test performance. The most appropriate approach or modality of assessment (i.e., bilingual, nonverbal, English, or native language) depends primarily on knowledge and integration of the individual's current age or grade, the type and nature of formal education he or she has received, and his or her current level of proficiency in both languages, not simply relative dominance. The first part of this chapter focuses on the delineation of an approach that has been intentionally designed to address these issues directly and that can provide practitioners with the necessary structure and guidance in determining the most appropriate modality of assessment for individuals in specific cases and situations.

---

This chapter is by Samuel O. Ortiz and Salvador Hector Ochoa.

The second fundamental question facing practitioners, once the modality of assessment has been determined, is whether the obtained test results were influenced primarily by the individual's cultural or linguistic difference than by actual or true ability. Having found an appropriate avenue for data collection does not automatically establish the validity of the results. In order to have confidence in the conclusions or interpretations that may be drawn from a particular constellation of test scores, practitioners must be reasonably certain, and able to defend the proposition, that what was measured in the individual, as reflected by test scores, was not primarily level of acculturation or English-language proficiency but real ability. Accordingly, the latter portion of this chapter revolves around discussion of an approach that was designed specifically to address the relative influence of cultural and linguistic factors on test performance, namely the CHC culture–language classifications and interpretive matrix (Ortiz & Flanagan, 1998; Flanagan et al., 2000; Flanagan & Ortiz, 2001; Ortiz, 2001). This approach provides practitioners with some guidance regarding test selection; however, its main purpose is to allow a systematic evaluation of the basic question presented at the outset: To what extent are the obtained test scores more a reflection of acculturational level or English-language proficiency than true ability?

Before proceeding further, we wish to state clearly that although the approaches presented in this chapter are designed to make assessment fairer, our guidelines and recommendations should not be viewed as a complete or comprehensive solution to all the potentially discriminatory aspects of assessing multilingual–multicultural populations. Comprehensive nondiscriminatory assessment involves the collection of multiple sources of data under the direction of a broad, systematic framework that uses the individual's cultural and linguistic history as the ultimate and most appropriate context from which to derive meaning and conclusions. Delineation of such a framework is well beyond the scope of this chapter, and the reader is referred elsewhere for a more detailed discussion (Ortiz & Flanagan, 2002; Ortiz, 2002). The methods outlined in the following sections are mainly intended to address how standardized tests can be utilized with diverse populations and how results obtained from their use may be interpreted in a nondiscriminatory manner. We believe that when standardized tests are chosen for use in any given assessment, the following recommendations will ensure that the obtained results are evaluated and interpreted in a systematic and defensible manner that helps to reduce bias related to issues of validity.

## THE OCHOA AND ORTIZ MULTIDIMENSIONAL ASSESSMENT MODEL FOR BILINGUAL INDIVIDUALS

One of the most important decisions facing practitioners in the evaluation of culturally and linguistically diverse individuals relates to selecting the most appropriate mode and language(s) of assessment. Making these decisions is complicated by the wide variety of factors that must be considered carefully and integrated simultaneously. At the very least, practitioners must balance at least four significant variables: (1) the current grade of the student; (2) the mode of assessment (reduced culture/language, native language, English, or both languages); (3) the current and previous types of educational program; and (4) the individual's current degree of language proficiency in both English and the native language. Given the wide range of variability inherent in some of these factors, the combinations that can result are rather daunting—and not surprisingly can quickly overwhelm even seasoned evaluators.

In recognition of the complexity of managing these variables, we have developed a method that can assist practitioners in selecting the most appropriate type and language of assessment for any particular case. Figure 11.1 illustrates our attempt to integrate these issues in a manner that accounts for the four major variables noted previously. We call this guiding framework the Multi-dimensional Assessment Model for Bilingual Individuals (MAMBI); it is the first systematic integration of these variables in the context of evaluating bilingual populations. Figure 11.1 is an initial attempt to integrate the most important variables that affect the decision to engage in assessment: (1) language profile, (2) instructional programming/history, (3) current grade level, and (4) assessment modality.

## Language Profile

As discussed in Chapter 9, the issues related to language proficiency in both languages form a critical foundation for determining the most appropriate method of assessment of the bilingual student. Table 9.1 contained a description of the various combinations of language proficiency that can be evaluated in terms of CALP level (1–5) in both languages, which must be considered simultaneously. As noted in that table, a CALP level of 1–2 is considered "minimal" proficiency, a CALP level of 3 is operationally defined as an "emergent" level of proficiency, and a CALP level of 4–5 is operationally defined as a "fluent" level of proficiency. The level of CALP, as discussed in Chapter 9, is determined by multiple sources of data, including, but not limited to, the CALP score obtained from the Woodcock–Muñoz Language Survey (WMLS), along with other informal measures of language functioning and proficiency. Practitioners must recognize that no single score or procedure should be used as the sole criterion for determining level of language proficiency or CALP. The limitations of existing tests (i.e., norm-sample representation) and the relative lack of theoretical specification underlying the concept of CALP necessitate the collection of a wide range of data on language before any conclusions regarding proficiency can be drawn.

English-language learners are most likely to be characterized by language profiles 1, 2, 3, 4, 5, 6, and 9. Profile 9 (fluent L1/fluent L2) will most likely reflect the experience of English-language learners who were enrolled in maintenance or dual-language bilingual programs, or of those who recently immigrated to the United States after receiving an appropriate and consistent education in their native country through at least the fifth grade and who have received at least 1 or 2 years of English-language development, aided by their native language CALP.

Profiles 7 (minimal L1/fluent L2) and 8 (emergent L1/fluent L2) are unlikely to characterize the typical English-language learner. The pattern of fluency in English prior to, or instead of, equivalent fluency in the native language suggests that these students have atypical or very unusual linguistic histories. For example, a child in a foreign country who begins learning a native language prior to being adopted by the age of 2 or 3 by monolingual English-speaking parents from the United States could conceivably achieve this pattern by the fifth grade. Likewise, fourth- and possibly some third-generation children being raised or cared for during the day partly by grandparents who have limited or no English proficiency, but with parents who have fluent English abilities, may also display this unusual pattern. The rarity of this type of linguistic profile, coupled with the fact that fluency in English has been obtained in a way and to a degree that closely resembles that of their monolingual English-speaking peers (i.e., nearly from birth, with monolingual English-speaking parents in a monolingual English-speaking environment), suggests that such students may be assessed in the same manner as a native English speaker.

## OCHOA AND ORTIZ MULTIDIMENSIONAL ASSESSMENT MODEL FOR BILINGUAL INDIVIDUALS

| Instructional program/history | Currently in a bilingual education program in lieu of, or in addition to, receiving ESL services | | | | | | | | Previously in bilingual education program, now receiving English-only or ESL services | | | | | | | | All instruction has been in an English-only program, with or without ESL services | | | | | | | |
|---|---|---|---|---|---|---|---|---|---|---|---|---|---|---|---|---|---|---|---|---|---|---|---|---|
| Current grade | K–4 | | | | 5–7 | | | | K–4 | | | | 5–7 | | | | K–4 | | | | 5–7 | | | |
| Assessment mode | NV | L1 | L2 | BL | NV | L1 | L2 | BL | NV | L1 | L2 | BL | NV | L1 | L2 | BL | NV | L1 | L2 | BL | NV | L1 | L2 | BL |
| Language profile 1 (L1 minimal/L2 minimal) | Ⓥ | √ | | √ | Ⓥ | √ | √ | √ | Ⓥ | √ | | √ | Ⓥ | | √ | √ | Ⓥ | √ | √* | √ | Ⓥ | | √ | √ |
| Language profile 2 (L1 emergent/L2 minimal) | Ⓥ | √ | | √ | Ⓥ | √ | √ | √ | Ⓥ | √ | | √ | Ⓥ | | √ | √ | Ⓥ | √ | √* | √ | | | | |
| Language profile 3 (L1 fluent/L2 minimal) | | Ⓥ | | | | Ⓥ | √ | | | Ⓥ | | | | Ⓥ | √ | | | | | | | | | |
| Language profile 4 (L1 minimal/L2 emergent) | Ⓥ | Ⓥ | | √ | Ⓥ | √ | √ | √ | Ⓥ | √ | √ | √ | Ⓥ | | √ | √ | Ⓥ | √ | √# | √ | Ⓥ | | √ | √ |
| Language profile 5 (L1 emergent/L2 emergent) | Ⓥ | √ | | √ | Ⓥ | √ | √ | √ | Ⓥ | √ | √ | √ | Ⓥ | √ | √ | √ | Ⓥ | √ | √# | √ | | | | |
| Language profile 6 (L1 fluent/L2 emergent) | | Ⓥ | | | | Ⓥ | √ | | | Ⓥ | √ | | | Ⓥ | √ | | | | | | | | | |
| Language profile 7 (L1 minimal/L2 fluent) | | | | | | | | | | | | | | | | | | | | | | | | |
| Language profile 8 (L1 emergent/L2 fluent) | | | | | | | | | | | | | | | | | | | | | | Ⓥ | | |
| Language profile 9 (L1 fluent/L2 fluent) | | | | | | Ⓥ | | | | | | | | Ⓥ | | | | | | | | | | |

FIGURE 11.1. The Ochoa and Ortiz Multidimensional Assessment Model for Bilingual Individuals (MAMBI). *Notes:* CALP level 1–2 = minimal proficiency; CALP level 3 = emergent proficiency; CALP level 4–5 = fluent proficiency. See Chapter 9 for more information. NV, assessment conducted primarily in a nonverbal manner with English-language–reduced/acculturation-reduced measures; L1, assessment conducted in the first language learned by the individual (i.e., native or primary language); L2, assessment conducted in the second language learned by the individual, which in most cases refers to English; BL, assessment conducted relatively equally in both languages learned by the individual (i.e., the native language and English); ■, combinations of language development and instruction that are improbable or due to other factors (e.g., Saturday school, foreign-born adoptees, delayed school entry); Ⓥ, recommended mode of assessment that should take priority over other modes and which is more likely to be the most accurate estimate of the student's true abilities; √, secondary or optional mode of assessment that may provide additional valuable information but which will likely result in an underestimate of the student's abilities; √*, mode of assessment not recommended for students in K–2, but may be informative in 3–4, although results will likely be an underestimate of true ability; √#, mode of assessment not recommended for students in K–1, but may be informative in 2–4, although results will likely be an underestimate of true ability.

## Instructional Programming/History and Current Grade Level

The second and third variables depicted in Figure 11.1 are related to the nature and type of instructional programming a pupil has received as well as his or her current grade level. Assessment would include careful analysis of experiences and histories of the child's educational programming. In general, English-language learners will most likely fall into one of three different educational circumstances. The first such circumstance involves whether the pupil currently participates *in a well-implemented bilingual education program, in lieu of, or in addition to, any ESL services* he or she may be receiving. Moreover, it must be known whether the pupil is currently in grade K–4 or 5–7. This point is important to ascertain because the research (see Chapter 4) is clear on the issue that the length of instruction in the native language is highly related to the development of the various linguistic proficiencies required for academic success (attainment of CALP). Students currently in this educational circumstance could be receiving a wide variety of instruction, ranging from transitional, maintenance, to dual-language, which will directly affect the development of CALP. Students who are in this educational circumstance and who are in grades 5–7 will likely be enrolled in a maintenance program or dual-language program that usually provides native-language instruction through grade 6 (long enough to firmly establish CALP in the native language.

The second educational circumstance—one of the more common histories encountered by English-language learners—is characterized by *students who have previously been in bilingual education but who are now receiving English-only instruction or ESL services*. Again, related to this consideration is the variable of current grade placement. Students in this educational circumstance who are in grades K–4 are likely to have been in a transitional type of bilingual program that typically force-exits students by the second or third grade (long before CALP has had time to develop adequately). Similarly, students in this educational circumstance who are in grades 5–7 have long since left native-language instruction behind, likely having also been in a transitional program, and therefore have not had the opportunity to attain sufficient levels of CALP to ensure academic success. For students in this educational circumstance, it should be emphasized that BICS not be equated with CALP. Such students will not only sound like native English speakers (due to lack of any perceptible accent), but they will also probably have suffered from the phenomenon known as language loss or deterioration (also described as subtractive bilingualism; see Chapter 4). The differences in language proficiency between the native-language and English speakers are often evaluated in terms of dominance—but then misinterpreted as indications of normal development, rather than of developmental processes that were altered by misguided or inappropriate pedagogy (sometimes known as program "casualties").

In the third educational circumstance—which is probably the most common situation in which the English language learner will find him- or herself—*all instruction has occurred in an English-only program with or without ESL services*. For students in both grade levels (K–4 and 5–7) no attention has been given, at any time, to the development of the native language and no opportunity to develop or acquire CALP in L1 to a degree that would generally ensure academic success. As these students progress through the educational system (i.e., K–12), the gap between the developmental level of their English language proficiency and the demands and expectations of the academic curriculum will widen and make it increasingly more difficult for them to succeed or compete academically. As noted in Chapter 4, these students may make adequate progress up to about third or fourth grade but will then begin to show a pattern of marked decline in achievement in English (Thomas & Collier, 1997, 2002).

The discussion of these three educational circumstances has been related primarily to the experiences of students who began their academic career (K–1) in the United States. We recognize, however, that some students enter the U.S. public school system at a later point (e.g., late elementary or junior high/high school). If these students received a normal and consistent education while residing in their native country, we would expect that they would have either already developed, or nearly developed, CALP in their native language (usually those students who come to the United States after grade 4). Indeed, the work of Cummins (1984) has demonstrated that the learning of English as a second language is greatly facilitated by the development of advanced fluency in the native language (i.e., CALP). For those students who come to the United States and enter the school system between grades K–4, CALP is not likely to have emerged or been established to a degree that is commensurate with academic expectations, and academic difficulties may result. Students who come to the United States from grade 5 or higher are much less likely to encounter academic problems, particularly after they have acquired BICS in English which takes only 1–3 years at the most. In these situations, it is important to obtain careful information about the nature and quality of instruction received in the student's native country. To the extent that the educational experience was appropriate, consistent, and well implemented, a reasonable expectation of CALP development can be determined.

## SELECTION OF ASSESSMENT MODALITY AS A FUNCTION OF LANGUAGE PROFILE, INSTRUCTIONAL PROGRAM/HISTORY, AND CURRENT GRADE LEVEL

When school-based practitioners are faced with assessing English-language learners, they must consider what is the most appropriate method for conducting the evaluation. The assessment can take the form of one or more of the following four approaches: (1) nonverbal assessment (NV); (2) assessment in the native language (L1); (3) assessment in English (L2); and (4) true bilingual assessment (BL). It should be noted that the first three modalities represent assessment practices that are in keeping with the definition we have specified regarding assessment of bilingual individuals, whereas the fourth modality refers to the definition and practices we have defined as the newer field of bilingual assessment. Despite our attempts to clarify and specify these approaches, we recognize that the significant limitations in current tools, instruments, and procedures will affect practitioners' ability to generate completely fair and equitable estimates of performance. Therefore, practitioners should not assume that after following the guidelines presented in this section and chapter, unbiased or nondiscriminatory results are inevitable. To the contrary, our efforts in specifying approaches to the selection of assessment modality, instruments, and an interpretive framework are meant to assist in reducing the current potential discriminatory aspects of assessment with bilingual individuals. The entire elimination of discriminatory aspects remains an unrealistic goal.

Our cautionary statements regarding the presumed validity of obtained results are represented graphically in Figure 11.1, where circled checkmarks indicate the recommended mode of assessment that should take priority over other modes. An underlined checkmark represents a secondary or optional mode of assessment that may provide additional valuable information but which will likely result in an underestimate of the student's abilities. The figure also contains blacked-out cells to indicate that these combinations of language development and instruction are either illogical, improbable, or could only occur with outside schooling (e.g., Saturday school, yeshiva, after-school programs). In addition, grey-shaded cells indicate that students who (1) display language profiles of these types (language profiles 1, 2, and 4), (2) are currently in, and have always been educated in, a bilingual education program, and (3) are now in 5th through 7th grades form a particular group of individuals whose language and academic development is most unexpected, given their background experiences and education.

## Nonverbal Assessment

The first modality, nonverbal (NV) assessment, is conducted primarily in a nonverbal manner with English-language-reduced and acculturation-reduced measures or instruments. Examples of instruments commonly used in this manner for this purpose include the Universal Nonverbal Intelligence Test (UNIT), the Leiter-R, selected tests from the Differential Abilities Scale (DAS), and the nonverbal components of the Stanford–Binet, 5th Edition (SB-5). Other instruments are often used, for example, those involving matrices; however, they tend to be less comprehensive in their measurement of the broad range of cognitive abilities compared to these instruments. We wish to emphasize that although nonverbal tests reduce the oral-language requirements expected of the examinee, the need for *communication* and receptive nonverbal comprehension remains unchanged. Whether prompted by signs, physical gestures, or short, abbreviated verbal prompts, the examinee must understand several important aspects of the process, in all testing situations, including what must be done, what is the expected correct response, when to begin, how quickly to work, and when to stop. The reduction or elimination of the oral-language requirement assists in overcoming the linguistic barrier that may exist between the examiner and the examinee, but it does not eliminate the influence of both the need for effective communication during the testing or the individual's level of acculturation with regard to the tasks being implemented and their respective degree of cultural loading. Although the examinee is not required to use oral- or expressive-language abilities, the tasks may nevertheless require some type of receptive language ability in order to fully comprehend the nature of the task at hand. The level of receptive language ability required will vary across nonverbal measures from none (i.e., the use of gestures 100% of the time) to comprehension of shortened/simplified verbal commands.

Although there have been previous recommendations for the use of nonverbal measures for all types of English-language learners, we advocate the use of nonverbal tests primarily for individuals who have not acquired CALP in either their native language or English (i.e., minimal or emergent in L1 or L2). These students fall under language profiles 1, 2, 4, and 5. The use of this modality is highly recommended for all students, irrespective of educational placement and grade level.

Our advocacy is cautious by design because we recognize that instruments classified as nonverbal approaches to the measurement of intelligence or cognitive ability vary considerably in the range of abilities that may be measured as well as those that comprise the composite scores that represent general intelligence with regard to the Cattell–Horn–Carroll (CHC) theory of cognitive abilities. For example, the Leiter-R provides adequate representation of only three broad abilities: *Gf* (Fluid Intelligence), *Gv* (Visual Processing), and *Glr* (Long-Term Retrieval). It underrepresents

*Gs* (Processing Speed), and other broad abilities, such as *Ga* (Auditory Processing), *Gsm* (Short-Term Memory), and *Gc* (Crystallized Intelligence), are not represented within the Leiter-R battery. In summary, there are no commercially available instruments that measure the full range of human cognitive abilities in a nonverbal manner.

The use of nonverbal instruments with English-language learners who have acquired a more advanced level of CALP (i.e., fluent in L1 or L2) may not be the optimal approach. These are students who fall under the language profiles 3, 6, and 9. Our recommendation is based on the fact that these students have developed CALP in either L1 or L2, which greatly reduces or eliminates the attenuating influence of the linguistic demands of any given test. Therefore, a better representation of their general cognitive functioning can be obtained via the use of instruments classified for use in either L1 or L2 assessment modalities, which provide a broader range of coverage with regard to broad abilities (vis-à-vis CHC theory). In fairness to the developers of these instruments, it should be noted that some cognitive abilities (e.g., auditory processing) may be extremely difficult, if not impossible, to measure independent of language and without the use of some type of oral-language requirement.

## Assessment in the Native Language

The second modality shown in Figure 11.1 is assessment in the native language (L1). Assessment of cognitive abilities or intelligence in L1 is rather limited because of the dearth of instruments available to assess in any language other than Spanish. The purpose of this modality is to provide a measure of functioning along particular cognitive abilities or general intelligence in the individual's native or primary language.

### Currently Participating in Bilingual Program, Grades K–4

Students in a well-implemented bilingual education program in grades K–4 would be expected to display language profiles 1 (L1 minimal/L2 minimal), 2 (L1 emergent/L2 minimal), or 5 (L1 emergent/L2 emergent). Although CALP has not been attained due to insufficient native-language instruction, use of this modality is recommended as a secondary-assessment option because it is important to collect information related to the language and cognitive development of the student. This information helps educators understand the potential factors that may affect a student's ability to function, in general, and in this specific academic setting. In addition, native-language assessment is relevant to the normal course of development expected of a student's age or grade-related peers, particularly with regard to the eventual emergence and attainment of CALP. Although this information is quite helpful, it should be noted that the obtained data may still underrepresent the student's true ability, because the degree of comparability (i.e., goodness of fit) between the student's cultural and linguistic background and the cultural and linguistic demands of the test remains questionable. To reinforce the fact that the obtained score may underrepresent the student's broad abilities or intelligence, this modality is checked but underlined in Figure 11.1.

It is possible that students currently in a bilingual education program in third or fourth grade may display language profiles 3 (L1 fluent/L2 minimal) or 6 (L1 fluent/L2 emergent). Students who are developmentally very advanced, have enriched home environments, or receive additional native-language instruction outside the public school system might develop a fluent level of

CALP slightly before the expected age for most children. Given that these students have attained a fluent CALP level in their native language, assessment in the native language is the preferred modality.

Another possible outcome for children attending bilingual programs in grades K–4 is language profile 4 (L1 minimal/L2 emergent). In this case, the student is actually more proficient in English and has developed relatively little proficiency in the native language, despite apparent enrollment in a "bilingual" program. When such a profile is encountered, it is imperative that practitioners obtain data regarding the percentage of L1 versus L2 instructional time across all grades attended by the student. It is most likely that this profile results from a poorly implemented or incorrectly structured bilingual program. In this situation, primary assessment in the native language is not recommended.

### Currently Participating in Bilingual Program, Grades 5–7

Native-language assessment is particularly appropriate for students in grades 5–7 who are currently participating in a well-implemented bilingual education program and who display language profiles 3 (L1 fluent/L2 minimal), 6 (L1 fluent/L2 emergent), and 9 (L1 fluent/L2 fluent) because CALP has been established in the native language. In these situations, the obtained composite scores may be a more accurate representation of these students' cognitive abilities and general intellectual functioning precisely because the pattern and development of CALP make them more comparable to the individuals on whom the test was normed. For these reasons, this modality is checked in Figure 11.1.

Students who are currently in bilingual education in grades 5–7 would be expected to have developed CALP. However, there are situations in which children educated under this circumstance will display development reflected by language profile 1 (L1 minimal/L2 minimal), 2 (L1 emergent/L2 minimal), 4 (L1 minimal/L2 emergent), or 5 (L1 emergent/L2 emergent). These are not the linguistic patterns that would be typically expected and suggest that some factors have attenuated the normal course of language development. Students with language profiles 2 or 5 may not have received sufficient or appropriate native-language instruction to attain CALP, or they may have some type of dysfunction related to the acquisition of language. Students with language profiles 1 or 4 show a significantly arrested degree of development, given the nature, amount, and length of instruction received in L1; this minimal level of CALP would be of considerable concern. For students educated under these circumstances and displaying these four profiles, measurement of their abilities in the native language will most likely result in an underestimate of their true functioning. However, given that the majority and amount of instruction received in the native language (which should have been sufficient to attain a fluent level of CALP) has not resulted in the level of linguistic development that would be predicted or expected, these students must be assessed in L1 in order to examine any potential causes for the observed delays.

### Previously Participated in Bilingual Program, Now in Grades K–4

For students who were previously in a bilingual education program but are now receiving English-only instruction (including ESL), a critical issue is the length of time they received such services. We have noted repeatedly that the longer a pupil receives native-language instruction, the more benefit derived and the more likely the chance that CALP may emerge or develop. Students in this educational circumstance will vary in terms of instruction received in L1 and L2, which, in turn, will significantly affect their language profiles as reflected in their respective CALP levels. For example, students currently in grades K–4 who are no longer in any type of bilingual education program could only have received from 1 to 4 years of native-language instruction—an amount that is insufficient to promote the full emergence or development of CALP. Students educated under these circumstances would most likely be English-language learners characterized by language profiles 1 (L1 minimal/L2 minimal), 2 (L1 emergent/L2 minimal), or 5 (L1 emergent/L2 emergent). English-language learners who have been educated in this educational circumstance and are characterized by these three language profiles should be assessed in their native language.

The use of this modality is recommended because it is important to recognize that these students have received some of their education in their native language—a fact that has implications for their developmental level in both languages with regard to the emergence and attainment of CALP. Although this information is quite helpful, it should be noted that the obtained data may still underrepresent the student's true ability because the degree of comparability (i.e., goodness of fit) between the student's cultural and linguistic background and the cultural and linguistic demands of the test remains questionable. To reinforce the fact that the obtained score may underrepresent the student's broad abilities or intelligence, this modality is checked and underlined in Figure 11.1.

It is possible, but not common, for students who were in bilingual education only until the third grade and exited before entry into fourth grade to have begun to develop CALP. Students educated under these circumstances might display language profile 3 (L1 fluent/L2 minimal) or language profile 6 (L1 fluent/L2 emergent). Students would fall into language profile 3 or 6 depending on the amount of L2 instruction that was provided while they were in bilingual education. It is recommend that students whose education has resulted in this pattern of linguistic development (i.e., language profiles 3 or 6) be assessed in their native language, because they have, in fact, attained CALP despite their limited or marginal level of instruction in the native language.

## Previously Participated in Bilingual Program, Now in Grades 5–7

For students who were previously in bilingual education but are now receiving English-only instruction or ESL services in grades 5–7, this most important issue is the length of time they received bilingual education services prior to being exited to English-only or ESL services. The longer a pupil receives native-language instruction, the more benefit derived and the more likely that CALP has emerged or developed. For example, those students who were exited toward the latter part of the elementary grades (end of fourth grade) will most likely have acquired a fluent or nearly fluent CALP level and display language profiles 3 (L1 fluent/L2 minimal), 6 (L1 fluent/L2 emergent), or 9 (L1 fluent/L2 fluent). Given the fact that these students have developed CALP in their native language, the preferred modality of assessment is the native language (L1), except for language profile 9. A student who received a bilingual education program through the fourth grade and is now in the seventh grade will have had sufficient time to develop CALP in his or her first language and transfer that learning to English to attain CALP in English as well (Profile 9). Given the equivalent levels of proficiency (i.e., CALP level of fluency in both L1 and L2), the recommended modality of assessment is either English or the native language.

However, students in grades 5–7 who were exited earlier in their elementary education (at or before third grade) will most likely have not acquired a fluent level of CALP. Across their entire elementary education, these students probably have received the greater portion of their instruction in English (L2), despite having had some native-language instruction. Consequently, they tend to display language profiles 4 (L1 minimal/L2 emergent) or 5 (L1 emergent/L2 emergent). These patterns may reflect the language loss or deterioration that would occur in the native language following premature cessation of instruction in that language in favor of English-only instruction. In these cases, English development tends to outpace native-language development, leading to either equivalent or greater proficiency in English. It should be noted, however, that the dominance of English is not an indicator or measure of native-like proficiency, as evidenced by the failure to obtain a fluent CALP level in English. Thus, it is recommended that students in this educational circumstance who display language profile 4 *not* be assessed in their native language, given that they have only obtained a minimal level of CALP in their native language and because the majority of their instruction has not been in their native language. Students in this educational circumstance who display language profile 5 have attained at least an emergent level of CALP fluency in both their native language and in English. Therefore, assessment in the native language is a secondary assessment option, but will likely result in an underrepresentation of true ability or functioning.

Students who were previously in bilingual education in grades K–4 but are now in grades 5–7 receiving English-only instruction most likely will not display a fluent level of CALP if they were exited at an early point in their elementary education (approximately first or second grade). Children educated under this circumstance could possibly display development reflected by language profile 1 (L1 minimal/L2 minimal) or 2 (L1 emergent/L2 minimal). These are the linguistic patterns that result from instructional programming factors (i.e., premature cessation of native-language instruction) and that attenuate the normal course of language development. Given that such students who display these two profiles probably have received the majority of their instruction in English and were not accorded the amount of time and instruction necessary to develop CALP in the native language, assessment in the native language is not recommended.

### English-Only Instruction, Grades K–4

Students who have received instruction in English solely throughout their early schooling (grades K–4) would most likely display language profiles 1 (L1 minimal/L2 minimal) or 2 (L1 emergent/L2 minimal). In the first case, students have not been given the benefit of any instructional programming that builds upon the foundation of the language with which they entered the school system (i.e., the native language). As a consequence, these students have not received the opportunity to develop any degree of advanced linguistic fluency. In addition, these students have received English-only instruction, which immediately places them at a developmental disadvantage compared to their monolingual English-speaking peers and makes them seem to be much less linguistically developed—through no fault of their own. Thus, we recommend that native-language testing be avoided because of the extreme interruption in the development of their native language.

For students who have received English-only instruction in grades K–4, it is expected that their English-language development would have developed at least to the emergent CALP level.

Their native-language development depends primarily upon the literacy environment in the home or community. Those students with opportunity and access to language-rich environments may develop an emergent level of native-language proficiency, despite receiving no type of native-language instruction. These students are likely to be characterized by language profile 5 (L1 emergent/L2 emergent). Students with little or no access to language-enriched environments would most likely display language profile 4 (L1 minimal/L2 emergent), wherein the native language has not been given sufficient opportunity to develop further since entering the school system. For students with language profile 5, some testing in the native language would be reasonable as a secondary option, albeit likely an underrepresentation. Students characterized by language profile 4 should not be tested in their native language because they have developed only minimal proficiency due primarily to lack of instruction or opportunity for informal development.

### English-Only Instruction, Grades 5–7

For students whose educational circumstances include an English-only instructional program and who are now in grades 5–7, we would expect a minimal level of native-language development primarily because of a lack of any native-language instruction and the process of language loss or deterioration due to disuse. Moreover, given that these students have received at least 5 or more years of academic instruction in English, in lieu of native-language instruction, we recommend they not be tested in their native language. As noted previously, the preferred modality of assessment in these cases would be a nonverbal approach, with testing in English as the secondary option.

## Assessment in English

The third assessment modality shown in Figure 11.1 is assessment in English (L2). Assessment of cognitive abilities or intelligence in L2 is much easier to accomplish than L1 assessment and is a routine part of training for psychologists and other school-based practitioners. Numerous instruments are available to practitioners for the assessment of cognitive abilities and intelligence in English; however, as is the case with native-language tests, none have norms that are entirely appropriate for use with English-language learners, even those who have become English dominant. As such, these instruments often yield results that tend to underrepresent the true abilities of English learners, except in cases where students have been accorded the benefit of primary-language instruction and education. Even those students who have been given an appropriate educational program in their native language may not have become fully acculturated, and performance could be adversely affected by this developmental variable as well. Instruments selected for use in this modality should provide a comprehensive assessment of the full range of human cognitive abilities, in accordance with a modern theoretical conceptualization of intelligence (e.g., CHC theory).

### Currently Participating in Bilingual Program, Grades K–4

Students in this educational circumstance generally do not come from households where English is the primary language. Even when English is spoken part of the time at home, it is often infrequent, limited, and may not follow the common grammatical or syntactical structures of standard English. Moreover, these students are in bilingual programs where they receive native-language instruction throughout most of their day. In such situations, we would not expect the student to display significant levels of CALP in English (i.e., fluent). Thus, the use of this assessment modality (assessment in English—L2) is not recommended.

## Currently Participating in Bilingual Program, Grades 5–7

Students in grades 5–7 currently in a well-designed and well-implemented bilingual program would be expected to display language profile 6 (L1 fluent/L2 emergent) or 9 (L1 fluent/L2 fluent), because it would be expected that CALP has been established in the native language. Testing in English is appropriate for students with language profile 9, because their level of CALP in English makes them more comparable to the individuals on whom the test was normed. Of course, these students could also be tested appropriately in their native language for the very same reasons. Testing in English is a secondary option for students with language profile 6, whereas this testing may yield useful information, it will likely result in an underrepresentation of true cognitive ability or functioning, given the fact that CALP in English has yet to be attained.

Students who are currently in bilingual education in grades 5–7 would be expected to have developed CALP in their native language and English. However, there are situations in which children educated under this circumstance display development reflected by language profile 3 (L1 fluent/L2 minimal) or 5 (L1 emergent/L2 emergent). These are not the linguistic patterns that would be typically expected and suggest some factors have attenuated the normal course of language development. Students with language profile 5 may not have received sufficient or appropriate English-language instruction necessary to attain CALP in English. If the bilingual education program was well implemented and designed appropriately, this profile may reflect the possibility of some type of dysfunction in the student related to the acquisition of language, as evidenced by the relatively equal patterns of delay in both the native language and English. Students with language profile 3 have also achieved a fluent level of CALP in their native language, as expected by their native-language instructional program, but have developed very little proficiency in English. Such a pattern is often the result of a bilingual program that has failed to provide adequate English-language instruction or any curriculum that promotes English-language development. Indeed, we are familiar with programs that have mistaken native-language-*only* instruction for "bilingual" education. In these situations, language profile 3 would be predicted and would not be a reason for concern. In either case, the levels of English language CALP for language profiles 3 and 5 (minimal and emergent, respectively) suggest that assessment in English is, at best, a secondary option and will also likely result in an underrepresentation of true ability.

For students currently in a well-implemented and well-designed bilingual education program in grades 5–7, very low levels of CALP in their native language and in English are not expected but may occur. Students in this educational circumstance characterized by language profiles 1 (L1 minimal/L2 minimal), 2 (L1 emergent/L2 minimal), or 4 (L1 minimal/L2 emergent) would be a cause for concern. However, assessment in English is not recommended because the student has not attained a fluent level of CALP in English, even though ample opportunity for its development has been provided. Moreover, these students have also failed to attain a fluent level of CALP in their native language, despite sufficient native-language instruction. Thus, if assessed in English, the cognitive abilities that might be adversely affecting the student's development of CALP in the native language and in English cannot be reliably identified and are confounded by the relative absence of English-language instruction.

### Previously Participated in Bilingual Program, Now in Grades K–4

As noted previously, students who have had this type of educational circumstance usually display language profiles 1 (L1 minimal/L2 minimal), 2 (L1 emergent/L2 minimal), or 5 (L1 emergent/L2 emergent). Moreover, it was previously noted that it is possible, but not common, that students who were only in bilingual education until the third grade and exited before entry into fourth grade could have begun to develop CALP. Students educated under these circumstances might display language profile 3 (L1 fluent/L2 minimal) or 6 (L1 fluent/L2 emergent), depending on the amount of L2 instruction that was provided while in the bilingual education setting.

Given that the time of exit from bilingual education will greatly impact the development of both languages, especially when the exiting occurs in the early elementary grades, language profiles (e.g. 1, 2, and 3) characterized by a minimal level of proficiency in English dictate that assessment *not* be conducted in English. When the level of CALP in English reaches the emergent level (e.g., language profiles 4, 5, and 6) assessment in English is a secondary option, although it will also likely result in an underrepresentation of true ability. For second-language learners who are educated in this circumstance and who evidence language profiles 1–6, other assessment modalities (e.g., nonverbal [profiles 1, 2, 4, and 5] or assessment in the native language [profiles 3 and 6]) are preferred, as noted in Figure 11.1.

### Previously Participated in Bilingual Program, Now in Grades 5–7

As noted in a previous section, a rationale for the possibility of language profiles 1–6 and 9 was provided. Given that only second-language learners who are educated in this circumstance and display profile 9 (L1 fluent/L2 fluent) have attained fluent CALP in English (L2), this is the only situation in which assessment in English can be considered a preferred approach, along with assessment in the native language. When the level of CALP in English reaches the emergent level (e.g., language profiles 4, 5, and 6), assessment in English is a secondary option, although it will also likely result in an underrepresentation of true ability. An additional reason why students with language profiles 4, 5, or 6 should be assessed in English is that they have likely received a substantial portion of their instruction in this language.

Given that the time of exit from bilingual education, especially in the early elementary grades, greatly affects the development of both languages, language profiles (e.g., 1, 2, and 3) characterized by only a minimal level of proficiency in English should be investigated because of the length of time that English instruction has been provided. Even in cases where students were exited from a bilingual program summarily (by first or second grade), English-only instruction from that point to the current grade placement (fifth to seventh grade) should have been sufficient to allow for the development of at least an emergent level of CALP in English. The fact that this has not occurred is an area of concern and merits further evaluation. However, because CALP in English has not been attained, assessment in English is mostly a secondary option, and the results are likely to underrepresent true ability or functioning. As noted in Figure 11.1, the preferred modality of assessment for language profiles 1 and 2 in this educational circumstance is nonverbal

(NV). The preferred modality of assessment for language profile 3 in this educational circumstance is the native language (L1), because CALP has been achieved.

## English-Only Instruction, Grades K–4

A rationale for the possibility of language profiles 1 (L1 minimal/L2 minimal), 2 (L1 emergent/L2 minimal), 4 (L1 minimal/L2 emergent), and 5 (L1 emergent/L2 emergent) was provided in a previous section. We would expect that students in this educational circumstance would most likely display language profiles 1 (L1 minimal/L2 minimal) or 2 (L1 emergent/L2 minimal), given that they have received instruction only in English and have not been afforded the opportunity to develop their native language. Language profiles 4 (L1 minimal/L2 emergent) or 5 (L1 emergent/ L2 emergent) can be seen in students in this educational circumstance in the latter grades in this level (i.e., grades 3 or 4). Students in this situation will most likely display language profile 4 (L1 minimal/L2 emergent) when they are not afforded the opportunity to develop their native language at home or in their community and have received instruction solely in English at school. If students are given access to language-enriched environments (in their native language) at home, church, or in their community and simultaneously receive instruction solely in English at school for several years, they may demonstrate language profile 5 (L1 emergent/L2 emergent).

School-based practitioners assessing second-language learners who are in this educational circumstance and who evidence one of these four language profiles need to consider two critical factors when determining whether to assess these students in English. The first factor is the student's current level of proficiency in English. The second factor is the number of years that the student has received English-only instruction. Both of these factors are incorporated in our MAMBI in Figure 11.1 and denoted by the use of an asterisk for language profiles 1 and 2 and the pound sign for language profiles 4 and 5.

We recommend that students with language profiles 1 or 2 who are currently in grades K–2 and who are being educated in this format *not* be tested in English. It is important to acknowledge that although these students have been educated in an English-only environment for a few years, the fact remains that they still have minimal proficiency in English—which is not unusual, given the limited number of years that they have received instruction in an English-only academic environment. Simultaneously, the majority of their language development across their life span (birth to grades 1 or 2) has been in their native language, not in English, and an extreme interruption in the development of their native language has occurred. For students who evidence language profiles 1 or 2 and are in grades 3 and 4, some testing in English would be reasonable as a secondary option, although it is likely to produce an underrepresentation.

Students who display language profiles 4 (L1 minimal/L2 emergent) or 5 (L1 emergent/L2 emergent) and are educated in this format differ from those with language profiles 1 or 2 in that they have obtained an emergent level of proficiency in L2. However, we recommend that students who demonstrate language profiles 4 or 5 and are currently in kindergarten or first grade *not* be tested in English. Even though students with language profile 4 have a higher level of proficiency in English than in their native language, these students still have not attained CALP in English. Moreover, they would not be expected to have attained CALP if educated in this educational circumstance. As noted previously, the majority of their language development across their life span has been in their native language, whereas they have had a mere 1–2 years in an English-only academic environment. For students with language profiles 4 or 5 in grades 2–4, some testing in English would be reasonable as a secondary option, albeit likely to produce an under-representation. As noted previously, the preferred assessment modality for pupils educated in this format and who evidence any one of the four aforementioned language profiles would be a non-verbal approach.

### English-Only Instruction, Grades 5–7

For students whose educational circumstances have included an English-only instructional program for at least 5 years, it would not be uncommon to find that they evidence language profiles 4 (L1 minimal/L2 emergent) or 5 (L1 emergent/L2 emergent). Given the number of years that they have received an English-only academic program in this format, we would expect that they would have attained an emergent level of proficiency in English. The level of proficiency in their L1 would depend on many factors in their home, church, and community (see Chapters 4 and 9).

Given that these students have received at least 5 years of education in an English-only in-structional setting, testing in English is a secondary option that is recommended as possibly yield-ing useful information but will likely result in an underrepresentation of true cognitive ability. The fact remains that for most of these students in this particular situation, CALP in English has yet to be attained.

## Bilingual Assessment

As noted in Chapter 10, the ideal method with which to test second-language learners is bilingual assessment. Very few instruments are currently available to assess English-language learners with this type of assessment modality. The recommendations included for this testing modality in Fig-ure 11.1 are made in the context of the measures that are currently available. When the pioneer work of Muñoz-Sandoval et al. (1998) and the current standard set by Alvarado (1999) are further developed and enhanced, respectively, the recommendations made in Figure 11.1 will most likely change.

Given the context of the measures that are currently available, this testing modality need not be considered for second-language learners who evidence language profiles 3 (L1 fluent/L2 mini-mal), 6 (L1 fluent/L2 emergent), or 9 (L1 fluent/L2 fluent). Students with one of these three lan-guage profiles have obtained CALP in their native language, and in the case of students with lan-guage profile 9, have also obtained CALP in English. Thus, as noted in Figure 11.1, the recommended testing modality for students with language profiles 3 or 6 is assessment in the native language (L1), and for individuals with language profile 9, assessment in the native lan-guage (L1) and in English (L2).

Once again, given the context and structure of the measures that are currently available, using a bilingual modality should be considered when testing second-language learners who evi-dence language profiles 1 (L1 minimal/L2 minimal), 2 (L1 emergent/L2 minimal), or 5 (L1 emer-gent/L2 emergent). Students who evidence one of these three language profiles have yet to develop CALP in their native language. Depending on the instructional program they have received (e.g., currently in bilingual education, previously in bilingual education, English-only in-struction, as noted in Figure 11.1), these students' verbal abilities can vary across L1 and L2. In other words, second-language learners may know some vocabulary words in both languages, some only in English, and others only in the native language. As noted previously, the BVAT is comprised of three subtests (Picture Vocabulary, Oral Vocabulary, and Verbal Analogies). Given that the BVAT requires administration in English first and then readministration in the native language only for those items missed in English, the child is given the opportunity to demonstrate his or her verbal cognitive abilities by using both of his or her linguistic repertoires. Thus, we could expect a "gain score" on the BVAT for students who evidence language profile 2, because these students' level of proficiency is higher in their L1 than in their L2. Students who evidence language profiles 1 or 5 have commensurate levels of proficiency in both languages. These students may or may not demonstrate a gain score on the BVAT when tested in their native language depending on what they know in one language and not the other. As noted in Figure 11.1, the use of this testing modality with students who have language profiles 1, 2, or 5 and who (1) are currently enrolled in a bilingual education program, (2) were previously enrolled in bilingual education but are now receiving English-only instruction, or (3) who have received English-only instruction (grades K–7) would be reasonable as a secondary option, although it is likely to produce an underrepresentation. This modality is recommended as a secondary option, because the BVAT only measures one broad ability, Crystallized Intelligence ($Gc$), and because the child has yet to attain CALP in either language.

## Caveats for Special Linguistic and Educational Circumstances

Although we have endeavored to cover the more common educational circumstances in the preceding discussion, we recognize that exceptions may arise that are not directly addressed in these guidelines. For example, on occasion, students enter the school system at a point other than kindergarten and may or may not have received any formal education in their native country. Moreover, when such students enter the school system in the United States, they may or may not receive native-language instruction. Factors such as the student's age and the types of programs available at different levels within the district where the student enrolls are additional variables that must be considered in determining the most appropriate manner in which to characterize the student's prior and current educational experience. When faced with making such determinations, the most relevant factors will be (1) whether or not the student received formal instruction, for how long, and of what quality before coming to the United States; (2) in what language the student received instruction in the core subjects, if schooling did take place; and (3) in what type of instructional program the student was placed, and in what language was instruction given upon arriving in the United States.

For students who did not enter the U.S. school system at the kindergarten or first-grade level, we suggest that the "current grade" categories be viewed alternatively as corresponding to the number of "years in school" in the United States. In addition, whereas the guidelines described above take into account both L1 and L2 simultaneously, determining the modality for assessment of students entering school well after kindergarten or first grade needs to be prioritized separately. For example, consider the case of a newly arrived 10-year-old, José, who has been placed in a fifth-grade classroom in an English-only or ESL program. If José has received a solid education in his native language, his CALP level would be most similar to other fifth-grade students under the classification of "currently in a bilingual education program in lieu of, or in addition to, receiving ESL services" (see Figure 11.1). Bilingual education is most similar to all-native-language instruction, in that they both use the primary language for instruction in the core subjects and for about the same length of time. Thus, assessment relative to the native language would follow the "5–7" recommendations section for this category, depending on the student's L1 proficiency level. However, if the student has not received much or any native-language instruction, linguistic development in L1 will be most similar to the "K–4" category and the recommendations in that section would be most appropriate for guiding the assessment modality.

Regardless of whether the student received native-language instruction prior to coming to the United States, instruction in English has only recently begun, and the services being received are also solely in English. Thus, the student's L2 linguistic development is most similar to other fifth-grade students under the classification of "all instruction has been in an English-only program, with or without ESL services" shown in Figure 11.1. Thus, assessment relative to English (L2) would follow the "K–4" section for this category, depending on the student's English language proficiency (likely to be minimal in L2). For the most part, the recommendations suggest a nonverbal approach; a language-reduced format is appropriate because English is just being learned. By following the logic and rationale outlined here, it should be possible to determine the most appropriate modality of assessment for most of those students whose educational and linguistic backgrounds are not reflected in the descriptions provided in Figure 11.1.

## Cultural and Linguistic Extensions of the CHC Cross-Battery Approach

The MAMBI assists practitioners in making rational and defensible choices regarding the best approach to a particular evaluation. Being able to select the most appropriate approach to the evaluation is key for the successful collection of the data and information necessary to answer the referral questions. Once the method with which data will be gathered has been determined, practitioners still face the problem of deciding which tests or battery is best and how the data can be interpreted in a nondiscriminatory manner.

Fortunately, the manner in which cultural or linguistic bias may operate in the use of standardized tests, as well as the implications of such bias, have been formally operationalized via the development of the cultural and linguistic extensions of the CHC cross-battery approach (Flanagan et al., 2000; Flanagan & Ortiz, 2001; Ortiz & Flanagan, 1998). These extensions are achieved through classification of standardized, norm-referenced tests—not by the usual grouping (i.e., according to the cognitive construct they are presumed to measure), but by (1) the degree to which each subtest is culturally loaded and (2) the extent of its inherent linguistic demands. Classification of tests along these two dimensions creates a new frame of reference from which to view test performance and assists in assigning meaning to results in a much less discriminatory manner.

In 1990 Figueroa recommended the application of empirically supported theoretical frameworks of intelligence to guide the assessment of culturally and linguistically diverse individuals and admonished practitioners to pay particular attention to cultural and linguistic dimensions. Building upon these notions, Ortiz and Flanagan (1998), Flanagan and Ortiz (2001), and Flanagan et al. (2000) developed a classification system for tests of intelligence and cognitive ability, as well as some special-purpose tests based on the inherent properties of the tests with regard to degree of cultural loading and degree of linguistic demand. An example of the classifications for the various WJ III subtests is presented in Table 11.1, which is adapted from the comprehensive classifications found in Flanagan and Ortiz (2001). A thorough discussion of the CHC cross-battery

**TABLE 11.1. Test Classifications by Degree of Cultural Loading and Linguistic Demand for the WJ III**

| Degree of linguistic demand | Age | Subtests | CHC ability |
|---|---|---|---|
| | | *Degree of cultural loading: Low* | |
| Low | 4–85+ | **SPATIAL RELATIONS** | *Gv* (Vz, SR) |
| Moderate | 4–85+ | **NUMBERS REVERSED** | *Gsm* (MW) |
| | 4–85+ | **VISUAL MATCHING** | *Gs* (P, R9) |
| High | 4–85+ | **CONCEPT FORMATION** | *Gf* (I) |
| | 4–85+ | **ANALYSIS–SYNTHESIS** | *Gf* (RG) |
| | 4–85+ | **AUDITORY WORKING MEMORY** | *Gsm* (MW) |
| | | *Degree of cultural loading: Moderate* | |
| Low | 4–85+ | **Picture Recognition** | *Gv* (MV) |
| | 4–85+ | **PLANNING** | *Gv* (SS) |
| | 4–85+ | **PAIR CANCELLATION** | *Gs* (R9) |
| Moderate | 4–85+ | **VISUAL–AUDITORY LEARNING** | *Glr* (MA) |
| | 4–85+ | **Visual Auditory Learning—Delayed** | *Glr* (MA) |
| | 4–85+ | **RETRIEVAL FLUENCY** | *Glr* (FI) |
| | 4–85+ | **RAPID PICTURE NAMING** | *Glr* (NA) |
| High | 2–85+ | **INCOMPLETE WORDS** | *Ga* (PC-A) |
| | 4–85+ | **SOUND BLENDING** | *Ga* (PC-S) |
| | 4–85+ | **MEMORY FOR WORDS** | *Gsm* (MS) |
| | 4–85+ | **AUDITORY ATTENTION** | *Ga* (UR) |
| | 4–85+ | **DECISION SPEED** | *Gs* (R7) |
| | | *Degree of cultural loading: High* | |
| High | 2–85+ | **VERBAL COMPREHENSION** | *Gc*(VL, LD) |
| | 2–85+ | **GENERAL INFORMATION** | *Gc* (K0) |

*Note.* With respect to the broad and narrow CHC abilities, tests printed in **BOLD UPPERCASE** letters are strong measures as defined empirically; tests printed in **bold upper- and lowercase** letters are moderate measures as defined empirically (see Flanagan, McGrew, & Ortiz, 2000; McGrew & Flanagan, 1998). Data from Flanagan and Ortiz (2001, pp. 233–242).

approach and the complete theoretical and empirical rationale behind the cultural–linguistic classifications are well beyond the scope of this chapter. Nevertheless, the information in Table 11.1 is used to illustrate the manner in which the cultural and linguistic classifications of a particular test or collection of tests can serve as a systematic method for reducing many of the discriminatory aspects of the assessment of bilingual individuals.

## Cultural Loading Classifications

As noted in Table 11.1, "degree of cultural loading" refers to the degree to which a given subtest from the WJ III requires specific knowledge of, or experience with, mainstream U.S. culture. The WJ III subtests in Table 11.1 were classified in terms of several culturally related characteristics, including (1) whether there was an emphasis on a particular thought or conceptual process, (2) the actual content or materials involved in the task, and (3) the nature of an expected response. Attention was also given to aspects of the communicative relationship between examinee and examiner (i.e., culturally specific elements, apart from actual oral language, such as affirmative head nods, pointing, etc.; see McCallum & Bracken, 1997). These characteristics were chosen in accordance with the findings of various researchers (e.g., Jensen, 1974; Valdés & Figueroa, 1996) who suggest that tests that are more process oriented and contain more novel stimuli and less communicative requirements tend to yield less discriminatory estimates of functioning or ability. Classification is divided into three levels (high, moderate, and low) reflecting the continuum-like nature of these culture-related variables.

## Linguistic Demand Classifications

The heading "degree of linguistic demand" refers to the amount of linguistic facility required by a given test and is based on three factors: (1) verbal versus nonverbal language requirements on the part of the examiner (in administration of the test); (2) receptive language requirements on the part of the examinee; and (3) expressive language requirements on the part of the examinee. Similar to the structure of classifications based on degree of cultural loading, the subtests from the WJ III are organized according to degree (i.e., high, moderate, and low). Knowledge of the degree to which any given test requires language ability and proficiency provides yet another means of selecting tests in a systematic way that reduces potential bias and helps to establish a defensible basis for interpretation.

Although only nine possible combinations comprise Table 11.1 (i.e., three levels of cultural loading by three levels of linguistic demand), the information remains a bit unwieldy when presented in a linear fashion, which makes it difficult to introduce additional notions beyond the basic classifications. To facilitate use of the information, and to allow for later interpretation of the influence of culture and language on test performance, Flanagan and Ortiz (2001) recommend use of the culture–language classification matrix that places the categories for degree of linguistic demand along the horizontal axis and the categories for degree of cultural loading down the vertical axis. The resulting matrix of WJ III subtests is presented in Figure 11.2.

Figure 11.2 contains the subtests from the WJ III arranged and classified in much the same manner as in Table 11.1 but in a format that allows the intersection of the two dimensions to be better perceived visually. As such, the information regarding classification along the dimensions of cultural loading and linguistic demand are more readily apparent. The ability to evaluate quickly the extent of cultural loading and degree of linguistic demands of the various WJ III subtests assists practitioners in deciding the suitability of any given subtest for use with individuals from diverse backgrounds. As will be discussed, it also provides a method for ruling in or out the primary influence of language or culture on test performance. The ability to determine the extent to which test results from the WJ III are, or are not, influenced by factors such as acculturation or English-language proficiency is a significant accomplishment that provides a strong basis for evaluating test results and their meaning fairly. The information in Figure 11.2 and Table 11.1 should not, however, be relied upon as the only guide for decisions related to test selection or interpretation. Rather, the information is intended primarily to supplement selection and interpretation within the context of a broader, defensible system of nondiscriminatory assessment. Nevertheless, when used in conjunction with other relevant assessment information (e.g., direct observations, review of records, interviews, language-proficiency testing, socioeconomic status, developmental data, family history), these classifications may lead to a significant decrease in bias of standardized testing practices.

Degree of Linguistic Demand

| | Low | Moderate | High |
|---|---|---|---|
| **Low** (Degree of Cultural Loading) | **SPATIAL RELATIONS** (*Gv*—VZ, SR) | **VISUAL MATCHING** (*Gs*—P, R9)<br>**NUMBERS REVERSED** (*Gsm*—MW) | **CONCEPT FORMATION** (*Gf*—I)<br>**ANALYSIS SYNTHESIS** (*Gf*—RG)<br>**AUDITORY WORKING MEMORY** (*Gsm*—MW) |
| **Moderate** | Picture Recognition (*Gv*—MV)*<br>PLANNING (*Gv*—SS)<br>PAIR CANCELLATION (*Gs*—R9) | **VISUAL–AUDITORY LEARNING** (*Glr*—MA)<br>Visual Auditory Learning—Delayed (*Glr*—MA)<br>**RETRIEVAL FLUENCY** (*Glr*—FI)<br>**RAPID PICTURE NAMING** (*Glr*—NA) | **MEMORY FOR WORDS** (*Gsm*—MS)<br>**INCOMPLETE WORDS** (*Ga*—PC)<br>**SOUND BLENDING** (*Ga*—PC)<br>**AUDITORY ATTENTION** (*Ga*—US/U3)<br>**DECISION SPEED** (*Gs*—R4) |
| **High** | | | **VERBAL COMPREHENSION** (*Gc*—VL, LD)<br>**GENERAL INFORMATION** (*Gc*—K0) |

**FIGURE 11.2.** Matrix of cultural loading and linguistic demand classifications of the WJ III. Tests printed in **BOLD UPPERCASE** letters are strong measures, as defined empirically; tests printed in **bold upper- and lowercase** letters are moderate measures, as defined empirically (see also Flanagan, McGrew, & Ortiz, 2000; McGrew & Flanagan, 1998). Adapted from Flanagan and Ortiz (2001, p. 248). Copyright 2001 by John Wiley & Sons, Inc. Adapted by permission.

## Bias Reduction via the WJ III Culture–Language Classification Matrix

The CHC culture–language matrix for the WJ III depicted in Figure 11.2 provides two immediate benefits to practitioners engaged in assessment of bilingual and other individuals with diverse backgrounds: (1) the ability to quickly select tests that may provide more accurate or fairer estimates of true ability; and (2) the ability to systematically evaluate the relative influence of cultural or linguistic factors on test performance. In both cases, a reduction in potential bias, which could affect the validity of the results, leads to more confidence in conclusions and inferences drawn from the data.

### Reducing Bias in Test Selection

Application of the cultural and linguistic extensions for the WJ III subtests depicted in Figure 11.2 rests on the premise that selection of a set of tests known to assess a particular construct, combined with consideration of the relevant cultural and linguistic dimensions of such tests, provides more reliable, valid, and interpretable assessment data than what are obtained using traditional methods. As noted previously, individuals who are less acculturated or who have lower English proficiency, tend to perform lower than monolingual peers raised in the U.S. mainstream from birth (Figueroa, 1990a; Hamayan & Damico, 1991a; Jensen, 1974; Mercer, 1979; Valdés & Figueroa, 1996). Consequently, scores for diverse individuals would be expected to better approximate their true ability on tests that are lowest in cultural loading and linguistic demand, and vice versa. By examining factors relevant to the background of the diverse individuals to be assessed (e.g., level of English- and other-language proficiency, language of instruction, educational and familial history, degree of acculturation), practitioners can select the tests that are the most suitable and least discriminatory. Although there will be individual considerations due to variation in experience and proficiency, *in general tests with the lowest cultural loadings and lowest linguistic demands should be selections of first choice.* Thus, administration of the Visual Matching subtest is expected, according to the literature, to be a truer estimate of ability (in this case, of *Gs*) than would administration of Decision Speed (which also measures *Gs*) because Visual Matching is lower in terms of both cultural loading and linguistic demand. Acculturation and language proficiency play a larger role in the subtest of Decision Speed; therefore, the results are less accurate or fair measures of true ability than for the subtest of visual matching.

## Reducing Bias in Test Interpretation

By making the relevant cultural loading and linguistic demands of tests more accessible and straightforward, the culture–language classification matrix for the WJ III in Figure 11.2 provides a reasonable framework for reducing discriminatory attributions to test performance in still another way. Research has already revealed the manner in which cultural and linguistic variables attenuate performance. Thus, when coupled with information regarding cultural and linguistic experience, defensible interpretation can be accomplished through analysis of the patterns formed by test data. Levels of acculturation and language proficiency operate as attenuating variables—that is, the greater the difference between an individual's background and the background of the norm group, the more likely the test will measure lower performance as a function of the lack of comparability in experience. Thus, cultural and linguistic differences serve to depress the scores of diverse individuals. These well-known and understood effects are illustrated in Figure 11.3.

The smaller arrow at the top, pointing to the right in Figure 11.3, indicates the increasing effect that language differences are likely to have on test performance as a function of the increasing linguistic demands of the tests. Use of tests that have relatively heavy language demands is likely to adversely affect the performance of linguistically different individuals to a relatively large degree as a function of their own level of proficiency. Individuals with near-native-English-language proficiency, as compared to their same-age monolingual English-speaking peers, would likely not show any difference on tests, irrespective of their linguistic loading. However, individuals who have only moderate or low levels of English-language proficiency, as compared to their monolingual English-speaking counterparts, will show only a slight or no difference on tests that have low linguistic demands, a marked difference on tests with moderate demands, and a profound difference on tests with high demands. Thus, use of tests that are more language reduced is likely to have less adverse effects and lead to fairer results.

Similarly, the small arrow on the left side pointing to the bottom in Figure 11.3 represents the increasing effect that cultural differences are likely to have on test performance as a function of the increasing cultural loadings of the tests. As before, tests that are highly culturally loaded tend to affect the performance of diverse individuals more than culturally reduced tests. The large arrow pointing diagonally from the upper-left cell to the bottom-right cell indicates the combined, overall effect that culture and language have on test performance. In general, performance of culturally and linguistically diverse individuals tends to be least affected by tests that are classified

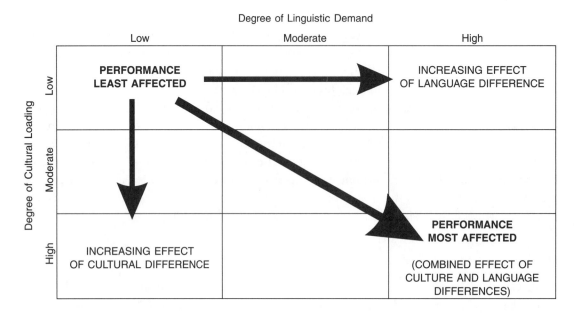

**FIGURE 11.3.** Pattern of expected test performance for culturally and linguistically diverse individuals. Adapted from Flanagan and Ortiz (2001, p. 260). Copyright 2001 by John Wiley & Sons, Inc. Adapted by permission.

more to the left and top of the matrix, and most affected by tests that are classified closer to the right and bottom of the matrix.

In sum, the arrows provide a graphical representation of the general patterns of expected performance for individuals with diverse cultural and linguistic backgrounds. This pattern is based on consistent findings from decades of research regarding the lower performance of individuals from diverse cultural and linguistic backgrounds on English-language tests. To the degree that the pattern of scores obtained by individuals from diverse backgrounds matches the expected decline in performance (i.e., from the upper left cell to the bottom right cell), it can be concluded that what has been measured is level of acculturation or English-language proficiency or both. When the expected pattern for diverse individuals is not found, then it can be said that some other factor (e.g., a disability) apart from culture and language has influenced the results. In such cases, although cultural and linguistic factors may be contributing somewhat to the pattern of obtained scores, it could not be concluded that they were the primary or only factors operating on the results. When the expected pattern is observed, then it can be reliably concluded that cultural or linguistic factors (often both) systematically influenced performance, more so than actual or true ability.

## A Worksheet for Nondiscriminatory Interpretation of Test Scores

To engage in nondiscriminatory interpretation of test results, practitioners need to make a few minor calculations. These computations can be facilitated by use of a worksheet developed specifically for this purpose, depicted in Figure 11.4. Practitioners must first insert the names of any tests that were used during the course of evaluation (note that additional spaces are provided in the event that other tests for which classifications exist were also utilized). The test names should

Name of Examinee: _____     Date: _____

## Degree of Linguistic Demand

| | Low | | Moderate | | High | |
|---|---|---|---|---|---|---|
| **Low** (Degree of Cultural Loading) | Test Name: _____ | Score: ( ) ( ) ( ) ( ) ( ) Cell Average = ___ | Test Name: _____ | Score: ( ) ( ) ( ) ( ) ( ) Cell Average = ___ | Test Name: _____ | Score: ( ) ( ) ( ) ( ) ( ) Cell Average = ___ |
| **Moderate** | Test Name: _____ | Score: ( ) ( ) ( ) ( ) ( ) Cell Average = ___ | Test Name: _____ | Score: ( ) ( ) ( ) ( ) ( ) Cell Average = ___ | Test Name: _____ | Score: ( ) ( ) ( ) ( ) ( ) Cell Average = ___ |
| **High** | Test Name: _____ | Score: ( ) ( ) ( ) ( ) ( ) Cell Average = ___ | Test Name: _____ | Score: ( ) ( ) ( ) ( ) ( ) Cell Average = ___ | Test Name: _____ | Score: ( ) ( ) ( ) ( ) ( ) Cell Average = ___ |

Degree of Cultural Loading

FIGURE 11.4. Culture–language matrix worksheet. From Flanagan and Ortiz (2001, p. 263). Copyright 2001 by John Wiley and Sons, Inc. Reprinted by permission.

be written in the cells that correspond to their respective cultural and linguistic dimensions, as listed in Table 11.1 or Figure 11.2. Next, to evaluate and compare patterns of performance across the matrix, the standard scores (converted to a common matrix, e.g., deviation IQ) obtained for each individual test should be written in the space next to the test name. Then for each set of tests grouped together according to their degree of cultural loading and degree of linguistic demand (i.e., for each cell), an overall mean or average is calculated. Note that the cell average has no meaning beyond an arithmetical representation of composite performance on tests that have been classified together on the basis of characteristics they possess and not on the ability they are intended to measure. Apart from representing overall performance on tests that share similar levels of cultural loading and linguistic demand, there is no inherent meaning or implied construct for the cell average, and it should not be interpreted in any other manner or ascribed any other meaning.

### General Guidelines for Interpretation

Once all cell averages have been calculated, interpretation is accomplished by examining *the degree to which the averages form a pattern that is either consistent or inconsistent with the pattern of expected performance*, as depicted in Figure 11.3. Generally speaking, when the overall pattern of scores obtained for a given individual approximates one or more of the three patterns expected for diverse individuals (decline in performance due to cultural loading, linguistic demand, or both), the results may be reasonably interpreted as reflecting the systematic attenuating effect of cultural or linguistic differences, or both, on performance. Scores that decrease vertically, from upper to lower cells, indicate the effect of cultural differences. Scores that decrease horizontally, from left to right, indicate the effect of language differences. Scores at or near the lower-right corner of the matrix, which tend to be lower than scores at or near the upper-left corner of the matrix, reflect the combined effect of culture and language differences. When any one or more of these patterns emerge from review of the data, support is provided for the notion that the individual's scores are more a reflection of cultural or linguistic differences (or both) than they are a true measure of actual ability or skill. When examination of the data reveals patterns that are not consistent with those expected or predicted for diverse individuals (i.e., any pattern that deviates from the three described), it is reasonable to assume that other factors, including the possibility of a disability, are playing a primary role in affecting test performance. Failure to find an expected pattern of performance (as depicted in Figure 11.3), however, does not automatically imply that measured performance is entirely valid or reliable. Interpretations of dysfunction or disability should be bolstered by a wide range and multiple sources of evidence that converge and support professional opinion and inferences drawn from the collected data. It should also be noted that culture and language are highly correlated and as such, singular effects of one or the other will be rare. The most common pattern will be that which shows the combined effect of both.

## APPLICATION OF THE TWO-STEP MODEL: CASE ILLUSTRATION

In order to illustrate how the MAMBI (step 1) and the culture–language classification matrix (step 2) can be used in actual practice, we provide a sample case illustration of the process, using a composite study of a child named Vianey.

## Background Information

Vianey is a female of Mexican American descent who is currently in seventh grade, where she receives English-only instruction in the general education setting. Her parents were born in Mexico and immigrated to the United States, where Vianey was born shortly thereafter. Both parents speak Spanish well but have had little and inconsistent education; they have very limited English-language skills. Vianey's primary language is Spanish; she did not attend any preschool or day-care program before entering kindergarten in the local public elementary school. Vianey was enrolled in a transitional bilingual program (early exit) with traditional pullout ESL services while in K–1, but then her family moved and she entered a different elementary school, where she was placed in an English-only program beginning in the second grade. Thus, she has been receiving English-only instruction for over 5 years and is beginning her 6th year of English instruction now that she is in seventh grade.

Vianey was referred for evaluation by her language arts teacher, who stated that although she speaks English well, she displays problems in reading and writing. The teacher feels that Vianey's performance, on the whole, is significantly below that of her classmates, despite the fact that her ability to communicate in English appears intact and that her speech is clear and accent free. Based on the collected language proficiency assessment data using the Woodcock–Muñoz Language Survey (WMLS) and other informal language assessment methods, Vianey was found to have a "minimal" CALP level in L1 (Spanish) and an "emergent" CALP level in L2 (English).

## Step 1: Selection of Modality of Assessment via the MAMBI

Step 1 requires that examiners ascertain what assessment modality would be the most appropriate for Vianey, given her linguistic development and proficiency in L1 (Spanish) and L2 (English). When viewed within the context of the MAMBI, Vianey's linguistic development and proficiency are best characterized by language profile 4 (L1 minimal/L2 emergent). According to the recommendations contained in the MAMBI chart, the preferred modality for assessment of Vianey's linguistic and educational background, current grade, and current language proficiency would be nonverbal, with English (L2) testing as a secondary or optional mode of assessment that may provide additional valuable information (although, it would likely result in an underrepresentation of her true ability).

Nonverbal assessment of Vianey's cognitive abilities is the preferred modality for evaluation, because she has yet to achieve a fluent level of CALP in L1 (Spanish) or in L2 (English)—that is, her language development is not comparable to her monolingual peers. Use of nonverbal methods and tools is one way in which the language demands can be reduced, albeit not eliminated entirely. Testing in L2 (English) is a secondary option in this case because Vianey has received over 5 years of English-language instruction, compared to 2 years of combined instruction in her native language and English in the transitional program she attended from kindergarten to second grade. In this instructional arrangement, Vianey was not allowed to reach the level of CALP that would be necessary to establish a foundation in her native language and which could serve to facilitate and enhance her English-language development. Moreover, given that she has received the majority of her instruction in English, it is not surprising that her CALP level in English is slightly more developed than her native-language proficiency—especially because Vianey has also been subject to the phenomenon known as language loss or language deterioration, wherein the lack of or interruption in instruction in the native language impedes its development and leads to loss through lack of use. Thus, evaluation of her cognitive abilities in English might prove to be of some value to the assessment because it will assist in determining the extent to which Vianey's development has proceeded in comparison to native English speakers. However, given that Vianey's linguistic (and cultural) background is at least moderately different from that of her monolingual English-speaking peers, the results from testing in L2 are likely to underrepresent her true cognitive ability.

## Step 2: Test Selection and Interpretation via the Culture–Language Classification Matrix

Because Vianey was reported to have broad-ranging difficulties in reading and writing, it was determined that the assessment should include evaluation of the full range of cognitive abilities with emphasis on nonverbal testing. As such, the UNIT was selected as the primary instrument because it can generate a full-scale IQ and because it allows for measurement in a nonverbal manner. The four subtests of the UNIT, which comprise the full-scale IQ score, are shown in matrix form in Figure 11.5.

As can be seen in this illustration, the nonverbal nature of the UNIT does not completely resolve issues related to linguistic demand (communication) or cultural loading. Of the four tests used, one is classified as high in cultural loading (Analogic Reasoning), one is classified as moderate in cultural loading (Symbolic Memory), and one is classified as moderate in linguistic demand (Spatial Memory). Nonetheless, all scores on the UNIT are within normal limits; however, there is

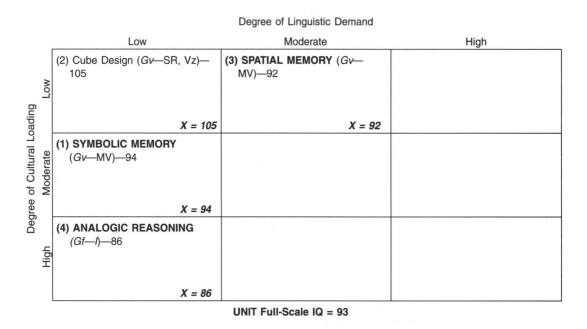

FIGURE 11.5. Matrix of cultural loading and linguistic demand classifications for Vianey's UNIT subtests. Tests printed in **BOLD UPPERCASE** letters are strong measures, as defined empirically; tests printed in **bold upper- and lowercase** letters are moderate measures, as defined empirically.

a clear degradation of performance as a function of cultural loading (SS = 105, 94, 86) and, to a certain extent, linguistic demand (SS = 105, 92). Moreover, Vainey's general cognitive ability as measured by the UNIT Full-Scale IQ was SS = 93, which falls well within the average range of intellectual functioning. It is important to recognize, however, that this global ability score is comprised of three tests of visual processing (Cube Design, Spatial Memory, and Symbolic Memory) and one test of fluid intelligence (Analogic Reasoning). The CHC theory of cognitive abilities integrates 10 broad abilities, of which 7 are typically measured, to one extent or another, by existing tests. Thus, in order to generate a broader picture of Vianey's general cognitive ability, it is necessary to assess other cognitive abilities not represented on the UNIT. Unfortunately, because nonverbal tests tend to offer a similarly narrow range of abilities, it is not possible to measure the full range of cognitive functioning that Vianey possesses without resorting to the secondary or optional modality in this assessment (i.e., testing in L2—English).

Given Vianey's current linguistic development and educational history, we recognize that this mode of testing will likely result in an underrepresentation of her true ability. As such, a decision was made to utilize the first seven subtests from the WJ III, which would provide a broader assessment of the range of her cognitive abilities as well as another global ability score based on a greater breadth of types of intellectual functioning. Results from testing conducted on Vianey with the WJ III are illustrated in matrix form in Figure 11.6.

A review of the patterns of performance reflected by Vianey's scores in the illustration reveal a clear tendency toward lower scores as a function of increasing demands in cultural loading and linguistic skills. A review of the scores in the columns (from left to right) shows that Vianey's performance decreases as the linguistic demands of the subtests increased (SS = 101, 91, 86; SS =

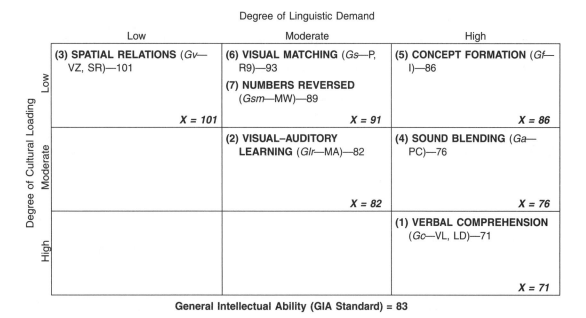

**FIGURE 11.6.** Matrix of cultural loading and linguistic demand classifications for Vianey's WJ III subtests. Tests printed in **BOLD UPPERCASE** letters are strong measures, as defined empirically; tests printed in **bold upper- and lowercase** letters are moderate measures, as defined empirically.

82, 76). Similarly, when the scores are examined from top to bottom (evaluation of the effects of cultural loading), it is evident that Vianey's performance also decreases as a function of increased cultural loading on the subtests (SS = 91, 82 and SS = 86, 76, 71). Vianey's general ability, as measured by the General Intellectual Ability (GIA) on the WJ III, was SS = 83, or about 10 standard score points lower than what she obtained on the UNIT. This decline in performance is expected, however, given the fact that Vianey's linguistic abilities in English are only at the emergent level. Because the WJ III battery, as a whole, tends to be based more on an individual's language abilities, achieving a representative performance requires a developmentally appropriate command or mastery of the language—a level that is not usually held by the typical English-language learner. As such, a lower global ability score than that which was obtained on the nonverbal administration of the UNIT is to be expected.

Thus far, interpretation of the results of cognitive testing with the UNIT and the WJ III has been described independently. Ideally, data from cognitive testing should be analyzed and interpreted in an integrated manner. Accordingly, Figure 11.7. provides a graphic representation of the combined results obtained from the UNIT and WJ III and serves as the best platform upon which interpretations should be made.

Because there is little overlap between the UNIT and WJ III subtests in the matrix (i.e., they occupy different cells), interpretation remains straightforward and indeed is made rather obvious by the resulting patterns. A review of the patterns seen in the data in Figure 11.7 (moving left to right across the matrix) indicates that as the linguistic demands of the tests administered to Vianey increase, her performance decreases accordingly (SS = 103, 91, 86; SS = 94, 82, 76; and SS = 86,

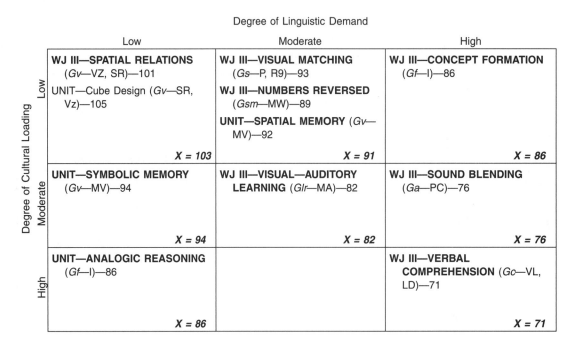

**FIGURE 11.7.** Matrix of cultural loading and linguistic demand classifications for Vianey's WJ III and UNIT subtests. Tests printed in **BOLD UPPERCASE** letters are strong measures, as defined empirically; tests printed in **bold upper- and lowercase** letters are moderate measures, as defined empirically.

71). This pattern indicates that Vianey's scores are more reflective of the linguistic demands of the subtests than of her actual cognitive ability. Similarly, when the data in Figure 11.7 are examined for cultural loading (moving from top to bottom in the matrix), the same type of pattern emerges: As the cultural loading of the tests increases, Vianey's performance decreases (SS = 103, 94, 86; SS = 91, 82; and SS = 86, 76, 71). Again, this pattern provides clear evidence that Vianey's performance decreased primarily in response to the influence of the increasing cultural loading of the subtests, relative to her level of acculturation, than to poor or deficient ability. This pattern is reinforced when considering the diagonal pattern of the data in the illustration. Data that appear along the top-left to lower-right diagonal in the matrix can be used to examine the combined effect of cultural loading and linguistic demand upon performance. Often, the combined effects are more robust than the effects of either influence alone. In this case, it can be seen that Vianey's performance again decreases markedly as the level of cultural loading and linguistic demand increase simultaneously (SS = 103, 82, 71).

Because the observed patterns of performance in Vianey's case are in line with what would be expected of individuals who are not fully acculturated to the U.S. mainstream and whose English language proficiency is not commensurate with their same age or grade peers, the only reasonable, and the least discriminatory, interpretation of these data is that Vianey's performance, as measured by the subtests given nonverbally and in English, is primarily due to these cultural and linguistic differences and is unlikely to reflect actual deficits in ability. With regard to general functioning or ability, Vianey's scores on the subtests that have the lowest cultural loadings and linguistic demands (e.g., nonverbal tests from the UNIT) were the highest overall and, in fact, were within normal limits. This pattern indicates that Vianey's global intellectual ability is most likely within the average range; however, this conclusion cannot be entirely verified, because the full range of cognitive abilities cannot yet be measured in a nonverbal manner or any other testing modality that greatly reduces the effects of language and cultural differences.

Were the patterns of performance observed in the data, as illustrated in Figure 11.7, inconsistent with what would be expected regarding the inhibitory influence of cultural or linguistic factors, then the most that could be said would be that cultural loading and linguistic demand represent contributory, but not primary, factors in determining performance. In such cases, this finding would mean that some other influence had produced the observed patterns. Of course, one possibility is the influence of a particular cognitive deficit or a weakness in one or more of the individual's intellectual abilities, and there could well be other possibilities (e.g., lack of motivation, fatigue, incorrect administration). Moreover, in these situations the overall cognitive ability, as measured by a full-scale score, could be considered a more accurate estimate of general or global functioning. If there is no reason to suspect noncognitive factors then it would be appropriate to consider whether a disability may be present. Interpretation of results from cognitive testing may then be conducted in the manner usually employed when conducting assessment in general. In order to lend more defensibility and validity to such interpretations, however, it is recommended that practitioners apply an empirically supported theoretical framework (e.g., CHC theory) to the data. Current guidelines for best practices in intellectual assessment advocate strongly for theoretically and empirically based interpretations of cognitive ability data. The following discussion utilizes CHC theory and CHC cross-battery principles (Flanagan & Ortiz, 2001; McGrew & Flanagan, 1998; Flanagan et al., 2000).

Although the subtests given from both the UNIT and the WJ III produce global ability scores, from a psychometric stance this combination of tests does not ensure that all of the broad cognitive abilities were properly or adequately measured (i.e., each construct is comprised of at least two measures or subtests). Indeed, a review of the CHC broad and narrow ability classifications of the subtests makes it clear that the only broad ability that is well represented (i.e., comprised of two qualitatively distinct narrow abilities that underlie the broad ability) is visual processing ($Gv$—which is comprised of Cube Design, Symbolic Memory, and Visual Memory from the UNIT and Spatial Relations from the WJ III). Each of the other six constructs ($Gc$, $Ga$, $Gsm$, $Glr$, $Gs$, and $Gf$) are represented by a single subtest (inadequate with which to make interpretations) or by two subtests, in the case of $Gf$, that measure the very same narrow ability (i.e., induction) when combined with the Analogic Reasoning subtest from the UNIT.

In order to make appropriate interpretations of the data collected on Vianey, additional testing needed to be conducted. The existing subtests would be supplemented in a way that would create defensible and valid broad ability clusters represented by qualitatively distinct narrow ability measures. Figure 11.8 provides an illustration of the combined UNIT and WJ III subtests originally administered along with the additional WJ III subtests that were selected to supplement the representation of the full range of cognitive abilities. Additional subtests (boxes) from the WJ III supplemental battery included Retrieval Fluency ($Glr$), Analysis–Synthesis ($Gf$), Auditory Attention ($Ga$), Decision Speed ($Gs$), Memory for Words ($Gsm$), and General Information ($Gc$). It should be noted that, so far, interpretation of the tests used to evaluate Vianey's abilities has been based on an alternative conceptualization—aggregation by shared subtest characteristics (cultural loading and linguistic demand)—rather than the traditional conceptualization—aggregation by construct measured. Thus, rather than using the CHC culture–language matrix to organize the results from initial and supplemental testing, the results are now organized according to the broad ability constructs specified by CHC theory. As noted, use of theory is crucial to the derivation of valid and defensible inferences and interpretations from the collected data. Figure 11.8 shows the organization of the UNIT and WJ III subtests according to the constructs measured.

Two points are of particular importance in Figure 11.8. First, when the data are aggregated according to the cognitive abilities they measure, it becomes clear that Vianey's performance (under the current assumption that culture and language are not operating here and were set aside) is problematic in the areas of $Gc$ (Crystallized Intelligence) and $Ga$ (Auditory Processing), as noted by the gray shading. All her other abilities (no shading) are well within the average range. Second, this interpretation is made on the basis of composite scores (i.e., based on two or more subtests), which are mathematical representations of real "things"—in this case, specific cognitive abilities. This methodology contrasts with the composite scores (mean or average scores obtained for each cell) used in the CHC culture–language matrix, which are only abstractions of performance on tests with shared characteristics and are not to be construed as having any inherent meaning. Composite scores drawn from the use of tests derive meaning only when couched within an empirically supported theoretical framework. As can be seen in Figure 11.8, the areas of functioning that create concern are $Gc$ and $Ga$. Although not conclusive in and of itself, Vianey's performance in these areas is low, and examination from this perspective leads to the conclusion that these cognitive deficits merit further investigation as the possible primary cause of her observed academic difficulties. For a more detailed explanation regarding application of CHC theory and the principles and procedures of the CHC cross-battery approach to measurement and interpretation, the reader should refer to the original sources (e.g., Flanagan et al., 2000; Flanagan & Ortiz, 2001; Flanagan, Ortiz, Alfonso, & Mascolo, 2002).

| CHC Broad Ability | UNIT and WJ III Subtests |
|---|---|
| **Gf—Fluid Intelligence** | **UNIT—ANALOGIC REASONING** (*Gf*—I)—86<br>**WJ III—CONCEPT FORMATION** (*Gf*—I)—86<br>**WJ III—ANALYSIS–SYNTHESIS** (*Gf*—RG)—92<br><div align="right">*X* = 88</div> |
| **Gc—Crystallized Intelligence** | **WJ III—VERBAL COMPREHENSION** (*Gc*—VL, LD)—71<br>**WJ III—GENERAL INFORMATION** (*Gc*—K0)—75<br><div align="right">*X* = 73</div> |
| **Gv—Visual Processing** | **WJ III—SPATIAL RELATIONS** (*Gv*—VZ, SR)—101<br>UNIT—Cube Design (*Gv*—SR, Vz)—105<br>**UNIT—SYMBOLIC MEMORY** (*Gv*—MV)—94<br>**UNIT—SPATIAL MEMORY** (*Gv*—MV)—92<br><div align="right">*X* = 98</div> |
| **Gsm—Short-Term Memory** | **WJ III—NUMBERS REVERSED** (*Gsm*—MW)—89<br>**WJ III—MEMORY FOR WORDS** (*Gsm*—MS)—91<br><div align="right">*X* = 90</div> |
| **Glr—Long-Term Retrieval** | **WJ III—VISUAL—AUDITORY LEARNING** (*Glr*—MA)—82<br>**WJ III—RETRIEVAL FLUENCY** (*Glr*—FI)—94<br><div align="right">*X* = 88</div> |
| **Ga—Auditory Processing** | **WJ III—SOUND BLENDING** (*Ga*—PC)—76<br>**WJ III—AUDITORY ATTENTION** (*Ga*—US/U3)—74<br><div align="right">*X* = 75</div> |
| **Gs—Processing Speed** | **WJ III—VISUAL MATCHING** (*Gs*—P, R9)—93<br>**WJ III—DECISION SPEED** (*Gs*—R4)—91<br><div align="right">*X* = 92</div> |

**FIGURE 11.8.** CHC broad ability classifications for Vianey's WJ III and UNIT subtests. Boxed subtests indicate those selected to supplement the full range of cognitive abilities; shading indicates areas of problematic performance. Tests printed in **BOLD UPPERCASE** letters are strong measures, as defined empirically; tests printed in **bold upper- and lowercase** letters are moderate measures, as defined empirically. Tests in regular case are logically classified.

# SUMMARY

The primary purpose of this chapter was to elucidate the major issues that form the foundation of nondiscriminatory assessment with regard to the use of standardized, norm-referenced tests of cognitive ability. There are, however, numerous other substantive issues that fall beyond the limits of this narrative and that could not be discussed. Fair and equitable cognitive assessment of culturally and linguistically diverse individuals rests primarily on a thorough understanding of the manner in which tests of intelligence or cognitive ability may be affected by acculturation and language proficiency. Although the current array of tests available today tends to be quite sophisticated, the use of these tests (including native-language tests) with diverse individuals continues to be hampered by factors that can result in discriminatory results. These difficulties are not inherent defects of particular tests but rather ubiquitous problems embedded in the very methods of test development and construction.

Primary among these potentially discriminatory aspects is the assumption of comparability across the experiential backgrounds of individuals that comprise the norm samples. Bias is less a function of technical inadequacies in the tests, than it is a function of differences in the experience between individuals in the norm group and the individuals to whom the test may be given. By virtue of their emerging bilingualism and often blended cultural backgrounds, the culturally and linguistically diverse individuals being considered for evaluation every day are not adequately represented by any existing norm sample. Therefore, if individuals from diverse populations are to be evaluated fairly, alternative methods must be employed in order to render test results more equitable or subject to less discriminatory interpretation. Given the complexities that would be involved in creating representative norm groups for individuals with varying levels of acculturation and English-language proficiency, it is unlikely that tests will be developed in the future that would obviate the need for this type of nondiscriminatory approach. According to Sattler:

> Probably no test can be created that will entirely eliminate the influence of learning and cultural experiences. The test content and materials, the language in which the questions are phrased, the test directions, the categories for classifying the responses, the scoring criteria, and the validity criteria are all culture bound. (1992, p. 579)

The distinction between bilingual assessment and assessment of bilingual individuals demonstrates that there are two avenues that can be pursued when standardized, norm-referenced tests are used in evaluation. When bilingual assessment is conducted, the bilingual evaluator has particular competencies and skills that allow for use of instruments such as the BVAT (Muñoz-Sandoval et al., 1998), the Batería-R COG (should the language of assessment be Spanish), as well as methods for deriving what may be fairer estimates of global functioning (e.g., via the BCA-Bil and GIA-Bil). Their limitations and validity concerns aside, these techniques represent a new wave of research that has only just begun to examine the complexities involved in evaluating the bilingual mind in a truly bilingual way.

The remainder of the chapter focused on assessment of bilingual individuals because this approach does not require the linguistic competency of bilingual assessment. Methods and procedures outlined included the MAMBI and the cultural and linguistic extensions of the CHC cross-battery approach organized as the culture–language classification matrix. These procedures represent perhaps the first comprehensive assessment model that provides an integration of the major variables involved in the evaluation of culturally and linguistically diverse populations. Because practitioners are competent in the administration of tests in English, they now have the means to deal with some of the more difficult tasks facing them: notably, the determination as to whether the obtained results can be interpreted as valid estimates of ability or, more reasonably, as measures of acculturation and English-language proficiency. Used in conjunction with other sources of information and data, the comprehensive model outlined in this chapter can help practitioners to overcome the central obstacles involved in conducting equitable assessment and make defensible and educated decisions. Ultimately, these procedures assist in addressing the most fundamental question in the assessment of bilingual individuals: the need to differentiate *difference* from *disorder*.

Whenever standardized, norm-referenced tests are used with culturally and linguistically diverse individuals, the possibility that what is actually being measured is degree of acculturation (or lack thereof) or English-language proficiency rather than ability always exists. True bilingual assessment may be limited to the few who possess the requisite skills, knowledge, and training to conduct it, but fair and equitable assessment of bilingual individuals remains within the scope of virtually any practitioner willing to learn about and comprehend the basic issues. Without question, use of the comprehensive procedures discussed in this chapter (i.e., the MAMBI and the cultural loading/linguistic demand classifications underlying the culture–language classification matrix) represent viable methods for reducing many of the most central aspects that lead to discriminatory results and inferences in the assessment of diverse individuals. These methods adhere to current standards of best practice and can be easily adopted.

# 12

# Assessment of Academic Achievement

## *Practical Guidelines*

The purpose of academic achievement measurement is to assess the skills and abilities children have acquired through direct intervention or instruction (Stetson, Stetson, & Sattler, 2001). Common areas of academic achievement measurement include reading, mathematics, spelling, and writing. Additional areas of measurement may include general subject areas such as science and social studies as well as specific skill areas such as proof reading, punctuation, and capitalization. Accurate assessment of each of these areas is critical to the development of appropriate instructional programming and eligibility determination for students exhibiting academic delays.

Several aspects of academic achievement measurement must be considered in order to accurately assess the academic progress of a child. For example, school-based practitioners attempting to measure academic achievement must consider the impact of previous educational and environmental experiences on skill acquisition. Because academic achievement is based on experientially dependent skills and abilities, a child's previous educational and environmental circumstances will greatly impact his or her performance on achievement measures. Similarly, children from culturally and linguistically diverse backgrounds may have life experiences and skills that are unique in comparison to the normative population on which many commonly used measures of academic achievement are based.

Overall, the measurement of academic achievement is an exceedingly complex process. The decision to use a norm-referenced assessment, curriculum-based assessment, or combination of assessment approaches must be based upon the individual needs of each student. The complexity of the process is multiplied when culture, language, and unique life experiences are considered.

The previous two chapters provided an extensive description of issues and concerns related to the assessment of culturally and linguistically diverse students. The reader is referred to these chapters for a discussion of culture bias, language bias, norm-sample representation, nonverbal

---

This chapter is by Robert L. Rhodes.

assessment, bilingual assessment, and the assessment of students with various degrees of English-language proficiency. The purpose of this chapter is to examine the issues and concerns associated with academic achievement measurement of students who are culturally and linguistically diverse, to provide an overview of the advantages and disadvantages of various assessment strategies and techniques, and to provide a summary of practical strategies and procedures.

## ACADEMIC ACHIEVEMENT ASSESSMENT OF CULTURALLY AND LINGUISTICALLY DIVERSE STUDENTS: ISSUES AND CONCERNS

The U.S. Department of Education's Office of Civil Rights, charged with the enforcement of laws that prohibit discrimination on the basis of race, color, or national origin in programs and activities that receive federal financial assistance (Title VI of the Civil Rights Act of 1964), issued the following guideline in an effort to address the inappropriate assessment and placement of culturally and linguistically diverse students:

> If students are not proficient in speaking, reading, writing, or understanding English, testing them in English may not demonstrate their ability or achievement skills. Steps must be taken so that students are not assigned to special education classes because of their lack of English language proficiency, rather than because they have a disability. (U.S. Department of Education, 2000a)

In a separate resource guide, the U.S. Department of Education (2000b) identified several factors that are particularly salient in ensuring accuracy in testing for students who are culturally and linguistically diverse. These factors include language proficiency, culture, and schooling. Table 12.1 provides a summary of factors related to the assessment of LEP students.

---

**TABLE 12.1. Factors Related to Accurately Testing Limited English Proficient Students**

Language proficiency

- The student's level of oral and written proficiency in English
- The student's proficiency in his or her home language
- The language of instruction

Cultural issues

- Background experiences
- Perceptions of prior experiences
- Value systems

Schooling issues

- The amount of formal elementary and secondary schooling in the student's home country, if applicable, and in U.S. schools
- Consistency of schooling
- Instructional practices in the classroom

---

*Note.* From U.S. Department of Education (2000b).

These factors have particular relevance for the assessment of academic achievement. As noted by Duran (1989), until a student is proficient in English, measures of achievement may really only be a crude test of English competence rather than an accurate assessment of academic growth and development. Likewise, the cultural background and culture-related perception of a child may not be represented in the standardization sample of many norm-referenced measures of academic achievement (Overton, 1996). Additionally, the unique educational and background experiences of a student, including variations in the amount, type, and location (home country and United States) of formal elementary and secondary schooling, as well as interrupted and multilocation schooling, affect language literacy, the contextual content of items, and the academic knowledge base necessary to appropriately interpret the results of norm-referenced measures of academic achievement (U.S. Department of Education, 2001).

It is important to note, however, that although language proficiency, culture, and schooling are three of the most salient issues related to the measurement of academic achievement, they are not the only issues requiring careful attention and consideration. Cole, D'Alonzo, Gallegos, Giordano, and Stile (1992, p. 219) identified several additional factors that should be considered in order to increase the accuracy of the assessment process:

1. Do sensory or communicative impairments make portions of the test inaccessible?
2. Do sensory or communicative impairments limit students from responding to questions?
3. Do test materials or methods of responding limit the student's ability to respond?
4. Does the content of the classroom instruction limit students from responding?
5. Is the examiner familiar to the student?
6. Are instructions explained in a familiar fashion?
7. Is the recording technique required of the student on the test familiar?

School-based practitioners selecting instruments and procedures for the assessment of academic achievement must evaluate these issues as well as method-specific advantages and disadvantages before selecting an assessment strategy that is appropriate for an individual child. The following section provides an overview of the advantages and disadvantages of using standardized or norm-referenced measures of academic achievement with students who are culturally and linguistically diverse.

## STANDARDIZED OR NORM-REFERENCED MEASURES OF ACADEMIC ACHIEVEMENT

There are two general types of individual achievement tests: screening tests and comprehensive tests. Screening tests are typically brief in nature and may contain just one subtest or component for each area assessed. Comprehensive tests usually contain more than one subtest per subject area and attempt to cover the subject areas in depth. Both screening and comprehensive tests are typically administered in a standardized fashion and are based upon the typical performance of standardization sample participants. Overton (2000) points out that a good sample population should include a large number of students (hundreds or thousands, depending on the nature of the test) who represent diverse groups. Proportional representation of students from all cultures and linguistic backgrounds targeted for comparison should be included in the norming process.

## Advantages of Using Norm-Referenced Measures of Academic Achievement

Norm-referenced measures of academic achievement offer several potential advantages as a component of a comprehensive assessment process. Sattler (2001) delineates several of these advantages, including the following:

1. Quantification of a child's functioning through the
   a. Description of a child's present functioning in reference to his or her peer group.
   b. Delineation of specific strengths and deficits.
   c. Provision of a baseline for measuring progress during and after treatment or intervention.
2. Economical and efficient use of time and energy
   a. Permitting a sample of achievement within a short period of time.
   b. Requiring less time and labor than most curriculum-based assessment procedures.
3. Provision of an objective standard through
   a. A prescribed administration and scoring format that is potentially less influenced by subjective judgment.
   b. Measures that typically have a high degree of reliability and validity.

These potential advantages are predicated on several critical assumptions (Figueroa & Hernandez, 2000). It is assumed, for example, that the individual participating in the assessment will have had similar experiences to individuals in the norming sample. It is also assumed that individuals will have had similar opportunity to learn the content measured by the test, the language used by the test, and the skills demanded by the test. Figueroa and Hernandez state that standardized achievement measures are particularly dependent on meeting these assumptions in order to reasonably assess academic ability. When these assumptions are not met, the estimate of an individual's academic achievement may be inaccurate and biased. The next section provides a discussion of some of the potential disadvantages of using norm-referenced measures of academic achievement with students who are culturally and linguistically diverse.

## Disadvantages of Using Norm-Referenced Measures of Academic Achievement

As previously mentioned, individuals who are culturally and linguistically diverse are often unique in comparison to the sample population of many norm-referenced measures of achievement. The use of such measures for this population has several potential disadvantages that could lead to an unfair or biased assessment. In order to avoid this costly outcome, it is important to understand what a fair or unbiased assessment involves. Lam (1995) identifies two antithetical views of fairness in assessment: equality and equity. The *equality viewpoint* of fairness proposes that all students be assessed in a standardized fashion, using the same assessment procedures, administration, scoring, and interpretation. Within this approach, bias will exist when using norm-referenced measures if the individual being assessed is somehow uniquely different from the norm group.

The *equity viewpoint* of fairness, in contrast, proposes that assessment be tailored to the individual student's instructional background and experiences, including prior knowledge, cultural experience, language proficiency, cognitive style, and interests. When the opportunity for a population to learn is not equal or fair (either because of linguistic, cultural, or experiential barriers), measures of achievement may unintentionally reflect a student's *opportunity* to learn rather than his or her *ability* to learn (Moreno, 1999). Bias is minimized and fairness is maximized when these extraneous and inhibitory factors are taken into consideration (Lam, 1995).

Unfortunately, efforts to take factors such as language, culture, and educational experience into consideration when using norm-referenced measures of achievement may inadvertently result in critically altered or inappropriate methods of assessment. Nonverbal tests, translated tests, or tests that are normed in the student's primary language are often utilized in order to assess students who are culturally and linguistically diverse. Substitution of the test format of choice (in the case of nonverbal measures) or test content (in the case of translated tests) may introduce unintentional sources of error. Likewise, utilizing a test that is in the student's primary

---

### TABLE 12.2. Standards for Testing Individuals of Diverse Linguistic Backgrounds

- Testing practice should be designed to reduce threats to the reliability and validity of test score inferences that may arise from language differences.

- When testing an examinee proficient in two or more languages for which the test is available, the examinee's relative language proficiencies should be determined. The test generally should be administered in the test taker's most proficient language, unless proficiency in the less proficient language is part of the assessment.

- Inferences about test takers' general language proficiency shall be based on tests that measure a range of language features, and not a single linguistic skill.

- Linguistic modifications recommended by test publishers, as well as the rationale for the modifications, should be described in detail in the test manual.

- When a test is recommended for use with linguistically diverse test takers, test developers and publishers should provide the information necessary for appropriate test use and interpretation.

- When a test is translated from one language to another, the methods used in establishing the adequacy of the translation should be described, and empirical and logical evidence should be provided for score reliability and the validity of the translated test's score inferences for the uses intended in the linguistic groups to be tested.

- When an interpreter is used in testing, the interpreter should be fluent in both the language of the test and the examinee's native language, should have expertise in translating, and should have a basic understanding of the assessment process.

*Note.* Data from American Educational Research Association, American Psychological Association, and National Council on Measurement in Education (1999).

language but normed in another country (e.g., Mexico) may help alleviate the issue of language while perpetuating the issue of inappropriate norm-group comparison.

The American Educational Research Association, the American Psychological Association, and the National Council on Measurement in Education (1999) issued a revision of the *Standards for Educational and Psychological Testing*, which includes a specific section related to standards for testing individuals of diverse linguistic backgrounds. Table 12.2 provides a summary of some of the recommended standards.

Figueroa and Hernandez (2000) comment that although the revised "Standards for Testing Individuals of Diverse Linguistic Backgrounds" break new ground along several dimensions, many concerns still remain, one of which is the continued use of translated tests and the linkage of test accommodations appropriate for bilingual learners with those appropriate for students with disabilities. Of additional concern is the provision of standards for the use of interpreters when there are no data to substantiate the assumption that it is possible to use an interpreter without severely and negatively affecting the standardization requisites, psychometric properties, and the interpretation of test scores. On a positive note, Figueroa and Hernandez note that the omission from the new standards of the historical accommodation of simply using more tests when there are no appropriate tests available is a welcome change.

## Commonly Used Norm-Referenced Measures of Academic Achievement

The following section provides a brief description of some of the most commonly used norm-referenced measures of academic achievement and the advantages and disadvantages of their use with students who are culturally and linguistically diverse.

### Woodcock–Johnson III Tests of Achievement

The Woodcock–Johnson III Tests of Achievement (WJ III; Woodcock, McGrew, & Mather, 2001b) is an individually administered battery of achievement tests for individuals from 2 to over 90 years of age. There are a total of 22 different tests, although not all of the tests are administered at the younger age levels. The Standard Battery is comprised of 12 tests, and the Extended Battery includes an additional 10 tests. The Standard Battery tests include Letter–Word Identification, Reading Fluency, Math Fluency, Spelling, and Writing Fluency. The Extended Battery generally includes more specific skill tests such as Editing, Word Attack, Spelling of Sounds, and Punctuation and Capitalization. The standardization sample of the WJ III included over 8,000 individuals and was stratified based on race, ethnicity, and Hispanic origin.

#### Advantages
- Current standardization sample reflecting race, ethnicity, and Hispanic origin.
- Broad-based, comprehensive approach in a well-designed and attractive format.

#### Disadvantages
- Emphasis on speed of performance on Reading Fluency, Writing Fluency, and Math Fluency tests may penalize students who are processing information in a second language.

- Although the administration manual provides general guidelines for English-language learners, no provision for alternate language administration is provided.
- Unable to be hand scored; must be computer scored.

## Kaufman Test of Educational Achievement—Second Edition

The Kaufman Test of Educational Achievement—Second Edition (KTEA-II; Kaufman & Kaufman, 2004) is designed to assess reading, mathematics, written language, and oral language. It is an untimed, individually administered test of achievement. The KTEA-II Comprehensive Form can be used with individuals from preschool through young adulthood who are between 4½ and 25 years of age. There are seven subtests in the standard battery: Letter and Word Recognition, Nonsense Word Decoding, Reading Comprehension, Math Concepts and Applications, Math Computation, Written Expression, and Spelling. The new standardization sample was stratified based on race, ethnicity, and Hispanic origin.

### Advantages
- Normed on the same standardization sample as the KABC-II, which allows for more accurate across-test comparison.
- Extended age range through 25 years of age (90+ years of age for the Brief Form).
- Error analysis procedure available for in-depth analysis of academic performance and instructional recommendations.
- Listening comprehension, oral expression, and written expression addressed in new version.

### Disadvantages
- Limited reliability and validity information available for newly revised version.
- No alternate language format is available.

## Wechsler Individual Achievement Test—Second Edition

The Wechsler Individual Achievement Test—Second Edition (WIAT-II; Psychological Corporation, 2001) is a comprehensive, individually administered battery for assessing the academic achievement of individuals from 4 years of age through adulthood, including norms for college students. Subtests include Oral Language, Listening Comprehension, Written Expression, Spelling, Pseudoword Decoding, Word Reading, Reading Comprehension, Numerical Operations, and Mathematics Reasoning. The WIAT-II was reportedly standardized on a large representative sample, including individuals with learning disabilities, intellectual disabilities, emotional disturbance, hearing impairment, gifted and talented, and at-risk preschoolers.

### Advantages
- Newly updated measure with expanded norm sample and age groups.
- Provides norm-referenced information related to each of the seven areas required by the Individuals with Disabilities Education Act.
- Empirically linked with the Wechsler Intelligence Scales for achievement and ability comparison.

*Disadvantages*

- As with other Wechsler measures, the WIAT-II places a heavy emphasis on language skills and verbal ability.
- No alternate language format is available.

## Batería Woodcock–Muñoz—Revisada: Pruebas de Aprovechamiento

The Batería Woodcock–Muñoz—Revisada (Woodcock & Muñoz-Sandoval 1996) is the parallel Spanish version of the Woodcock–Johnson Psychoeducational Battery—Revised. It contains a series of individually administered standardized tests designed to measure academic achievement and Spanish oral-language achievement of Spanish-speaking individuals. The Batería was standardized on over 4,000 individuals from 2 to over 90 years of age. The standardization process took place in several countries, including the United States. The Pruebas de Aprovechamiento assesses reading, mathematics, written language, and knowledge. The skills assessed in reading include *destrezas basicas en lectura* (basic reading skills) and *comprension de lectura* (reading comprehension). In mathematics *destrezas basicas en matematicas* (basic mathematics skills) are measured, as is *razonamiento en matematics* (mathematical reasoning). For written language, *destrezas basicas en escritura* (basic writing skills) are tested.

*Advantages*

- Comprehensive, broad-based approach in Spanish.
- Preliminary Language Use Survey is available to enhance the interpretation of test results.
- Comparative Language Index is available for students who complete both the Batería and the Woodcock–Johnson—Revised to examine individual strengths in Spanish versus English and norm-based levels of proficiency in each language.

*Disadvantages*

- The standardization sample is drawn from both within and outside of the United States and, as a result, does not allow for direct norm-referenced comparison to same-age individuals living within the United States.
- Conversely, although the standardization sample is drawn from several countries, numerous items maintain a U.S.-based focus (e.g., U.S. ZIP codes, U.S. currency, U.S. time zones, and the English system of measurement). This is especially evident in the Social Studies subtest and limits the utility of the Batería for students whose educational experience is not based in the United States (Frary, 1998).

## Aprenda: La Prueba de Logros en Español, Segunda Edición

The second edition of the Aprenda (Aprenda 2; Psychological Corporation, 1997) assesses Spanish-speaking students' academic achievement in reading, language arts, and mathematics. It is designed for students in grades K–12 and mirrors the content and processes measured by the Stanford Achievement Test—Ninth Edition. A multiple-choice battery is available for fall or spring testing and includes Reading, Mathematics, Language, Listening, and English subtests. An optional open-ended battery is also available for year-round testing and includes Reading, Mathematics, and Writing subtests. An optional English component is also available for 4th through 12th grade. The standardization sample was selected to represent the United States Spanish-speaking population in relation to U.S. region and country of origin.

*Advantages*
- Norm-referenced measure of achievement designed and created in Spanish.
- The first Spanish-language achievement measure to include an English component to assess the progress of Hispanic bilingual students in their acquisition of English as a second language.
- The first Spanish-language achievement measure to offer criterion-referenced Performance Standards that reflect bilingual teachers' expectations of what students should know and be able to do in the classroom.
- Assesses reading and listening with selections written and illustrated by well-known Hispanic authors.

*Disadvantages*
- The processes by which students were "identified by their school districts as being equally proficient in English and Spanish" are not included. Ochoa (1998) notes that this omission is a critical limitation, given the difficulty of finding individuals who are truly balanced bilingual students across the reading, writing, listening, and speaking domains.
- The various regions of the United States and countries of origin seem to be under-represented in the current standardization sample.
- Norm-based comparison of students who were educated outside of the United States with the Aprenda 2 standardization sample is inappropriate.

The diversity of cultural, linguistic, and educational experiences represented in the school-age population precludes the selection of any one instrument as an "instrument of choice." Although each successive generation of tests appears to be more sensitive to, and representative of, students who are culturally and linguistically diverse, potential disadvantages remain with the genre of currently available measures. In response to the limitations and the very real potential for biased and unfair results, alternative procedures for assessing academic achievement have been explored.

## INFORMAL MEASURES OF ACADEMIC ACHIEVEMENT

Numerous authors have advocated for the use of alternative procedures to assess the skills and abilities children have acquired through either direct intervention or instruction (e.g., Shinn, 2002; Fuchs & Fuchs, 1997). Because of the difficulties inherent the use of norm-referenced measures of academic achievement with students who are culturally and linguistically diverse, criterion-referenced and curriculum-based assessment procedures have generated a great deal of interest. The next section provides an overview of some of the advantages and disadvantages of using criterion-referenced and curriculum-based assessment with students who are culturally and linguistically diverse.

## Criterion-Referenced Assessment of Academic Achievement

Criterion-referenced assessment is designed to compare the performance of a student to a specific criterion rather than to the performance of students in a norm group. The criterion used for comparison may be a specific objective written by the teacher, a school-, district-, or statewide standard, or a skill or sequential task included in a scope-and-sequence chart of a published curriculum (Overton, 2000). Salvia and Hughes (1990) recommend the following steps for conducting a criterion-referenced assessment of academic achievement: (1) specify reasons for decisions; (2) analyze the curriculum; (3) formulate the behavioral objectives; (4) develop appropriate assessment procedures; (5) collect data; (6) summarize data; (7) display the data; and (8) interpret data and make decisions. Most criterion-referenced measures are informal, nonstandardized instruments that are created or adapted by the teacher or evaluator. A limited number of commercially produced criterion-referenced measures is available. The Brigance Diagnostic Assessment is an example of a commonly used, commercially available criterion-referenced measure designed for use with Spanish-speaking students.

### *Brigance Diagnostic Assessment of Basic Skills, Spanish*

The Brigance Diagnostic Assessment of Basic Skills, Spanish (Brigance–Spanish; Brigance & Messer, 1984) is designed for students in kindergarten through sixth grade for whom Spanish is a first language. The stated purpose of the Brigance–Spanish is to determine whether a student is performing at grade level in academic subjects in his or her native language, and to help distinguish whether or not a student's weaknesses are due to limited English proficiency or to a specific learning disability. The Brigance–Spanish has the following sections: Readiness, Speech, Functional Word Recognition, Oral Reading, Reading Comprehension and Word Analysis, Listening, Writing and Alphabetizing, Numbers and Computation, and Measurement. Not all parts of the test are administered to every student; the teacher/evaluator is encouraged to check off skills that he or she knows the student has mastered. The test is administered individually, and some test items have illustrations. Scoring guidelines for most items allow for a variety of appropriate answers. In addition to Spanish, the Brigance is also available in Portuguese.

## Curriculum-Based Assessment of Academic Achievement

Curriculum-based assessment (CBA) is the process of determining a student's instructional needs within a curriculum by directly assessing specific curriculum skills (Poteet, 1995). CBA is generally considered a type of criterion-referenced measurement in which a standard or criterion is designated within a set of items to indicate mastery of instructional content (Poteet, 1995). A recent study by Shapiro, Angello, and Eckert (2004) indicates that curriculum-based assessment has increasingly become a staple of school psychology and assessment practice. Shapiro et al. report that the number of school psychology training programs including curriculum-based assessment procedures as part of their graduate program of study, and the number of practitioners utilizing curriculum-based assessment in their day-to-day activities have both increased significantly in the past decade. It is important to note, however, that nearly half of all school psychologists surveyed by Shapiro et al. indicated that they do not typically use curriculum-based assessment procedures as part of the assessment process.

*Curriculum-Based Measurement*

There are various forms and approaches to CBA; one of the most widely used forms is curriculum-based measurement (CBM; Deno, 1985). CBM was initially developed in response to a recognized limitation of other CBA measures: the absence of a uniform approach to item selection and test development (Shinn, 1989). CBM follows standardized administration and scoring procedures, including (1) the selection of one long-term goal instead of a series of short-term curricular steps; (2) use of prescribed measurement methods; and (3) incorporation of rules that allow for the systematic summary and evaluation of information (Fuchs & Fuchs, 1990). Computer software is available to assist in charting student performance across time. CBM's standardized administration and scoring and broad sample of performance allow the teacher or evaluator to identify discrepancies in performance levels between individuals and peer groups (Fuchs & Fuchs, 1997).

Fuchs (2004) states that two curriculum-based measurement approaches have typically been used to identify measurement tasks that simultaneously integrate the various skills required for competent year-end performance. The first is the identification of a task that correlates highly with the component skills of an academic domain: for example, the identification and measurement of passage-reading fluency as a robust indicator of skill in other academic domains such as reading comprehension, decoding, word identification, and vocabulary. The second approach to the identification of measurement tasks related to expected year-end performance involves systematic sampling of skills constituting the annual curriculum to ensure that each weekly CBM represents the curriculum equivalently. For example, in math each weekly test would incorporate the same problem types in the same proportion: addition, subtraction, multiplication, and division. The total test score serves as an indicator of overall math competence in the annual curriculum and would be graphed to depict the rate of learning (Fuchs, 2004).

## Advantages and Disadvantages of Using Informal Measures of Academic Achievement

The advantages and disadvantages of using informal measures, such as criterion-referenced assessment and curriculum-based assessment, to assess the academic achievement of students who are culturally and linguistically diverse are listed for quick reference:

*Advantages*
- Direct comparison to instructional content and demands of the classroom environment.
- Unlimited in nature; may generate any desired criterion and corresponding items.
- Criterion and item selection may be individualized according to student's cultural, linguistic, and educational background.
- Ongoing documentation may be maintained to chart student progress toward meeting individual and classroom curricular goals.

*Disadvantages*
- Development and application of teacher-made criterion-referenced measures may vary widely from teacher to teacher.

- Student mobility will greatly affect utility of measures.
- Because of the individuality of teacher-made measures, comparison of a student's performance to settings outside of scope of the curriculum (e.g., class to class or district to district) is limited.
- Likewise, the use of scope-and-sequence charts from published curriculum as a criterion reference may not correspond with a student's actual classroom instruction and educational experiences.
- Although the more standardized approach of CBM assists in addressing the preceding limitations, the model's heavy reliance on decision making based on visual inspection of the data introduces other potential sources of error.
- Among both criterion-referenced and curriculum-based methods of assessment, teachers must guard against "teaching to the test" based upon the sample of curricular content selected for assessment.
- Finally, informal measures in isolation may not provide the requisite information necessary for eligibility determination and service provision in many states.

## Recommendations for Using Criterion-Referenced and Curriculum-Based Measures

Table 12.3 provides a summary of the various issues and concerns that should be considered when using criterion-referenced and curriculum-based measures as the means of assessing the academic achievement of students who are culturally and linguistically diverse.

---

**TABLE 12.3. The Use of Criterion-Referenced and Curriculum-Based Measures with Students Who Are Culturally and Linguistically Diverse**

---

Issues and concerns that should be carefully considered when using criterion-referenced and curriculum-based measures include:

- The extent to which the curricular content of the classroom or course is culturally representative of the student. Curricular additions and adjustments should be made as necessary.
- The student's previous or current participation in ESL and bilingual education programming and the outcome of program participation (see Chapters 4 and 5).
- Known or suspected sensory or communicative impairments (see Chapters 5 and 7).
- The amount, type, and location (home country and United States) of formal elementary and secondary schooling (see Chapter 5 and 7).
- The student's mobility and attendance pattern and the potential impact on academic progress (see Chapter 7).
- The student's current level of acculturation in relation to the appropriateness of assessment items and procedures (see Chapter 8).
- The student's level of English language proficiency in comparison to the language of the criterion-referenced or curriculum-based measures (see Chapter 9).
- Skills other than the target skill required to complete tasks or assignments.
- Experiences outside of the school setting that support or detract from academic success.

---

## CONCLUSION: TOWARD A COMPREHENSIVE MODEL
## OF ACADEMIC ACHIEVEMENT ASSESSMENT

Ascher (1990) provides a fitting synopsis of the issues related to the assessment of academic achievement among students who are culturally and linguistically diverse, stating that assessment should be

> sensitive to issues such as content and processing factors such as speed. Further, an assessment should be capable of comparing performance on tasks across two languages. No universal instruments currently exist for doing this in every domain of assessment. The school psychologist who relies heavily on existing tests in a single language ends up with many scores but no empirical or hypothetical direction for interpreting or diagnosing from them. (p. 4)

It is currently not, and most likely never will be, feasible to comprehensively assess the academic achievement of students who are culturally and linguistically diverse through one approach or technique. Norm-referenced measures of achievement often do not provide an accurate indication of a student's performance because of unique cultural, linguistic, and experiential factors that are not reflected in the standardization sample. This limitation of norm-referenced measures introduces varying degrees of error into the assessment process, depending upon the background and experiences of the individual student. Likewise, informal measures of academic achievement, such as criterion-referenced measurement and curriculum-based assessment, are helpful in assessing a student's academic performance according to the demands of a specific setting or published curriculum, but are limited in their application to other settings and may not provide the information necessary for eligibility determination and service provision. Neither norm-referenced nor curriculum-based measures are without specific limitations and, as a result, should be considered complementary points of comparison rather than mutually exclusive procedures.

Taken as a whole, interviews, observations, norm-referenced measures, and informal measures should be viewed as a menu of options through which more, not less, information is sought. For some students, certain procedures or techniques are clearly inappropriate and should be unconditionally discarded from the assessment process. For other students, careful selection of complementary procedures and techniques may allow for the evaluation of information generated from both formal and informal measures. A guiding directive of the assessment process (both legally and ethically) is that each component must be selected in relation to the individual needs of the student.

Just as it is overly simplistic and reckless to utilize norm-referenced measures of academic achievement with students who are culturally and linguistically diverse without first carefully considering the unique skills and experiences of individual students, it seems equally simplistic to exclude an entire group from participation in norm-referenced measurement of achievement based upon ethnicity or dual-language exposure. Rather, each student's individual cultural, language, schooling, and other applicable experiences must be weighed in order to determine the most appropriate method(s) of measuring academic achievement in students who are culturally and linguistically diverse.

# References

Algozzine, B., Christenson, S., & Ysseldyke, J. (1982). Probabilities associated with the referral to placement process. *Teacher Education and Special Education, 5*(3), 19–23.

Alvarado, C. G. (1999). *A Broad Cognitive Ability—Bilingual Scale for the WJ-R Tests of Cognitive Ability and the Batería Woodcock–Muñoz Pruebas de Habilidad Cognitiva—Revisada* (Research Report Number 2). Itasca, IL: Riverside.

Amado, A. J., Sines, M., & Garza, S. (1999, August). *School psychology training: Psychological assessment of Hispanic English proficient students.* Paper presented at the meeting of the American Psychological Association, Boston.

American Educational Research Association, American Psychological Association, & National Council on Measurement in Education. (1999). *Standards for educational and psychological testing.* Washington, DC: American Psychological Association.

American Psychological Association. (2002). *Ethical principles of psychologists and code of conduct.* Washington, DC: Author.

Anstrom, K. (1996). Defining the limited-English proficient student population. *National Clearinghouse of Bilingual Education: Directions in Language and Education, 1*(9).

Artiles, A. J. (1998). The dilemma of difference: Enriching the disproportionality discourse with theory and context. *Journal of Special Education, 32,* 32–36.

Artiles, A. J., Rueda, R., Salazar, J. J., & Higareda, I. (2002). English-language learner representation in special education in California urban school districts. In D. J. Losen & G. Orfield (Eds.), *Racial inequity in special education* (pp. 117–136). Cambridge, MA: Harvard Education Press.

Artiles, A. J., & Trent, S. C. (1994). Overrepresentation of minority students in special education: A continuing debate. *Journal of Special Education, 27,* 410–437.

Ascher, C. (1990). *Assessing bilingual students for placement and instruction.* New York: ERIC Document Reproduction Service (No. EDO-UD-90-5).

August, D., & Hakuta, K. (1998). *Educating language-minority children*. Washington, DC: National Academy Press.

Baker, K., & de Kanter, A. (1981). *Effectiveness of bilingual education: A review of the literature*. Washington, DC: U.S. Department of Education, Office of Planning, Budget, and Evaluation.

Baker, K., & de Kanter, A. (1983). Federal policy and the effectiveness of bilingual education. In K. Baker & A. de Kanter (Eds.), *Bilingual education: A reappraisal of federal policy* (pp. 33–86). Lexington, MA: Lexington Books.

Barona, A., & Santos de Barona, M. (1987). A model for the assessment of limited English proficient students referred for special education services. In S. H. Fradd & W. J. Tikunoff (Eds.), *Bilingual education and bilingual special education* (pp. 183–210). Boston: College-Hill.

Berry, J. W. (2003). Conceptual approaches to acculturation. In K. M. Chun, P. B. Organista, & G. Marín (Eds.), *Acculturation: Advances in theory, measurement, and applied research* (pp. 17–38). Washington, DC: American Psychological Association.

Bersoff, D. N., & Hofer, P. T. (1990). The legal regulation of school psychology. In C. R. Reynolds & T. B. Gutkin (Eds.), *The handbook of school psychology* (2nd ed., pp. 937–961). New York: Wiley.

Bialystok, E. (1991). *Language processing in bilingual children*. New York: Cambridge University Press.

Brigance, A. H., & Messer, P. (1984). *Brigance Diagnostic Assessment of Basic Skills: Spanish edition*. North Billerica, MA: Curriculum Associates.

Brown v. Board of Education, 347 U.S. 483 (1954).

Center for Applied Linguistics. (2001). *Two-way bilingual immersion tables*. Retrieved September 10, 2002, from *www.cal.org/twi/directory/tables.html*.

Chamberlain, P., & Medinos-Landurand, P. (1991). Practical considerations for the assessment of LEP students with special needs. In E. V. Hamayan & J. S. Damico (Eds.), *Limiting bias in the assessment of bilingual students*. Austin, TX: Pro-Ed.

Chinn, P. C., & Hughes, S. (1987). Representation of minority students in special education classes. *Remedial and Special Education, 8*, 41–46.

Chun, K. M., Organista, P. B., & Marín, G. (2003). *Acculturation: Advances in theory, measurement, and applied research*. Washington, DC: American Psychological Association.

Civil Rights Project. (2000). *Executive summary: Conference of minority issues in special education*. Retrieved June 23, 2001, from *www.law.harvard.edu/civilrights/conferences/SpecEd/exsummary.html*.

Cole, J., D'Alonzo, B., Gallegos, A., Giordano, G., & Stile, S. (1992). Test biases that hamper learners with disabilities. *Diagnostique, 17*, 209–225.

Cole, M., & Cole, S. R. (1993). *The development of children*. New York: Scientific American Books.

Collier, C., & Hoover, J. J. (1987). Sociocultural considerations when referring minority children for learning disabilities. *Learning Disabilities Focus, 3*(1), 39–45.

Collier, V. (1987). Age and rate of acquisition of second language for academic purposes. *TESOL Quarterly, 21*, 617–641.

Collier, V. (1989). How long? A synthesis of research on academic achievement in a second language. *TESOL Quarterly, 23*, 509–531.

Council for Exceptional Children. (1996). *The use of interpreters for linguistically diverse individuals*. Reston, VA: Author.

Council for Exceptional Children. (1997). *Code of ethics for educators of persons with exceptionalities*. Arlington, VA: Author.

Coutinho, M. J., & Oswald, D. P. (2000). Disproportionate representation in special education: A synthesis and recommendations. *Journal of Child and Family Studies, 9*, 135–156.

Crawford, J. (1995). *Bilingual education: History, politics, theory and practice* (3rd ed.). Los Angeles: Bilingual Educational Services.

Cummins, J. (1983). Bilingualism and special education: Program and pedagogical issues. *Learning Disability Quarterly, 6,* 373–386.

Cummins, J. (1984). *Bilingualism and special education: Issues in assessment and pedagogy.* San Diego: College-Hill.

Cummins, J. (1986). Empowering minority students: A framework for intervention. *Harvard Educational Review, 56,* 18–35.

Damico, J. S. (1991). Descriptive assessment of communicative ability in limited English proficient students. In E. V. Hamayan & J. S. Damico (Eds.), *Limiting bias in the assessment of bilingual students* (pp. 157–218). Austin, TX: Pro-Ed.

Damico, J. S., & Hamayan, E. V. (1991). Implementing assessment in the real world. In E. V. Hamayan & J. S. Damico (Eds.), *Limiting bias in the assessment of bilingual students* (pp. 303–316). Austin, TX: Pro-Ed.

Damico, J. S., & Oller, J. W. (1980). Pragmatic versus morphological/syntactic criteria for language referrals. *Language, Speech, and Hearing Services in Schools, 11,* 85–94.

Damico, J. S., Oller, J. W., & Storey, M. E. (1983). The diagnosis of language disorders in bilingual children: Surface-oriented and pragmatic criteria. *Journal of Speech and Hearing Disorders, 48,* 385–394.

Daniel R. R. v. Texas Board of Education, El Paso Independent School District, 874 F.2d 1036 (5th Cir. 1989).

Daniels, V. I. (1998). Minority students in gifted and special education programs: The case for educational equity. *Journal of Special Education, 32,* 4–13.

Danoff, M. (1978). *Evaluation of the impact of ESEA Title VII Spanish/English bilingual education programs: Overview of study and findings.* Palo Alto, CA: American Institutes for Research (ERIC Document Reproduction Service No. ED 154 634).

Daughtery, D. W. (1999). Disproportionality issues in the implementation of IDEA '97. *NASP Communique, 28*(4), 16–18.

Deno, S. L. (1985). Curriculum-based measurement: The emerging alternative. *Exceptional Children, 52,* 219–232.

de Valenzuela, J. S., & Cervantes, H. T. (1998). Procedures and techniques for assessing the bilingual exceptional child. In L. M. Baca & H. T. Cervantes (Eds.), *The bilingual special education interface* (3rd ed., pp. 168–187). Columbus, OH: Merrill.

Diana v. California. No. C-70-37 (N.D. Calif. 1970) (consent decree).

Diana v. State Board of Education, Civ. Act. No. C-70-37 (N.D. Cal., 1970, *further order,* 1973).

Donovan, M. S., & Cross, C. T. (2002). *Minorities in special and gifted education.* Washington, DC: National Research Council.

Drane, E. R. (2002). Sociocultural context effects on teachers' readiness to refer for learning disabilities. *Exceptional Children, 69*(1), 41–53.

Dunn, L. M. (1968). Special education for the mildly retarded: Is much of it justifiable? *Exceptional Children, 35,* 5–22.

Duran, R. P. (1989). Assessment and instruction of at-risk Hispanic students. *Exceptional Children, 56*(2), 154–158.

*Education for All Handicapped Children Act of 1975* (Public Law No. 94-142), renamed *Individuals with Disabilities Education Act* in 1990, 20 U.S.C. Chapter 33.

Ehrman, M. E. (1996). *Understanding second language learning difficulties.* Thousand Oaks, CA: Sage.

Esquivel, G. B. (1988). Best practices in the assessment of limited English proficient and bilingual children. In A. Thomas & J. Grimes (Eds.), *Best practices in school psychology* (pp. 113–123). Washington, DC: National Association of School Psychologists.

Family Educational Rights and Privacy Act (Public Law 93-380), 20 U.S.C. 1232g (1974).

Fierros, E. G., & Conroy, J. W. (2002). Double jeopardy: An exploration of restrictiveness and race in special education. In D. J. Losen & G. Orfield (Eds.), *Racial inequity in special education* (pp. 39–70). Cambridge, MA: Harvard Education Press.

Figueroa, R. A. (1983). Test bias and Hispanic children. *Journal of Special Education, 17,* 431–440.

Figueroa, R. A. (1990a). Best practices in the assessment of bilingual children. In A. Thomas & J. Grimes (Eds.), *Best practices in school psychology* (Vol. 2, pp. 93–106). Washington, DC: National Association of School Psychologists.

Figueroa, R. A. (1990b). Assessment of linguistic minority group children. In C. R. Reynolds & R. W. Kamphaus (Eds.), *Handbook of psychological and educational assessment of children: Intelligence and achievement* (pp. 671–696). New York: Guilford Press.

Figueroa, R. A., Delgado, G. L., & Ruiz, N. T. (1984). Assessment of Hispanic children: Implications for Hispanic hearing-impaired children. In G. L. Delgado (Ed.), *The Hispanic deaf: Issues and challenges for bilingual special education* (pp. 124–153). Washington, DC: Gallaudet College Press.

Figueroa, R. A., Fradd, S. H., & Correa, V. I. (1989). Bilingual special education and this special issue. *Exceptional Children, 56*(2), 174–178.

Figueroa, R. A., & Hernandez, S. (2000). *Testing Hispanic students in the United States: Technical and policy issues.* Washington, DC: President's Advisory Commission on Educational Excellence for Hispanic Americans.

Finn, J. D. (1982). Patterns in special education placement as revealed by the OCR survey. In K. A. Heller, W. H. Holtzman, & S. Messick (Eds.), *Placing children in special education: A strategy for equity* (pp. 322–381). Washington, DC: National Academy Press.

Flanagan, D. P., McGrew, K. S., & Ortiz, S. O. (2000). *The Wechsler Intelligence Scales and Gf–Gc theory: A contemporary approach to interpretation.* Boston: Allyn & Bacon.

Flanagan, D. P., & Ortiz, S. O. (2001). *Essentials of cross-battery assessment.* New York: Wiley.

Flanagan, D. P., Ortiz, S. O., Alfonso, V., & Mascolo, J. (2002). *The achievement test desk reference (ATDR): Comprehensive assessment and learning disability.* New York: Allyn & Bacon.

Flugum, K. R., & Reschly, D. J. (1994). Prereferral interventions: Quality indices and outcomes. *Journal of School Psychology, 32*(1), 1–14.

Ford, D. Y. (1998). The underrepresentation of minority students in gifted education: Problems and promises in recruitment and retention. *Journal of Special Education, 32,* 4–14.

Foster, G. C., Ysseldyke, J. E., Casey, A., & Thurlow, M. L. (1984). The congruence between reason for referral and placement outcome. *Journal of Psychoeducational Assessment, 2,* 209–217.

Frary, R. B. (1998). Review of the Batería Woodcock–Muñoz—Revisada. In J. C. Impara & B. S. Plake (Eds.), *The thirteenth mental measurements yearbook.* Lincoln, NE: University of Nebraska Press.

Fuchs, D. (1991). Mainstream assistance teams. A prereferral intervention system for difficult-to-teach students. In G. Stoner, M. R. Shinn, & H. W. Walker (Eds.), *Interventions for achievement and behavior problems* (pp. 241–267). Silver Spring, MD: National Association of School Psychologists.

Fuchs, L. S. (2004). The past, present, and future of curriculum-based measurement research. *School Psychology Review, 33*(2), 188–192.

Fuchs, L. S., & Fuchs, D. (1990). Curriculum-based measurement: A standardized long-term goal approach to monitoring student progress. *Academic Therapy, 25*(5), 615–632.

Fuchs, L. S., & Fuchs, D. (1997). Use of curriculum-based measurement in identifying students with disabilities. *Focus on Exceptional Children, 30*(3), 1–16.

Fugate, D. J., Clarizio, H. F., & Phillips, S. E. (1993). Referral-to-placement ratio: A finding in need of reassessment? *Journal of Learning Disabilities, 26*(5), 413–416.

Furlong, M. (1988). An examination of an implementation of the simple difference score distribution model in learning disability identification. *Psychology in the Schools, 25,* 125–132.

Glennon, T. (2002). Evaluating the Office of Civil Rights' minority and special education project. In D. J.

Losen & G. Orfield (Eds.), *Racial inequity in special education* (pp. 195–217). Cambridge, MA: Harvard Education Press.

Gonzalez, G. (2004). *Symposium addressing the needs of secondary LEP students: Texas Education Agency bilingual/ESL update.* Retrieved September 7, 2004, from *www.tea.state.tx.us?curriculum/bipresentations.html.*

Gould, S. J. (1996). *Mismeasure of man.* New York: Norton.

Greene, J. P. (1998). A meta-analysis of the effectiveness of bilingual education. Retrieved November 11, 2002, from *www.ourworld.compuserve.com/homepages/jcrawford.greene.htm.*

Grosjean, F. (1989). Neurolinguists beware! The bilingual is not two monolinguals in one person. *Brain and Language, 36,* 3–15.

Guadalupe Organization v. Tempe Elementary School District No. 3, Civ. No. 71-435 (D. Ariz., 1972).

Guajardo Alvarado, C. (2003). *Best practices in the special education evaluation of culturally and linguistically diverse students.* Retrieved May 22, 2003, from *www.updc.org/oldsite/pdf/best.pdf.*

Hakuta, K. (1986). *Mirror of language: The debate on bilingualism.* New York: Basic Books.

Hallberg, G. R. (1996). Assessing bilingual and LEP students: Practical issues in the use of interpreters. *NASP Communique, 25*(1), 16–18.

Hamayan, E. V., & Damico, J. S. (Eds.). (1991a). *Limiting bias in the assessment of bilingual students.* Austin, TX: Pro-Ed.

Hamayan, E. V., & Damico, J. S. (1991b). Developing and using a second language. In E. V. Hamayan & J. S. Damico (Eds.), *Limiting bias in the assessment of bilingual students* (pp. 39–76). Austin, TX: Pro-Ed.

Harris, J. D., Gray, B. A., Davis, J. E., Zaremba, E. T., & Argulewicz, E. N. (1988). The exclusionary clause and the disadvantaged: Do we try to comply with the law? *Journal of Learning Disabilities, 21,* 581–583.

Harry, B. (1994). *The disproportionate representation of minority students in special education: Theories and recommendations* (Project Forum). Alexandria, VA: National Association of State Directors of Special Education.

Harry, B., Klinger, J. K., Sturges, K. M., & Moore, R. F. (2002). Of rocks and soft places: Using qualitative methods to investigate disproportionality. In D. J. Losen & G. Orfield (Eds.), *Racial inequity in special education* (pp. 71–92). Cambridge, MA: Harvard Education Press.

Hearne, D. (2000). *Teaching second language learners with learning disabilities: Strategies for effective practice.* Oceanside, CA: Academic Communication Associates.

Heller, K. A., Holtzman, W. H., & Messick, S. (Eds.). (1982). *Placing children in special education: A strategy for equity.* Washington, DC: National Academy Press.

Heubert, J. P. (2002). Disability, race, and high-stakes testing of students. In D. J. Losen & G. Orfield (Eds.), *Racial inequity in special education* (pp. 137–166). Cambridge, MA: Harvard Education Press.

Holtzman, W. H. (1982). Preface. In K. A. Heller, W. H. Holtzman, & S. Messick (Eds.), *Placing children in special education: A strategy for equity* (pp. ix–xiii). Washington, DC: National Academy Press.

Hoover, J. J., & Collier, C. (1985). Referring culturally different children: Sociocultural considerations. *Academic Therapy, 20,* 503–509.

Hopstock, P., & Bucaro, B. (1993). *A review and analysis of estimates of LEP student population.* Prepared under contract for the U.S. Department of Education by Development Associates, Arlington, VA.

*Individuals with Disabilities Education Act* (Public Law No. 101-476), 20 U.S.C. Chapter 33 (1990).

*Individuals with Disabilities Education Act Revision* (Public Law No. 105-17), 20 U.S.C. Chapter 33 (1997).

Jacob-Timm, S., & Hartshorne, T. S. (1998). *Ethics and law for school psychologists* (3rd ed.). New York: Wiley.

Jensen, A. R. (1974). How biased are culture-loaded tests? *Genetic Psychology Monographs, 90,* 185–244.

Jensen, A. R. (1976). Construct validity and test bias. *Phi Delta Kappan, 58,* 340–346.

Jensen, A. R. (1980). *Bias in mental testing.* New York: Free Press.

Jitendra, A. K., & Rohena-Diaz, E. (1996). Language assessment of students who are linguistically diverse: Why a discrete approach is not the answer. *School Psychology Review, 25*(1), 40–56.

Kamphaus, R. W. (1993). *Clinical assessment of children's intelligence.* Boston: Allyn & Bacon.

Kaufman, A. S. (1994). *Intelligent testing with the WISC-R.* New York: Wiley.

Kaufman, A. S., & Kaufman, N. L. (2004). *Kaufman Test of Educational Achievement—Second Edition.* Circle Pines, MN: American Guidance Service.

Kauffman, J. M., Hallahan, D. P., & Ford, D. Y. (1998). Introduction to the special section. *Journal of Special Education, 32,* 3.

Kayser, H. (1989). Speech and language assessment of Spanish–English speaking children. *Language, Speech and Hearing Services in School, 20,* 226–244.

Kayser, H. (1993). Hispanic cultures. In D. Battle (Ed.), *Communication disorders in multicultural populations* (pp. 114–157). Boston, MA: Andover Medical Publishers.

Kea, C. D., & Utley, C. A. (1998). To teach me is to know me. *Journal of Special Education, 32,* 44–47.

Kindler, A. L. (2002). *Survey of the states' limited English proficient students and available educational programs and services 1999–2000 summary report.* Washington, DC: National Clearinghouse for English Acquisition and Language Instruction Educational Programs.

Kovaleski, J. F., & Prasse, D. P. (1999). Assessing lack of instruction. *NASP Communiqué, 28*(4), 24–25.

Krashen, S. D. (1985). *Inquiries and insights: Second language teaching, immersion and bilingual education, literacy.* Englewood Cliffs, NJ: Alemany Press.

Lam, T. C. (1995). *Fairness in performance assessment.* Greensboro, NC: ERIC Document Reproduction Service (No. EDO-CG-95-25).

Langdon, H. W. (1985, February). *Working with interpreters and translators in a school setting.* Paper presented at the Fordham University Bilingual Conference, New York, NY.

Langdon, H. W. (1994). *Interpreter/translator process in the educational setting: A resource manual.* Sacramento: Resources in Special Education.

Larry P. v. Riles, 343 F. Supp. 1306 (D.C. N.D. Cal., 1972), aff'd., 502 F.2d 963 (9th Cir. 1974), *further proceedings,* 495 F. Supp. 926 (D.C. N.D. Cal., 1979), aff'd., 502 F.2d 693 (9th Cir. 1986).

Lopez, E. C. (1995). Best practices in working with bilingual children. In A. Thomas & J. Grimes (Eds.), *Best practices in school psychology II* (pp. 1111–1121). Washington, DC: National Association of School Psychologists.

Lopez, E. (1992, April). *A survey of school interpreters: Implications for practice and research.* Paper presented at the National Association of School Psychologists Conference, Washington, DC.

Lopez, E. C. (1997). The cognitive assessment of limited English proficient and bilingual children. In D. P. Flanagan, J. L. Genshaft, & P. L. Harrison (Eds.), *Contemporary intellectual assessment: Theories, tests, and issues* (pp. 506–516). New York: Guilford Press.

Lopez, E. C. (2002). Best practices in working with school interpreters to deliver psychological services to children and families. In A. Thomas & J. Grimes (Eds.), *Best practices in school psychology IV,* (pp. 1419–1432). Washington, DC: National Association of School Psychologists.

Losen, D. J., & Orfield, G. (2002). Introduction: Racial inequity in special education. In D. J. Losen & G. Orfield (Eds.), *Racial inequity in special education* (pp. xv–xxxvii). Cambridge, MA: Harvard Education Press.

Lynch, E. W., & Hanson, M. J. (1996). Ensuring cultural competence in assessment. In M. McLean, D. B. Bailey, Jr., & M. Wolery (Eds.), *Assessing infants and preschoolers with special needs* (2nd ed., pp. 69–94). Englewood Cliffs, NJ: Prentice Hall.

Macias, R. F. (1998). *Summary report of the survey of the states' limited English proficient students and available educational programs and services 1996–97.* Washington, DC: National Clearinghouse for Bilingual Education.

MacMillian, D. L., & Reschly, D. J. (1998). Overrepresentation of minority students: The case for greater specificity or reconsideration of variables examined. *Journal of Special Education, 32,* 15–24.

Maldonado-Colon, E. (1986). Interpreting data of linguistically/culturally different students referred for disabilities or disorders. *Journal of Reading, Writing, and Learning Disabilities International, 2*(1), 73–83.

Marín, G., & Gamba, R. J. (1996). A new measurement of acculturation for Hispanics: The Bidimensional Acculturation Scale for Hispanics (BAS). *Hispanic Journal of Behavioral Sciences, 18*(3), 297–316.

Markowitz, J. (1996a). *Disproportionate representation: A critique of state and local strategies* (Policy Forum Report). Alexandria, VA: National Association of State Directors of Special Education.

Markowitz, J. (1996b). *Strategies that address the disproportionate number of students from racial/ethnic minority groups receiving special education services: Case studies of selected states and school districts.* Alexandria, VA: National Association of State Directors of Special Education.

Markowitz, J. (2002). *State criteria for determining disproportionality.* Alexandria, VA: National Association of State Directors of Special Education.

Matsumoto, D. (1994). *Cultural influences on research methods and statistics.* Pacific Grove, CA: Brooks/Cole.

Mattes, L. J., & Omark, D. (1991). *Speech and language assessment for the bilingual handicapped* (2nd ed.). Oceanside, CA: Academic Communication Associates.

Mattes, L. J., & Santiago, G. (1985). *Bilingual Language Proficiency Questionnaire.* Oceanside, CA: Academic Communication Associates.

McCallum, R. S., & Bracken, B. A. (1997). The Universal Nonverbal Intelligence Test. In D. P. Flanagan, J. L. Genshaft, & P. L. Harrison (Eds.), *Contemporary intellectual assessment: Theories, tests, and issues* (pp. 268–280). New York: Guilford Press.

McGrew, K. S., & Flanagan, D. P. (1998). *The Intelligence Test Desk Reference (ITDR): Gf–Gc Cross-Battery Assessment.* Boston, MA: Allyn & Bacon.

McKnight, A., & Antunez, B. (1999). *State survey of legislative requirements for educating limited English proficient students.* Washington, DC: National Clearinghouse for Bilingual Education. Retrieved September 3, 2002, from *www.ncela.gwu.edu.ncbepubs/reports/state-legislation/index.htm.*

Mercer, J. R. (1979). *System of multicultural pluralistic assessment: Technical manual.* New York: Psychological Corporation.

Mills v. Board of Education of District of Columbia, 348 F.Supp. 866 (1972); *contempt proceedings*, 551 Educ. of the Handicapped L. Rep. 643 (D.D.C. 1980).

Moreno, J. F. (1999). *The elusive quest for equality.* Cambridge, MA: Harvard Educational Review.

Muñoz-Sandoval, A. F., Cummins, J., Alvarado, C. G., & Ruef, M. L. (1998). *The Bilingual Verbal Ability Test.* Itasca, IL: Riverside.

National Association of School Psychologists. (1997). *Professional conduct manual for school psychologists containing the principles for professional ethics and the standards for the provision of school psychological services.* Bethesda, MD: Author.

National Association of School Psychologists. (2000). *Professional conduct manual.* Bethesda, MD: Author.

National Center for Educational Statistics (NCES). (1992). *Data Center Common Core of Data: CD-rom installation and technical guide.* Arlington, VA: CTMG Publishers.

National Center for Educational Statistics (NCES). (1997a). *1993–1994 schools and staffing survey: A profile of policies and practices for limited English proficient students: Screening, methods, program support and teacher training (NCES 97472).* Washington, DC: Author.

National Center for Educational Statistics (NCES). (1997b). *The condition of education 1997, supplemental table 4-1.* Retrieved September 3, 2002, from *nces.ed.gov.pubs/ce/c97040d01.html.*

National Center for Educational Statistics (NCES). (2001). *Statistics in brief: Public school student, staff, and graduate counts by state, school year 1999–2000.* Washington, DC: Author.

National Center for Educational Statistics (NCES). (2002). *Schools and staffing survey, 1999–2000: Overview of the data for public, private, charter, and Bureau of Indian Affairs elementary and secondary schools (NCES 2002-313).* Washington, DC: Author.

National Clearinghouse for English Language Acquisition and Language Instruction Educational Programs. (2002a). *States' elementary and secondary LEP enrollment growth and top languages, 1999–2000*. Retrieved August 13, 2002, from *www.ncbe.gwu.edu/ncebpubs/reports/states-data/2002/index.htm*.

National Clearinghouse for English Language Acquisition and Language Instruction Educational Programs. (2002b). *United States most commonly spoken languages*. Retrieved August 13, 2002, from *www.ncbe.gwu.edu/askncela/05toplangs.html*.

National Clearinghouse for English Language Acquisition and Language Instruction Educational Programs. (2002c). *United States' rate of LEP growth*. Retrieved August 13, 2002, from *www.ncbe.gwu.edu/states/stateposter.pdf*.

National Research Council (NRC). (2002). *Minority students in special and gifted education* (M. S. Donovan & C. T. Cross, Eds.). Washington, DC: National Academy Press.

National Registry of Interpreters for the Deaf. (2002). *Code of ethics*. Alexandria, VA: Author.

Neisser, U., Boodoo, G., Bouchard, T. J., Boykin, A. W., Brody, N., Ceci, S. J., Halpern, D. F., Loehlin, J. C., Perloff, R., Sternberg, R. J., & Urbina, S. (1996). Intelligence: Knowns and unknowns. *American Psychologist, 51*, 77–101.

Nuttall, E. V. (1987). Survey of current practices in the psychological assessment of limited-English proficient handicapped children. *Journal of School Psychology, 25*, 53–61.

Oakland, T. (Ed.). (1977). *Psychological and educational assessment of minority children*. New York: Brunner/Mazel.

Oakland, T., & Laosa, L. M. (1977). Professional, legislative, and judicial influences on psychoeducational assessment practices in schools. In T. Oakland (Ed.), *Psychological and educational assessment of minority children* (pp. 15–26). New York: Brunner/Mazel.

Ochoa, S. H. (1998). Review of the Aprenda: La Prueba de Logros en Español, Segunda Edición. In J. C. Impara & B. S. Plake (Eds.), *The thirteenth mental measurements yearbook*. Lincoln, NE: University of Nebraska Press.

Ochoa, S. H. (2003). Assessment of culturally and linguistically diverse children. In C. R. Reynolds & R. W. Kamphaus (Eds.), *Handbook of psychological and educational assessment of children: Intelligence and achievement* (2nd ed., pp. 563–583). New York: Guilford Press.

Ochoa, S. H., Galarza, A., & Gonzalez, D. (1996). An investigation of school psychologists' assessment practices of language proficiency with bilingual and limited-English-proficient students. *Diagnostique, 21*(4), 17–36.

Ochoa, S. H., Garza, S., & Amado, A. (1999, August). *School psychology training pertaining to psychological assessment of African Americans*. Paper presented at the meeting of the American Psychological Association, Boston.

Ochoa, S. H., Gonzalez, D., Galarza, A., & Guillemard, L. (1996). The training and use of interpreters in bilingual psycho-educational assessment: An alternative in need of study. *Diagnostique, 21*(3), 19–40.

Ochoa, S. H., Morales, P., & Hernandez, M. (1997, April). *School psychologists' concerns about assessing culturally and linguistically diverse pupils*. Paper presented at the meeting of the National Association of School Psychologists, Anaheim, CA.

Ochoa, S. H., Powell, M. P., & Robles-Piña, R. (1996). School psychologists' assessment practices with bilingual and limited-English proficient students. *Journal of Psychoeducational Assessment, 14*, 250–275.

Ochoa, S. H., Rivera, B. D., & Ford, L. (1997). An investigation of school psychology training pertaining to bilingual psycho-educational assessment of primarily Hispanic students: Twenty-five years after *Diana v. California. Journal of School Psychology, 35*(4), 329–349.

Ochoa, S. H., Rivera, B. D., & Powell, M. P. (1997). Factors used to comply with the exclusionary clause with bilingual and limited-English-proficient pupils: Initial guidelines. *Learning Disabilities Research and Practice, 12*(3), 161–167.

Ochoa, S. H., Robles-Piña, R., Garcia, S. B., & Breunig, N. (1999). School psychologists' perspectives on referrals of language minority students. *Multiple Voices for Ethnically Diverse Exceptional Learners, 3*(1), 1–14.

Office of Special Education and Rehabilitation Services, Office of Special Education Programs. (2000). *Twenty-second annual report to Congress on the implementation of the Individuals with Disabilities Education Act.* Retrieved May 11, 2001, from *www.ed.gov/offices/OSERS/OSEP/OSEP2000AnlRpt/ExecSumm.html.*

Office of Special Education and Rehabilitation Services, Office of Special Education Programs. (2001). *Twenty-third annual report to Congress on the implementation of the Individuals with Disabilities Education Act.* Retrieved August 1, 2002, from *www.ed.gov/offices/OSERS/OSEP/OSEP2000AnlRpt/ExecSumm.html.*

O'Malley, J. (1978). Review of the evaluation of the impact of ESEA Title VII Spanish/English bilingual education programs. *Bilingual Resources, 1,* 6–10.

Omark, D. R., & Watson, D. L. (1981). *Assessing bilingual exceptional children: Inservice manual.* San Diego, CA: Los Amigos Research Associates.

Ortiz, A. A. (1990). Using school-based problem solving teams for prereferral interventions. *The Bilingual Special Education Perspective, 10*(1), 3–5.

Ortiz, A. A. (1992). Assessing appropriate and inappropriate referral systems for LEP special education students. *Proceedings of the Second National Research Symposium on Limited English Proficient Student Issues: Focus on Evaluation and Measurement.* Washington, DC: U.S. Department of Education, Office of Bilingual Education and Minority Languages Affairs.

Ortiz, A. A. (1997). Learning disabilities occurring concomitantly with linguistic differences. *Journal of Learning Disabilities, 30*(3), 321–332.

Ortiz, A. A., & Kushner, M. I. (1997). Bilingualism and the impact on academic performance. *Academic Difficulties, 6*(3), 657–679.

Ortiz, A. A., & Maldonado-Colon, E. (1986). Recognizing learning disabilities in bilingual children: How to lessen inappropriate referrals of language minority students to special education. *Journal of Reading, Writing, and Learning Disabilities International, 2*(1), 43–56.

Ortiz, A. A., & Polyzoi, E. (1986). *Characteristics of limited English proficient Hispanic students in programs for the learning disabled: Implications for policy, practice and research—Part I: Report summary* (ERIC Reproduction No. ED 267578). Austin, TX.

Ortiz, S. O. (1999). "You'd never know how racist I was, if you met me on the street." *Journal of Counseling and Development, 77*(1), 9–12.

Ortiz, S. O. (2001). Assessment of cognitive abilities in Hispanic children. *Seminars in Speech and Language, 22*(1), 17–37.

Ortiz, S. O. (2002). Best practices in nondiscriminatory assessment. In A. Thomas & J. Grimes (Eds.), *Best practices in school psychology IV* (pp. 1321–1336). Washington, DC: National Association of School Psychologists.

Ortiz, S. O., & Flanagan, D. P. (1998). *Gf–Gc* cross-battery interpretation and selective cross-battery assessment: Referral concerns and the needs of culturally and linguistically diverse populations. In K. S. McGrew & D. P. Flanagan (Eds.), *The Intelligence Test Desk Reference (ITDR): Gf–Gc Cross-Battery Assessment* (pp. 401–444). Boston: Allyn & Bacon.

Ortiz, S. O., & Flanagan, D. P. (2002). Best practices in working with culturally diverse children and families. In A. Thomas & J. Grimes (Eds.), *Best practices in school psychology IV* (pp. 337–352). Washington, DC: National Association of School Psychologists.

Oswald, D. P., Coutinho, M. J., & Best, A. M. (2002). Community and school predictors of over-representation of minority children in special education. In D. J. Losen & G. Orfield (Eds.), *Racial inequity in special education* (pp. 1–14). Cambridge, MA: Harvard Education Press.

Oswald, D. P., Coutinho, M. J., Best, A. M., & Singh, N. N. (1999). Ethnic representation in special education: The influence of school-related and demographic variables. *Journal of Special Education, 32,* 194–206.

Overton, T. (1996). *Assessment in special education: An applied approach* (2nd ed.). Englewood Cliffs, NJ: Prentice Hall.

Overton, T. (2000). *Assessment in special education: An applied approach* (3rd ed.). Upper Saddle River, NJ: Prentice Hall.

Parrish, T. (2002). Disparities in the identification, funding, and provision of special education. In D. J. Losen & G. Orfield (Eds.), *Racial inequity in special education* (pp. 15–38). Cambridge, MA: Harvard Education Press.

PASE (Parents in Action in Special Education) v. Hannon, 506 F. Supp. 831 (N.D. Ill. 1980).

Peña, E., Quinn, R., & Iglesias, A. (1992). The application of dynamic methods to language assessment: A nonbiased procedure. *Journal of Special Education, 26,* 269–280.

Pennsylvania Association for Retarded Citizens (PARC) v. Commonwealth of Pennsylvania, 334 F. Supp. 1257 (D.C. E.D. Pa. 1971), 343 F. Supp. 279 (D.C. E.D. Pa. 1972).

Perez, R. J., & Ochoa, S. H. (1993). A comparison of planning and personnel factors in bilingual programs among exemplary, non-exemplary, and accreditation notice schools. *Bilingual Research Journal, 17,* 99–115.

Poteet, J. A. (1995). Educational assessment. In J. Choate, B. Enright, L. Miller, J. Poteet, & T. Rakes (Eds.), *Curriculum-based assessment and programming* (3rd ed.). Needham Heights, MA: Allyn & Bacon.

President's Commission on Excellence in Special Education Report. (2002). *A new era: Revitalizing special education for children ad their families.* Retrieved July 15, 2002, from *www.ed.gov/inits/commissionsboards/whspecialeducation/reports.html.*

Project Forum. (1995). *Disproportionate representation of culturally and linguistically diverse students in special education: A comprehensive examination.* Alexandria, VA: National Association of State Directors of Special Education.

Psychological Corporation. (1997). *Aprenda: La Prueba de Logros en Español, Segunda Edición.* San Antonio, TX: Author.

Psychological Corporation. (2001). *Wechsler Individual Achievement Test—Second Edition.* San Antonio, TX: Author.

Ramirez, J. D. (1992). Executive summary of volumes I and II of the final report: Longitudinal study of structured English immersion strategy, early-exit, and late-exit transitional bilingual education programs for language-minority children. *Bilingual Research Journal, 16,* 1–62.

Ramirez, J. D., Yuen, S. D., & Ramey, D. R. (1991). *Final report: Longitudinal study of structured English immersion strategy, early-exit, and late-exit transitional bilingual education programs for language-minority children: Executive summary.* San Mateo, CA: Aguirre International.

Randall-David, E. (1989). *Strategies for working with culturally diverse communities and clients.* Washington, DC: Association for the Care of Children's Health.

Reschly, D. J. (1981). Evaluation of the effects of SOMPA measures on classification of students as mildly mentally retarded. *American Journal of Mental Deficiency, 86*(1), 16–20.

Reynolds, C. R. (2000). *Consent decree.* In C. R. Reynolds & E. Fletcher-Janzen (Eds.), *Encyclopedia of special education.* New York: Wiley.

Reynolds, C. R., & Kaiser, S. M. (1990). Test bias in psychological assessment. In C. R. Reynolds & R. W. Kamphaus (Eds.), *Handbook of psychological and educational assessment of children: Intelligence and achievement* (pp. 611–653). New York: Guilford Press.

Rhodes, R. L. (1996). Beyond our borders: Spanish-dominant migrant parents and the IEP process. *Rural Special Education Quarterly, 15*(2), 19–22.

Rhodes, R. L. (2000). School psychology and special education in Mexico: An introduction for practitioners. *School Psychology International, 21*(3), 252–264.

Rhodes, R. L., Kayser, H., & Hess, R. (2000). Neuropsychological differential diagnosis of Spanish speaking preschool children. In C. R. Reynolds, E. Fletcher-Janzen, & T. L. Strickland (Eds.), *Handbook of cross-cultural neuropsychology* (pp. 317–334). New York: Plenum Press.

Rhodes, R. L., & Páez, D. (2000). Cultural attitudes towards special education. In C. R. Reynolds & E. Fletcher-Janzen (Eds.), *Encyclopedia of special education* (2nd ed., pp. 496–499). New York: Wiley.

Roid, G. H., & Miller, L. J. (1997). *Leiter International Performance Scales—Revised*. Wood Dale, IL: Stoelting.

Roseberry-McKibbin, C. (2002). *Multicultural students with special language needs* (2nd ed.). Oceanside, CA: Academic Communication Associates.

Rosenfield, S., & Esquivel, G. B. (1985). Educating school psychologists to work with bilingual/bicultural populations. *Professional Psychology: Research and Practice, 16*, 199–208.

Rossell, C. H., & Baker, K. (1996). The educational effectiveness of bilingual education. *Research in the Teaching of English, 30*(1), 7–74.

Rueda, R., Cardoza, D., Mercer, J., & Carpenter, L. (1985). *An examination of special education decision making with Hispanic first-time referral in large urban school districts: Longitudinal study I report, final report* (ERIC Reproduction No. ED 312 8100).

Salvia, J., & Hughes, C. (1990). *Curriculum-based assessment: Testing what is taught*. New York: Macmillan.

Salvia, J., & Ysseldyke, J. E. (1991). *Assessment* (5th ed.). New York: Houghton Mifflin.

Samuda, R. J., Kong, S. L., Cummins, J., Pascual-Leone, J., & Lewis, J. (1991). *Assessment and placement of minority students*. New York: C. J. Hogrefe/Intercultural Social Sciences Publications.

Sanchez, G. (1934). Bilingualism and mental measures: A word of caution. *Journal of Applied Psychology, 18*, 765–772.

Sandoval, J., Frisby, C. L., Geisinger, K. F., Scheuneman, J. D., & Grenier, J. R. (Eds.). (1998). *Test interpretation and diversity: Achieving equity in assessment*. Washington, DC: American Psychological Association.

Sattler, J. M. (1992). *Assessment of children (rev. 3rd ed.)*. San Diego, CA: Sattler.

Sattler, J. M. (2001). *Assessment of children: Cognitive applications* (4th ed.). San Diego, CA: Sattler.

Scarr, S. (1978). From evolution to Larry P., or what shall we do about IQ tests? *Intelligence, 2*, 325–342.

Schiff-Myers, N. B. (1992). Considering arrested language development and language loss in the assessment of second language learners. *Language, Speech, and Hearing Services in Schools, 23*, 28–53.

Schiff-Myers, N. B., Djukic, J., McGovern-Lawler, J., & Perez, D. (1993). Assessment considerations in the evaluation of second-language learners: A case study. *Exceptional Children, 60*(3), 237–248.

Schrag, J. (2000). *Discrepancy approaches for identifying learning disabilities*. Alexandria, VA: National Association of State Directors of Special Education.

Serna, L. A., Forness, S. R., & Nielsen, M. E. (1998). Intervention versus affirmation: Proposed solutions to the problem of disproportionate minority representation in special education. *Journal of Special Education, 32*, 48–51.

Shapiro, E. S., Angello, L. M., & Eckert, T. L. (2004). Has curriculum-based assessment become a staple of school psychology practice? An update and extension of knowledge, use, and attitudes from 1990 to 2000. *School Psychology Review, 33*(2), 249–257.

Shinn, M. R. (1989). *Curriculum-based measurement: Assessing special children*. New York: Guilford Press.

Shinn, M. R. (2002). Best practices in using curriculum-based measurement in a problem-solving model. *Best practices in school psychology IV* (pp. 671–697). Washington, DC: National Association of School Psychologists.

Stetson, R., Stetson, E. G., & Sattler, J. M. (2001). *Assessment of academic achievement*. In J. M. Sattler (Ed.), Assessment of children: Cognitive applications (4th ed., pp. 576–609). San Diego, CA: Sattler.

Telzrow, C. F., McNamara, K., & Hollinger, C. L. (2000). Fidelity of problem-solving implementation and relationship to student performance. *School Psychology Review, 29*(3), 443–461.

Texas A&M University System. (2002). *Teacher demand study 2001–2002*. Bryan, TX: Institute for School–University Partnerships. Retrieved September 3, 2002, from *www.partnerships.tamu.edu/yr2s&d.pdf.*

Texas Education Agency. (2004). *2003–2004 student enrollment: Statewide totals*. Retrieved September 17, 2004, from *www.tea.state.tx.us/cgi/sas/broker?-service=marykay?program=aoh.*

Therrien, M., & Ramirez, R. (2000). *The Hispanic population in the United States: March 2000, Current Population Reports* (P20-525). Washington, DC: U.S. Census Bureau.

Thomas, W. P., & Collier, V. P. (1996). *Language minority student achievement and program effectiveness*. Fairfax, VA: George Mason University, Center for Bilingual/Multicultural/ESL Education.

Thomas, W. P., & Collier, V. P. (1997). *School effectiveness for language minority students*. Washington, DC: National Clearinghouse for Bilingual Education.

Thomas, W. P., & Collier, V. P. (2002). *A national study of school effectiveness for language minority students' long-term academic achievement:* Retrieved September 4, 2002, from *www.crede.uscu.edu/research/llaa1.html.*

Urban Teacher Collaborative. (2000). *The urban teacher challenge: Teacher demand and supply in the great city schools*. Retrieved September 13, 2002, from *www.rnt.org/quick/utc.pdf.*

U.S. Bureau of the Census (2001). *Percent of persons who are foreign born: 2000*. Washington, DC: Author.

U.S. Department of Education. (1977). Assistance to states for education of handicapped children: Procedures for evaluating specific learning disabilities. *Federal Register, 42,* 65083.

U.S. Department of Education. (1999a). *Assistance to states for the education of children with disabilities: Early intervention program for infants and toddlers with disabilities, final regulations*. Washington, DC: Office of Special Education and Rehabilitative Services, U.S. Department of Education.

U.S. Department of Education. (1999b). *1997 elementary and secondary school civil rights compliance report*. Washington, DC: Author.

U.S. Department of Education. (2000a). *The provision of an equal education opportunity to Limited English Proficient students*. Washington, DC: Office for Civil Rights.

U.S. Department of Education. (2000b). *The use of tests as part of high-stakes decision-making for students: A resource guide of educators and policy-makers*. Washington, DC: Office for Civil Rights.

U.S. Department of Education. (2001). *The longitudinal evaluation of school change and performance in Title I schools: Final report*. Washington, DC: Planning and Evaluation Service, U.S. Department of Education.

Valdés, G., & Figueroa, R. A. (1996). *Bilingualism and testing: A special case of bias*. Norwood, NJ: Ablex.

Valles, E. C. (1998). The disproportionate representation of minority students in special education: Responding to the problem. *Journal of Special Education, 32,* 52–54.

Weaver, L., & Padron, Y. (1999). Language of instruction and its impact on educational access and outcomes. In A. Tashakkori & S. H. Ochoa (Eds.), *Reading on equal education: Volume 16. Education of Hispanics in the United States: Politics, policies, and outcomes* (pp. 75–92). New York: AMS Press.

Weber, W. K. (1990). Interpretation in the United States. *Annals of the American Academy of Political and Social Sciences, 511,* 145–158.

Wilkinson, C. Y., & Ortiz, A. (1986). *Characteristics of limited English proficient and English proficient learning disabled Hispanic students at initial assessment and reevaluation*. Handicapped Minority Research Institute on Language Proficiency. Austin, TX: The University of Texas at Austin.

Willig, A. (1985). A meta-analysis of selected studies on the effectiveness of bilingual education. *Review of Educational Research, 55*(3), 269–317.

Willig, A. (1986). Special education and the culturally and linguistically different child: An overview of issues and challenges. *Reading, Writing, and Learning Disabilities, 2,* 161–173.

Woodcock, R. W., & Johnson, M. B. (1989). *WJ-R Tests of Cognitive Ability*. Itasca, IL: Riverside.

Woodcock, R. W., McGrew, K. S., & Mather, N. (2001a). *The Woodcock–Johnson III Tests of Cognitive Abilities*. Itasca, IL: Riverside.

Woodcock, R. W., McGrew, K. S., & Mather, N. (2001b). *The Woodcock–Johnson III Tests of Achievement.* Itasca, IL: Riverside.

Woodcock, R. W., McGrew, K. S., Mather, N., & Schrank, F. A. (2003). *Woodcock–Johnson III Diagnostic Supplement to the Tests of Cognitive Abilities.* Itasca, IL: Riverside.

Woodcock, R. W., & Muñoz-Sandoval, A. F. (1993). *Woodcock–Muñoz Language Survey.* Chicago, IL: Riverside.

Woodcock, R. W., & Muñoz-Sandoval, A. F. (1996). *Batería Woodcock–Muñoz: Pruebas de habilidades cognitiva—Revisada.* Itasca, IL: Riverside.

Woodcock, R. W., & Muñoz-Sandoval, A. F. (2001). *Woodcock–Muñoz Language Survey Normative Update.* Chicago, IL: Riverside.

Ysseldyke, J. E., Algozzine, B., & Thurlow, M. L. (1992). *Critical issues in special education* (2nd ed.). Boston: Houghton Mifflin.

Ysseldyke, J. E., Vanderwood, M. L., & Shriner, J. (1997). Changes over the past decade in special education referral to placement probability: An incredibly reliable practice. *Diagnostique, 23*(1), 193–201.

Zappert, L., & Cruz, B. (1977). *Bilingual education: An appraisal of empirical research.* Berkeley, CA: Bay Area Bilingual Education League.

# Index